Praise for

ONE DOCTOR

"Dr. Brendan Reilly has done history a true service. . . . He is a good, fluent writer with a fine ear for dialogue, and his excursions from the particulars of his cases to broad medical, social, and economic principles are always on point. Dr. Reilly deserves a resounding bravo."
—*The New York Times*

"Powerful. . . . [W]atching him piece together a diagnosis, scrap by scrap, makes for riveting scenes—part mystery, part thriller."
—*The Wall Street Journal*

"Compassion, dedication, respect, professional competence, humility. All of these qualities shine through."
—*The Boston Globe*

"[N]icely intertwines true stories of challenging patients with valuable lessons. Empathy and thoughtfulness—*One Doctor* has oodles of it."
—*Booklist*

"[V]aluable insight into modern medicine. Gripping and compassionate."
—*New York Daily News*

"Heart-pounding pace and drama . . . remarkable . . . an intimate exploration of modern medicine and the human condition."
—*Publishers Weekly*

ONE DOCTOR

CLOSE CALLS, COLD CASES, AND THE MYSTERIES OF MEDICINE

BRENDAN REILLY, M.D.

ATRIA PAPERBACK

New York   London   Toronto   Sydney   New Delhi

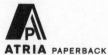

ATRIA PAPERBACK
A Division of Simon & Schuster, Inc.
1230 Avenue of the Americas
New York, NY 10020

First Atria Paperback edition November 2014

ATRIA PAPERBACK and colophon are trademarks of Simon & Schuster, Inc.

For information about special discounts for bulk purchases, please contact Simon & Schuster Special Sales at 1-866-506-1949 or business@simonandschuster.com.

The Simon & Schuster Speakers Bureau can bring authors to your live event. For more information or to book an event, contact the Simon & Schuster Speakers Bureau at 1-866-248-3049 or visit our website at www.simonspeakers.com.

Designed by Kyle Kabel

Manufactured in the United States of America

10 9 8 7 6 5 4 3 2 1

The Library of Congress has catalogued the hardcover edition as follows:

Reilly, Brendan M.
 One doctor : close calls, cold cases, and the mysteries of medicine / Brendan Reilly.
 p. ; cm.
 Includes index.
 Summary: "A first-person narrative that takes readers inside the medical profession as one doctor solves real-life medical mysteries"—Provided by publisher.
 I. Title.
 [DNLM: 1. Physician's Role—Personal Narratives. 2. Physician-Patient Relations—Personal Narratives. W 62]
 R690
 610.69'5—dc23   2013006739

ISBN 978-1-4767-2629-8
ISBN 978-1-4767-2635-9 (pbk)
ISBN 978-1-4767-2636-6 (ebook)

For: Brendan and Kristin (and Chi-town);
Caitlin and Christopher (and Beantown);
Colin and the wee one (and their tomorrows);
and
Janice, now and always.

CONTENTS

CONTENTS

INTRODUCTION

> Live a simple and temperate life, that you may give all your
> powers to your profession. Medicine is a jealous mistress;
> she will be satisfied with no less.
>
> —Sir William Osler (1904)

Despite this famous advice from a legendary physician, most doctors
don't live a simple life. All of us, seduced at an early age by Osler's
mistress, conduct our own lifelong affair with medicine. This book
is about mine.

One Doctor is a true story about real people—most of which took
place during two weeks in the winter of 2010. It recounts, in sometimes intimate detail, my doctoring of patients in the wards, emergency department, and intensive care unit of a renowned teaching
hospital in New York City. These experiences exemplify many of
the challenges doctors and patients face today in the dramatic, high-
tech world of modern medicine. But doctoring has changed, not
just since Osler's time but during my own time, too. For this reason,
my story flashes back to long ago when I worked as a primary care
physician in a small New England town. There, I did a different kind
of doctoring, now largely forgotten or obsolete, when physician-
patient relationships were deeper and more enduring than in today's
"provider-consumer" medical culture. This difference—the contrast
between doctoring then and doctoring now—lies at the heart of my
story. It is a cautionary tale, but a hopeful one, too.

My story is unusual in three ways. First and foremost, I am a dinosaur, an old-fashioned internist, a species of doctor on the verge of extinction. Although every doctor's perspective is unique, mine reflects the passing of a notable era in medicine. During my career, doctors like me served not only as their patients' primary care physician but also as an expert in the many subspecialties of internal medicine. As Osler did in his time, we cared for our patients whenever they needed us, day or night, and wherever they were—in the office or intensive care unit, in nursing homes and in their own homes. Such a task, daunting in the past, is impossible today. Medicine has changed irrevocably—on balance, I believe, for the better—and I harbor no hope of saving dinosaurs like me. But I am convinced that, as medicine continues to evolve, future doctors (and their patients) will do well to remember my medicine, my mistress. She is a goddess, her power and charms divine. But, like Osler's mistress, she is also a gadfly—a principled, perfectionist pain-in-the-ass—which my profession (and, I believe, modern society) can ill afford to lose. It is her spirit that I try to capture, and preserve, in this book.

Second, I tell my story in an unconventional way, in the first person in real time. I describe my own actual in-the-moment, minute-to-minute experiences as seen through my own eyes. With this you-are-there approach, I try to bring the reader "inside" one doctor's world; I try to show you—not merely tell you—what I do, how I do it, what it feels like. In recent years, many people have told stories—some with happy endings, some not—about their experiences as a patient in the U.S. health care system. This book tells the doctor's side of those stories, up close and personal.

Finally, an accident of timing motivated me to write this story. The events came together when disparate challenges in my own life—personal and professional, past and present—collided at one serendipitous point in time. This collision happened when challenges facing me mirrored similar ones facing my profession and my country. Most of the patients you will meet in these pages are older people with chronic diseases (including my own ninety-year-old parents) who don't have one doctor and who exemplify stormy issues roiling medicine today and for the foreseeable future. I focus on these patients (who, for various reasons, required urgent medical care) because most of us—you and I and our loved ones—will be one of them someday. Not only do these folks comprise the great majority of patients whom I (and most doctors) see today, they also "consume" the lion's share of all U.S. health care resources. One cannot begin to understand modern American medicine—or, increasingly, medicine around the globe—without understanding the challenges (and rewards) of doctoring such people.

I interrupt my story occasionally to comment briefly about its historical background or future implications. These commentaries claim no special expertise about their subjects (each of which could justify a book of its own); rather, their purpose is to deepen the reader's understanding of my story. To paraphrase Hamlet, in this book the story's the thing: What actually happened to me and my patients during the time described was the wellspring for everything written here. For this reason, just as one physician's experience could never embrace the full sweep and complexity of modern doctoring, this book addresses only some of the many contentious issues facing medicine today.

Whether my story will, as Hamlet hoped his own would, "catch the conscience of the King" is for you to decide. As I write this, politicians and policy makers in the United States are debating the form, function, and financing of smart new models of "accountable" health care. (Sadly, medicine has become increasingly unaccountable; today, it is often unclear who is responsible for the inexplicable way patients are treated.) Little good can come of these promising new ideas unless doctors step up, help to make them right, and take responsibility for implementing them well. But doctors can't do this alone. Ultimately, it is you—our patients, the body politic—who will be decisive in these matters. That's why I'd like you to meet my mistress and learn more about her kind of doctoring.

All true tales contain errors. I have tried hard to minimize my own. All persons, events, and settings depicted here are factual. Most names and a few details have been changed to protect individuals' privacy or their confidential medical information. Reproduction of conversations is approximate, not verbatim, as best my memory allows. Any other misrepresentation of actual fact is unintentional.

That said, let the story begin.

PART I

NOW

Not every patient can be saved, but his illness may be eased by the way the doctor responds to him—and in responding to him, the doctor may save himself. . . . It may be necessary to give up some of his authority in exchange for his humanity, but as the old family doctors knew, this is not a bad bargain. . . . The doctor . . . has little to lose and much to gain by letting the sick man into his heart.

—Anatole Broyard, "Doctor Talk to Me" (1990)

PROLOGUE

I had forgotten Manhattan has hills. I don't mean the ones Sinatra was talking about, the ones you climb so you can make it there, you'll make it anywhere. I mean the downhill run from Third to Second Avenue on Seventieth Street and then the gentler slope from First to York where the hospital rises up out of the river like a berthed ocean liner. When I was young, these ups and downs didn't matter much. Now, a New Yorker again after almost forty years away, I'm glad gravity is on my side as I slip-slide down the frosted sidewalk in the dark.

Dawn won't happen for another two hours. Even so, except for a final white dusting overnight, the streets are plowed and passable, last night's storm banked high along the curbs. I'm impressed. True, this is the Upper East Side, where Bloomberg and the bankers live; God only knows how the South Bronx looks this morning. But I have to hand it to them: I don't remember January cleaning up this fast in the old days. Today, in the city that never sleeps, the streets are empty, not a soul in sight. Huge darkened apartment towers snooze en masse as I trudge dutifully to work this Saturday morning, tired before I begin. I haven't had a day off in weeks but that's my own damned fault, as one of my patients, Mrs. Leavitt, a wisecracking eighty-year-old pistol, says. I'm well aware that my way, like Sinatra's, is on the way out. But what can I say? It's the only way I know.

Mrs. Leavitt's bad liver and worse kidneys landed her on 5 North, a medical ward at New York Presbyterian Hospital, a few days ago. On rounds yesterday morning, she asked who would be taking care of her over the weekend. Because my residents and interns all get at least one day off on the weekend—the legacy of Libby Zion, who died at this hospital—I, the senior attending physician, am the only one of my team who will see Mrs. Leavitt (and our other nineteen patients) on both Saturday and Sunday. I told her so.

Ha, ha, that's a good one, she said, winking.

Mmm.

No, really, Dr. Reilly, who will be here? My daughter is flying in from Miami.

I told her again.

She looked at the residents and interns around her bed, all of them younger than my children, none of them offering a different version of our weekend schedule. Incredulous, Mrs. Leavitt squinted at me hard.

Where are you from, doctor?

New York, originally. Why do you ask?

New York doctors don't work weekends.

She said this without a trace of irony or doubt. A simple statement of fact: It doesn't snow at the equator.

I told her that I cover my own weekends because, if you're sick enough to be a patient in the hospital, it's safer if you're seen every day by the doctor who knows you best.

In your case, Mrs. Leavitt, that's me.

She looked as if I'd just told her that the pope was going to be her new rabbi. But she bounced back fast.

So, I guess you're not married, huh?

The residents and I all laughed but her crack hit home. For many years now, whenever I'm on service at the hospital for weeks at a time—leaving and coming home in the dark, exhausted, sucked dry seven days a week—my wife leaves town. She visits our kids in Boston and Chicago or she travels with friends. I don't blame her a bit, not after putting up with my way for all these years. A perpetual intern, Janice would explain to Mrs. Leavitt, that's what he is, a perpetual intern. She doesn't mean it as a compliment.

Against the red, I cross the intersection at Seventieth and York, deserted now. During the daytime frenzy here, even native New

Yorkers tend to obey the traffic lights, a trauma center and five major medical institutions looming all around them. In addition to New York Presbyterian Hospital, where I'm headed now, this brief stretch of York Avenue houses Memorial Sloan Kettering Cancer Center; the Hospital for Special Surgery; Rockefeller University, whose leafy campus has nurtured Nobel Prize winners for decades; and Cornell University's medical school, where I and thousands of other doctors here serve as teaching and research faculty. These five world-class institutions, concentrated in a few square blocks, collaborate in various ways but, of course, they compete with each other, too. In U.S. health care, it's all about the money. Cutting-edge medical care—24/7, nonstop, even at 5:00 a.m. on a Saturday—doesn't come cheap, especially in this neighborhood.

That's why names are visible all around me. Even in the dark you can't miss them: Harkness and Payson, Niarchos and Helmsley, Weill and Greenberg, Hearst and Whitney, others, too. One of these names has been carved large into the massive stone façade of every hospital wing, every research building, every ivy tower here. Say what you will about the robber barons, a few of them give back, and it makes a difference.

I walk east on Seventieth Street, downhill again, toward the river. There, high above the churning waters, stands a memorial to hospital staff who died on 9/11. I can't see their names in the dark, but soon, when the sun rises, they will shine again. Facing east and writ large, their memorial's inscription—*Inspired to Care*—glows bright with every new day.

I turn right, into the hospital's northeast entrance. Here, in the graceful stone portico with leaded glass doors, a small brass plate reads: *Lying-In Hospital 1799 A.D.* Like all storied hospitals, New York Presbyterian is an ever-changing mosaic, its many parts added, connected, and modified over time. Decades have passed since this part of the hospital was used for mothers and babies. Now its grand cobblestoned rotunda—where horse-drawn carriages with footmen once arrived, the lady of the house ready for her confinement— is quarantined behind ugly chain-link fencing, its space a delivery site for the endless construction projects that plague all modern hospitals today. But, inside the lobby's marbled vestibule, a second brass plate still reminds all who enter: "This building is dedicated to the well-being of mothers and babies in memory of Laura Spelman Rockefeller, Anno Domini 1928."

I'm an internist, not a baby doctor. Even so, today, as on most days when I pass this dedication, I take some comfort from it. Not so long ago, childbirth was perilous, even if your name was Rockefeller. Back then, losing one or more of your kids to a childhood illness— measles, smallpox, diphtheria—was the *rule*, not the exception. The Rockefeller dedication reminds me that transformative progress in medicine doesn't happen overnight. The cancers and chronic de-generative diseases that kill most of my patients today probably will take me out, too, but they won't get my grandson. The new science is astonishing, galloping, closing in on cures. Remarkable things are happening, thanks in large part to academic medical centers like this one, and I'm proud to be here.

The elevator shushes open on the fifth floor. Around a corner, the Department of Medicine's "wall of fame" softly illuminates a long corridor. Here hang photographic portraits of every young doctor who has served as Cornell's chief medical resident since before World War II. Each of them a star, some are giants: David Rogers, chief resident in 1951–52, who became the first president of the Robert Wood Johnson Foundation; Tom Killip (1957–58), whose research about heart attacks laid the foundation for modern cardiac care; Tony Fauci (1971–72), the NIH AIDS researcher who, when I was a med-ical student here, seemed godlike as he prowled the wards teaching, day and night. I walk this corridor often in the course of my work-day, usually preoccupied by something when, suddenly, randomly, I turn and find one of these photos staring at me. Sometimes it's Tom Almy (1942–43), who recruited me to Dartmouth after he became chairman of medicine there (and where I served as chief resident myself). Spookier still, sometimes it's Bill Grace (1945–46), whom my father served as a chief resident before I was born. Dad is ninety-one now. He's not doing so well. But his blind blue eyes still flash with admiration when he reminisces about the eminent Dr. Grace.

Down the hall, in my office, I hang my coat and exchange it for a long white one. As I button it, the pockets stuffed with my trusty stethoscope and ophthalmoscope and other tools of the trade, my pulse quickens. It's a good thing, this brief flutter of fear, even after all these years. In Chicago, Michael Jordan used to say that if you're not nervous in the locker room before the game starts you've got no business going out there on the floor. I'm no Michael Jordan, but I know that today, like every day, will be a crapshoot: No matter how hard I work or how good I am, it might still turn out badly. Even when you do everything right, it still comes down to how the ball bounces.

And so, I do now what I do every day: I give a little salute to the beautiful blonde whose picture sits on my desk. Most people today don't recognize her, but when she disappeared, presumed but never proven dead, she was the most famous woman in the world. In time, the mystery of her loss became a cold case, forgotten by all but a few. I met one of those few, many years ago. While searching for her, he found me. He asked me to help him, to be his doctor. As it turned out, I couldn't help him. In fact, after you hear his story, you may think I did a lot worse than that. But that was then.

Now, as I head out to see my patients, the pretty lady in the picture is smiling. It's a wary smile, one that knows all about big risks and bad bounces. But it's a winning one, too, and I like to think she's smiling at me.

Chapter 1

LOST AND FOUND

> The difference between good and bad thinking . . . involves
> overcoming the inertia that inclines one to accept sugges-
> tions at their face value . . . it involves willingness to endure
> a condition of mental unrest and disturbance. Reflective
> thinking, in short, means judgment suspended during fur-
> ther inquiry; and suspense is likely to be somewhat painful.
>
> —John Dewey, *How We Think* (1910)

6:50 a.m. Saturday

I'm thinking maybe we got lucky.

Friday nights are cursed in big-city hospitals. No one knows why
exactly but mortality rates go up on the weekend. (You'd think we
would have figured this out by now, right? I mean, we're talking
about people's lives here.) So, if my team didn't get any new disasters last night—if we beat the Friday-night whammy—it's cause
for celebration. And from where I'm standing now, in the 10 Central corridor outside Mr. Warner's room, I'm thinking we caught
a break. I've seen my team's other eighteen patients, including the
first two of our three new overnight admissions from the ED, and
they're all looking pretty good. Mr. Warner is our last overnight
admission, and from what I can see as I enter his room, he's looking
pretty good, too.

This is doctor-talk, of course. My patient's "looking pretty good" is not anything you'd want to look like. Take Mr. Covinski, for example. When I saw him on 2 North a little while ago he was sleeping, thank God, because we had finally gotten his pain from his prostate cancer under control. His brother had flown him in here from Poland thirty-six hours ago and it had hurt just to watch this big, strapping, stoical guy grimace and groan and pace the room as we doubled, then redoubled, then doubled again the huge doses of morphine he needed to get any relief at all. When, at last, he murmured sleepily, *Dah, dah, no boli, no boli, thank you, doctor*, our work (and worry) had just begun. We don't know if we can rein in his galloping cancer, which has begun to invade his spinal cord. Mr. Covinski's just one bad break away from terminal paraplegia.

We worry even more about this because Mr. Rodriguez, another nice guy dealt a bad hand, lies paralyzed in the room next door to Mr. Covinski. Ten years ago, a drive-by shooting changed Mr. Rodriguez's life forever. Somehow he remains upbeat despite the wheelchair and the colostomy bags and the gigantic gaping wound where his lower spine and buttocks used to be. (Last week, when the new med students joined our team, one of them fainted dead away on the floor when we rolled Mr. Rodriguez over to examine his rear end.) Lately, he spends more time in the hospital than at home, one resistant wound infection after another, and it's probably just a matter of time before the bacteria finally win. Still, whenever we visit, he always asks us how *we're* doing.

Doc Steinberg, our patient on 5 West, always asks how we're doing, too, but he's a retired psychiatrist, so we figure it's just force of habit in his case. I'm the one who sounds like a shrink because I keep telling Doc Steinberg, *It's not your fault; it's not your fault.* He had a cold a few weeks ago, prescribed himself a broad-spectrum antibiotic that he didn't need, and now he's here, recovering from antibiotic-induced colitis that almost killed him. The bleeding in his colon has slowed but it caused his kidneys to stop working and now all four of his limbs look like tree trunks, so swollen with fluid he can't even get out of bed. The next few days will tell whether he spends the rest of his life on a dialysis machine. Still, he always smiles and makes jokes about the head-to-toe costumes we all wear for infection control—*You look like poltergeists,* Doc Steinberg says—whenever we come into his isolation room. And, every day, as we exit his room, he intones his lesson for our interns and medical students: *Remember, young doctors, the treatment can be worse than the disease.*

We could probably use Doc Steinberg's help with Ms. Jackson, our patient on 8 North who is homeless and crazy but refuses to speak with any social workers or Psychiatry. She's been here for more than a month now—no nursing home or shelter will take her—roaming the hallways day and night, even at five this morning, trying to engage anyone who will listen to her manic rants about how her liver problem was caused by Halley's Comet and why her breast cancer is actually good for her. Behind her psychosis, Ms. Jackson is a charming, intelligent woman, but her jaundice was caused by hepatitis C, not gamma rays, and we can't always tell which hallucinations are caused by her worsening liver disease and which by her manic depression. As if that weren't enough, her breast cancer has spread all through her body and we have no one to talk to about what to do when she starts to go downhill, as she soon will.

Looking "pretty good" in doctor-talk is all about *compared to what?* On first glance, though, Mr. Warner really does look pretty good, even compared to you or me. Seen from the doorway to his room, he might be meditating or listening closely to music he cares about. In his cranked-up hospital bed, he sits erect, as if doing yoga, his eyes closed but his chin held high, intensely attentive to something. My first impression—how sick can he be if he's so focused on something else?—would ring true to most casual observers, especially those not inured to the sensory assaults of a hospital ward. If, like Mr. Warner, I were held captive here—defenseless against the gurgle and flush of bedpans, the clatter of breakfast trays in the corridor, the caffeinated chatter at the nurses' station—I would try to tune it all out, too, find some peaceful personal space just for myself.

I want this to be true: I want Mr. Warner not to be sick. I don't want him to be like Mr. Atkins, the new patient I saw an hour ago who was helicoptered in last night with a belly full of cancer. (He doesn't qualify as a Friday-night disaster. The disasters are the ones we can still save. This poor guy's going to die and there's nothing we can do about it except make his passing a little easier for him and his family.) No, I want Mr. Warner to be more like Mr. Tosca, the patient I just left downstairs in the emergency department. He was admitted to our team last night and is still waiting for a bed, but we can probably send him home this morning. That's what I want for Mr. Warner, for his sake as well as mine.

Even if we get lucky this time, it won't last. My team, like all the medical teams here, is on call for new admissions every day all day, 24/7. Our next disaster may be waiting for us right now in the emergency department, one STAT page away. Even so, there's an ebb and flow to this business and you welcome the ebb as you brace for the flow.

But, of course, it doesn't matter what I want. On second glance, Mr. Warner doesn't look so good. His white-blond hair is damp, pasted down in random places, and I suspect, before I come closer to confirm it, that he's wet with sweat. One blue-stockinged foot sticks out from under his sheets at an odd, supinated angle and there is something odd about those sheets, rumpled and untucked, like maybe the night wasn't nearly as peaceful as he looks now.

These few odd facts, in the telling of them, sound simple enough, as if you just have to look to see them and know them to be so. But that's not the way it is. In real time, these observations don't register as discrete facts at all. I know them as I tell them now only upon reflection. In the moment, as I approach Mr. Warner's bedside, all that I experience is an uneasy awareness of dissonance: Something here is not what it seems. Somewhere in my subconscious, a red flag is flapping.

Consciously, all I know is that Mr. Warner is a seventy-six-year-old HIV-positive man admitted through the emergency department a few hours ago for treatment of a urinary infection. When I read this in his emergency department chart, two things came immediately to mind. First, elderly people with HIV are rare, even today. Most of the lifesaving advances in HIV treatment are relatively new; almost everyone infected twenty or thirty years ago is dead. This means either that Mr. Warner acquired his infection late in life or that he is one of a few very lucky ones. Second, most patients admitted to the hospital from our emergency department for treatment of a urinary infection don't have a urinary infection. (Or, if they do, that's not the main reason they need to stay in the hospital.) This fact—that diagnoses made in our ED are often incomplete—is no criticism of our ED docs; it happens in every hospital. There's only so much you can figure out in a busy emergency department during the few hours that sick, complicated patients stay there before being admitted to the hospital. In fact, the most important function of emergency departments today is identifying which patients are *really* sick (and must be hospitalized) and which ones are not (and can safely go home). The ED docs here at New York Presbyterian are very good at this: More than nine times out of ten, they're right.

All told, then, I know four things before I meet Mr. Warner. First, he's a rarity, an old man with HIV. Second, he's here—admitted to the inpatient medical service from our emergency department—so he's probably pretty sick. Third, whatever diagnostic testing has already been done in the ED, it's likely that no one knows yet what's really wrong with this guy. And, fourth, somewhere in my subconscious brain, that red flag is flapping. My gut is telling me: Be careful here.

Over the years I've learned to listen to my gut, but that doesn't mean I can trust it. So I know what I have to do now—and there's nothing subconscious about it. It's like working in an auto repair shop. You listen to what the car owner says; you ask him some questions; you listen carefully to his answers; and then you look under the hood. People today think medicine is all about technology—DNA tests and MRI scans and robotic surgery. But it isn't. There's an age-old, tried-and-true method to clinical medicine, and there's nothing mysterious or high-tech about it. It's grunt work. And, as the grease monkeys in the auto shops say, if you shortcut the grunt work you'll screw up the job.

I use my intuition—my gut—to make snap judgments every day. All doctors do. Occasionally, in a true emergency, there's no alternative: We must decide in a flash. Much more often, though, we make snap decisions and we're not even aware we're doing it. Experienced doctors, in particular, develop this habit; reflexively, we "just know" what to do, probably because we've encountered a particular clinical situation so many times before.

These snap decisions can backfire. Instinctive judgments—the ones we make in the blink of an eye—are subject to bias, error, and bad luck. Knowing this, expert decision-makers take pains "to combine the best of conscious deliberation and instinctive judgment," not an easy thing to do; indeed, learning how to do this, according to Malcolm Gladwell, author of *Blink*, is "one of the great challenges of our time." Had I appreciated the enormity of this challenge years ago, before I began doing research about it, I might have hesitated before taking it on. But, as it turned out, when Gladwell wrote in *Blink* about efforts to improve doctors' instinctive judgments, he was writing about me.

Together with a team of researchers in Chicago, I had published a series of studies in medical journals showing that use of a prediction rule—a guideline based on strong scientific evidence—improved doctors' intuitive judgments when deciding how to treat patients who arrive in emergency departments with symptoms that could indicate a possible heart attack. This prediction rule relies on just four "bits" of clinical information, so to most doctors it seemed overly simplistic. How could such an important (life-or-death) clinical decision depend on so few things? But it does. We found that doctors' intuitive decisions, unaided by the prediction rule, weren't nearly as good as the decisions they made when using the rule. This finding interested Gladwell because it exemplifies a successful effort to "thin-slice" a complex, high-stakes decision, boiling it down to the few critical factors known to affect its outcome. The important point wasn't that the prediction rule (an exemplar of "conscious deliberation") performed better than doctors' instinctive judgment. The point was that the *combination* of conscious deliberation and instinctive judgment is beneficial.

One might think doctors would welcome this kind of research, but most don't. In fact, many doctors resent the idea that their clinical judgment can be improved by consulting simple, step-by-step algorithms. (Derisively, doctors call this idea "cookbook medicine.") Expert clinical judgment, they protest, requires not only vast knowledge and long experience but also a finely tuned intuition that defies conscious, rational explanation.

The paradox here is obvious. We medical doctors acquire medical knowledge and validate it by the scientific method—by hyper-rational, deliberate, reproducible ways of knowing. And yet, many practicing doctors insist they know what to do for patients based on subconscious intuitions they can't begin to explain. They may be right. I don't know. Neither does Malcolm Gladwell or anyone else. But certainly Gladwell is right when he says we need to learn more about this. Because there's a lot riding on these decisions.

When I speak to Mr. Warner, he opens his eyes. They are the color of a calm Caribbean. I introduce myself. He replies, *How do you do?*, his diction precise, its tone patrician. I tell him I'm the senior physician who will be caring for him in the hospital and he seems to look me over before saying, *Oh, yes, how good of you to stop by*, and now I'm beginning to question my flapping red flag—maybe I'm wrong, maybe he really is just meditating, tuning us out, not sick at all.

Then I notice that he seems to be looking not at me but over my shoulder somewhere. *How are you feeling?* I ask, watching to see if he focuses on me. I'm standing on his right but his eyes drift left and now I'm not sure if he sees me at all. I repeat my question and he says, *Oh, yes, thanks very much, it's kind of you to ask*, as if he is addressing someone other than me.

And so he is.

According to Mr. Warner, he isn't in the hospital at all (*Oh, no, I never go to hospitals, how dreary they are*), he's visiting a friend for a week in the country (*Today is Wednesday, of course, what a strange question*) and it's not January of 2010, it's September of 1984 and Reagan is the president (*He still looks awfully good, don't you agree?*) and he says, *Now that you mention it, it is a bit stuffy in here*, but no, he hasn't had a fever or problems with urination or a headache or cough or anything else, and *Oh, yes, I take my pills, yes, indeed, I never miss my pills—what, my pills? The names of my pills? Oh, yes, that's a good one, ha ha ha, having names for pills . . .*

So much, then, for the first part of the grunt work: the listening and asking questions and listening some more. This guy's gonzo. I don't know whether he's always this confused—Alzheimer's or AIDS or another kind of dementia—or whether he's usually compos mentis but delirious now from acute illness. We'll have to find out for sure from someone who knows him.

In the old days, Mr. Warner would have had one doctor. The doctor taking care of him in the hospital would have been the doctor who already knew him: *his* doctor. But I don't know Mr. Warner and I can't rely at all on what he tells me. This is a big problem because, for experienced doctors, the history (what the patient tells you) is 90 percent of diagnosis.

So I do what I must in this situation: I become a veterinarian. Unable to rely at all on verbal communication, I depend entirely on what I can see and smell, what I can feel with my hands and hear with my stethoscope, the nonverbal signs and sounds his body makes. Even master clinicians can learn only so much from the patient's physical examination alone, but sometimes, like a mechanic looking under the hood, you can see right away what's wrong.

As any mechanic will tell you, though, you can see only what you're ready to see. For starters, your mind must be open, receptive to whatever sensory signals arrive, a sort of Zenlike "being there." In busy hospitals, this is easier said than done. Here, in addition to the racket in the corridor, the damned televisions, and that infernal *bleep-bleep-bleep* from behind the curtain where Mr. Warner's roommate lies, the distractions are olfactory and visual, too. That nauseating hospital smell—bodily effluvia mixed with medicinal vapors and bacterial decay. And what about these random personal items scattered around Mr. Warner's bed? An expensive-looking leather travel clock. Three different pairs of eyeglasses. An apricot-colored ascot. With practice, doctors learn to ignore many of these sensory distractions and focus selectively, "attending" exclusively to the task at hand.

When looking under the hood, doctors must also know what's normal and what's not. For car mechanics, the trick is knowing all the different makes and models and years; for doctors, it's knowing all the normal variants of the one make and model as it ages through the years. In the old days, many people had "routine" physical examinations performed by their doctors as part of an annual checkup. There are good (and bad) reasons why this practice has fallen out of favor today, but one unintended consequence is that recently trained doctors, when compared to dinosaurs like me, have examined relatively few normal people. The result is a less finely tuned diagnostic instrument, an examiner less able to know by looking at a spot on the skin, or feeling a lump in the breast, or hearing a murmur in the heart whether it's abnormal (and potentially serious) or just a variant of normal (and nothing to worry about). Examining all the different parts of thousands of different people takes time, but, in the process, you get pretty good at knowing what's within the normal human range and what isn't.

Finally, if you want to "see smart" you must know what you're looking for. In medicine, the symptoms and signs doctors look for are "context-specific," contingent on the particular clinical situation. (This is why the patient's history is so important: It tells the doctor what to look for.) In Mr. Warner's case, the clinical context is unclear. I know that he's HIV positive but I don't know whether the virus has seriously damaged his immune system. Blood tests in the emergency department showed an elevated white blood cell count, often an indicator of infection, but because Mr. Warner is new to our hospital—he has no previous encounters recorded in our electronic medical records—we don't know his CD4 lymphocyte count, the essential measure of HIV-infected patients' immune function. How doctors think about HIV patients—what kinds of complications they may develop—depends critically on this key contextual fact: Is the patient seriously immune-compromised or not?

Just as important in Mr. Warner's case, I don't know whether his confusion is new or old. (Nor, if new, how new. Weeks? Hours?) A CT scan of his brain in the ED was reported as normal but the diagnostic significance of this result in Mr. Warner's case depends critically on his history. Not knowing how long he's been "not himself"—a simple thing his family or friends or personal doctor would know—means I can't know yet how to process the information about his CT scan.

So, even though my mind is open as I begin to look under Mr. Warner's hood—and even though I have lots of experience in distinguishing abnormal from normal findings—I am well aware that I may miss something important even if it's right here in front of my nose. In this case, I don't know exactly what I'm *looking for*—because I don't know *him*.

He has a fever. I don't take his temperature with a thermometer but he's hot to the touch. This explains the beads of sweat on his forehead and the damp cling of his hospital gown. His pulse is strong and regular but it's fast, 120 beats per minute. His breathing seems normal and unlabored but I take the fifteen seconds to actually count his breaths because tachypnea (rapid breathing, faster than twenty breaths per minute) is an important sign of how sick someone is. If you don't take the trouble to count, you can miss this. Mr. Warner breathes six times in fifteen seconds. Twenty-four breaths per minute.

Almost certainly, then, he's infected: the combination of fever, a fast pulse, rapid breathing, and a high white blood cell count defines SIRS, the medical acronym for Systemic Inflammatory Response Syndrome, the body's typical physiological reaction to infection. Now the "context" for my looking is becoming clearer: *Where* is his infection? What's *causing* it? How bad is it?

Top to bottom, I don't find much. His scalp and eyes and ears are normal. His neck isn't stiff. There's no sign of thrush in his mouth—the sticky white plaques of fungus that often signify severely compromised immunity—and I feel no enlarged lymph glands in his neck, armpits, or groin. When I percuss with my fingers and listen with my stethoscope, his lungs sound healthy, not just in the back but in the front and sides, too. His belly is flat and nontender and all the organs there seem normal in size and shape. I had wondered about his left leg and foot when I first saw him from the doorway but he is able to move and bend them without difficulty, and I find no swelling or tenderness anywhere in his muscles or joints. His genitalia are normal and when I slide my gloved, lubricated finger into his rectum, he doesn't flinch and there's no sign of blood in his stool or swelling or tenderness of his prostate. The normal prostate exam and absence of any tenderness when I punch gently each of his kidneys make me doubt even more that he has a urinary infection, his preliminary diagnosis in the ED.

But I'm not finding an obvious alternative diagnosis, either. So far, I've found only two things that are not entirely normal. One is a small, bruised needle mark over his lower spine. This means he's had a spinal tap, something that wasn't mentioned in his ED chart. The second is his heart: The soft *Shhh!* I hear through my stethoscope when I lay it under his right collarbone tells me his aortic valve is a little stiff and the musical *Whoot!* I hear under his left nipple says his mitral valve leaks a little, too. But more than a few "normal" seventy-six-year-old hearts sing these same notes. So I don't make much of them yet.

Finally, I perform a neurological examination. For some doctors, this would seem superfluous in a patient who had a normal CT scan of his brain just a few hours ago. In fact, many non-neurologists today don't know how to do a competent neurological examination because they rely so heavily on CT and MRI scans to answer their neurological questions. But, in the old days, the neurological exam was all we had; CT scans and MRIs didn't exist. After these wondrous technologies were introduced in the 1980s and 1990s, old-timers like me learned how often our bedside neurological exam missed important findings. But we also learned that CTs and MRIs can miss important things, too, some of which are detectable *only* by a thorough bedside neurological exam.

This neurological examination, which requires the patient's cooperation, isn't easily done with Mr. Warner. His verbal facility is intact (*Yes, yes, I see it, that's a wristwatch you're wearing, rather a cheap one, actually . . .*), but his attention quickly wanders. He tends to drift off, not to sleep but somewhere else. He's hyperalert but he's listening to something or someone who isn't me. Even so, he manages to cooperate well enough for me to establish that his cranial nerves (visual acuity and eye movement, hearing, facial movement and sensation, swallowing and tongue movement) function well. He moves his arms and legs with apparently normal strength and coordination. His reflexes (muscle twitches elicited by tapping his knees and elbows and other places) seem normal and symmetrical. When I formally test his mental status, he's still completely out to lunch—disoriented to time and place, unaware of where he is or what he's doing here. In fact, I'm finding exactly what I expected to find before I formally examined his nervous system—he's confused and disoriented, with a waxing and waning attention span, but he has no "focal" abnormality of strength or perception or coordination. These are the findings one expects in an elderly patient delirious from infection. But none of this tells me what or where or how bad his infection is.

Except for one thing.

When I scratch the bottom of his foot with my thumbnail, dragging it slowly up the lateral side of his sole from his heel to the arch and then across the arch toward his big toe, his reaction is normal on the right foot but abnormal on the left. The normal response in this Babinski reflex is a curling down of all five toes, as most of us do when someone tickles our feet. But when I tickle Mr. Warner's left foot, his big toe doesn't curl down like his other toes. Instead, it stands up straight, archly erect, pointing back toward his face: *Hey, hey, look at me!*

I repeat this, several times, on both feet, to make sure. But every time the result is the same: unequivocally abnormal—and only on the left.

This is trouble. Big trouble.

It's the Friday-night curse. In spades.

No one knows how this happens—how the mind of an expert diagnostician works—but in an instant, I think I know exactly what's wrong with Mr. Warner. I can *see* his disease—it's like I'm looking at it, a full-color picture in a pathology textbook, his heart and brain cut open on an autopsy table. If I'm right, Mr. Warner's one priapic big toe means that even if we do everything we can to help him—and, in a great hospital like New York Presbyterian, we can do as much as anyone anywhere—the chance that he'll ever leave the hospital alive is less than fifty-fifty.

Diagnosing disease has something to do with patterns. Like grandmasters in chess who can play (and win) twenty matches simultaneously, always knowing the best move to make from patterns of the pieces on the board, expert clinicians recognize patterns of patients' symptoms and signs. Based on their prior experience with these patterns, expert doctors know what to do next. Research suggests that chess grandmasters store as many as fifty thousand different chessboard "patterns" in their working memory. It's likely that expert doctors can recognize a similar number of clinical scenarios.

Unfortunately, most doctors are not experts. Like grandmasters in chess, master clinicians are rare. Remarkably, the medical profession doesn't know much about its master clinicians.

How can this be? How can we not know more about medicine's grandmasters? The main reason is that hospitals and medical schools don't consider this a priority. Instead, hospitals focus on financial performance and meeting national accreditation standards; medical schools prioritize biomedical research and the training of competent (not expert) doctors. And, even if hospitals or universities considered it an important priority, how would they learn about master clinicians? Which "expert" doctors would they identify for study or emulation? Countless compendia list "best doctors" (in the United States, or New York, or wherever), but these rankings, much like the magazine ratings of "best" hospitals or "best" medical schools, are based as much on hype as on fact.

The truth is it's not at all obvious who the best doctors are. Unlike chess, where the best players acquire grandmaster status by beating everyone else, there's no objective way to identify the best players in medicine. This poses a real problem because the study of expertise in any field requires the study of its superstars. (K. Anders Ericsson, an expert on expertise, has noted: "Medicine has its legendary clinicians, but these are as rare as Olympic gold medalists and have not been systematically studied.") Finally, even if we could corral these "legendary" clinicians, *how* would we study them? One of the most remarkable things about master clinicians, like experts in many other fields, is that most of them, when asked, *can't explain* how they do what they do so well.

I suspect that the key to understanding this problem lies in learning more about how two different ways of human thinking complement each other. "System 1" thinking is fast, effortless, automatic, and nonconscious—the kind of thinking Malcolm Gladwell wrote about in *Blink*. Somewhat surprisingly, experts in many fields (including medicine) do much of their best work using System 1 thinking: They perform complex (cognitive and technical) operations effortlessly and fast, seeming not to think about them consciously at all. (This would explain why, when asked, experts can't explain themselves.) But such expertise is achieved only after long experience and repeated practice of skills whose acquisition requires "System 2" thinking—the slow, assiduous, controlled process characteristic of conscious, deliberate learning. After many years (and only in some people), the need for (conscious) System 2 thinking when performing these complex tasks goes away—and then (subconscious) System 1 thinking "takes over." How this happens is a mystery. But, just as grandmasters learn to recognize patterns of chess pieces and know instantly what to do, master clinicians learn to recognize patterns of symptoms and signs and know instantly what they mean.

One important difference between chess and medicine is that the grandmaster knows with certainty where all the pieces stand on the chessboard: The facts of each pattern are unambiguous. The grandmaster also knows that *all relevant facts* are there on the board to see, because the facts of chess are limited to thirty-two pieces on sixty-four squares. But in medicine, sometimes relevant clinical facts are missing and must be found. Even when all the facts are known, the pattern they make can be illusory because one or more of the "facts" may not be what it seems. Thus, unlike grandmasters in chess, master clinicians always "vet" the facts of the case—they make sure the pieces of information before them are factual and complete—before they allow themselves to "see" any pattern at all.

One upgoing toe. It seems such a trivial thing. But I can hang my hat—and maybe Mr. Warner's life—on what it means.

Mr. Warner's abnormal Babinski response on the left means that the motor pathways on the right side of his brain (which control muscle power on the left side of his body) are damaged. Just a moment ago, when I tested the muscle strength in his arms and legs, they had seemed normal to me, so I go back and test his strength again. Now, when he holds both of his arms up to shoulder height and I try to push them down against his resistance, maybe—but just maybe—his left is weaker than his right. And when I test his legs again, trying to push his knee down as he flexes it up hard toward his hip, I can talk myself into a left-right difference there, too. But it's subtle, very subtle, and I'm not sure if it's real.

I don't want it to be real. I want to talk myself out of it. I want my Friday-night disaster just to go away.

And so I do a more sensitive test, which I hadn't done before. I ask Mr. Warner to close his eyes and hold both of his arms up to shoulder height in front of him, palms up, and I watch to see what happens. He's so out of it that he has difficulty following my instruction, but, even so, there can be no doubt: His right arm and hand remain elevated a rock-solid ninety-degree angle above his torso, his palm parallel to the ceiling; but, after just a few seconds, his left hand begins to pronate, its palm turning slowly toward his right, and then his whole left arm, slowly, very slowly, begins to drift down—an inch, then three. This "pronator drift" means that he does indeed have slight motor weakness of the left side of his body, so slight that it's easy to miss.

Knowing this, now I put my face directly in front of his face and ask him to look me straight in the eyes. When he does this, I take my right hand and make a move as if to punch him hard on the left side of his face. I stop just short of hitting him but he doesn't even blink. When I make the same threatening move with my left hand toward the right side of his face, he does the normal thing: He flinches, defensively pulling his head back to protect himself.

Now I know why Mr. Warner tends to turn his head to the left. It's not that he sees something there that distracts him. In fact, it's just the opposite: He can't see *anything* in his left visual field. He is half blind and doesn't know it. By turning his head to his left, he is subconsciously using his intact right visual field to see more of what's in front of him.

Combined with his left-sided motor deficit, this visual field cut means one of two things: Either one lesion in Mr. Warner's brain is responsible for both his weakness and his visual loss—in which case, it must be a very large lesion in his right cerebral hemisphere—or he has two separate lesions in his brain, one in the right frontal (motor) area and another in the right occipital (visual) area. In either case, what's most important is that the CT scan of his brain just a few hours ago in the ED didn't show *anything* abnormal: no signs of infection or hemorrhage or tumor.

Most likely, this means that Mr. Warner has had a big stroke (or two smaller strokes) at some time within the past twenty-four hours. When an artery that delivers oxygen and nutrients to a part of the brain is blocked by a blood clot (the cause of most strokes), that part of the brain suddenly can't function, but the resulting brain damage may not be visible on a CT scan until twenty-four hours later. If diagnosed quickly, before the damage to oxygen-starved brain cells becomes permanent, strokes can be treated successfully with powerful clot-busting drugs, the same kind that are used to treat heart attacks. But clot-buster drugs help only if administered within three to six hours of the *onset* of the stroke, and because most stroke victims don't get to the hospital in time, these drugs don't help nearly as many people as they could.

Reflexively, I look at my watch. It's 7:04. I've been with Mr. Warner for less than fifteen minutes but, including his time in the emergency department last night, he's been here for more than ten hours. If Mr. Warner came to the ED with these neurological deficits, then it would be too late, our three-to-six-hour "therapeutic window" to use clot-buster drugs already closed. But if he didn't—if, instead, he had his stroke *after* he arrived at the hospital, right here under our noses—then we would still have a chance to treat him and prevent potentially devastating brain damage. Not knowing which of these scenarios is true, ordinarily I would STAT page the hospital's stroke team (on-site 24/7) to help me decide what to do, right now, no time to waste.

But I don't page the stroke team. And I'm relieved that no one else did either.

Most patients having a stroke don't have a fever and heart murmurs; they don't have Mr. Warner's *kind* of stroke. He probably has a blood clot in his brain, but if I'm right about what's wrong with him, he has the one kind of blood clot—the one rare kind—for which we *never* use clot-busting drugs. Because, if we did, we'd kill him.

Mr. Warner's kind of clot is called a vegetation. To the naked eye, it looks like a tiny piece of cauliflower. That's what I've been seeing in my head—tiny bushes on a stalk—ever since that one big toe stood up and announced, *Hey, hey, look at me!* just a minute ago. In my mind's eye I can see inside the cauliflower, too, as under a microscope, where bacteria, probably the virulent *Staphylococcus* species, are chewing—yes, literally chewing—on Mr. Warner's once pristine, sterile heart valve. Surrounding the swarms of killer bacteria is an army of white blood cells, thousands of them, fighting desperately to contain and kill the *Staph* before the *Staph* kill Mr. Warner.

This vegetation is a battlefield. And if the right antibiotics don't arrive in time to reinforce the army of white blood cells, the bacteria always win in cases like these. *Always.* There aren't many things that are always true in medicine, but this is one of them, a 100 percent certainty. Right now, the bacteria clearly have the upper hand. Part of the vegetation has broken off from Mr. Warner's heart valve, traveled through his circulation into his brain, and stuck there, closing off an artery.

That would be bad enough. A stroke is plenty bad enough.

But now those *Staph* bacteria are growing and multiplying— legions of them—not only in Mr. Warner's heart but also inside that artery in his brain. And, they are eating. That's what *Staph* bacteria do: They multiply and they eat. Unless Mr. Warner is a lucky man, unless we can kill all of the bacteria with huge doses of powerful intravenous antibiotics, those killer swarms will eat clear through the wall of that artery right into his brain.

Then the bleeding will start. The bleeding into his brain.

When that happens, there won't be a damned thing we can do to save him. Clot-buster drugs would only make it worse. Much worse.

I hustle out to the nursing station. There, surrounded by computer terminals, several nurses are huddled together for their change-of-shift meeting, the nurses coming off last night's eleven-to-seven shift "handing off" their patients to those starting the seven-to-three shift today. These hand-off meetings are crucially important to good patient care, the time when the nurses discuss what's happened overnight to their patients, what needs to be done for each one this morning, what to watch out for today. As a rule, then, no one—and I mean *no one*—interrupts nurses during their change-of-shift meeting.

But there's no time to waste. This can't wait.

I steel myself for an icy reception, but after I quickly explain the situation, the head nurse, Ms. Croft, understands immediately. She's a pro; she even thanks me. Whatever Mr. Warner's diagnosis—we haven't confirmed my own suspicions yet—he's delirious and nurses know better than anyone how dangerous delirium can be. Confused, agitated, or hallucinating, some delirious patients climb out of their hospital bed and fall, breaking a hip. Others bleed after ripping out their IVs, urinary catheters, or surgical drains. I've even known one who died after jumping out her hospital room window.

Knowing these things, Ms. Croft assigns an aide—*Now, Sylvia, do it now, please*, she says urgently—to go into Mr. Warner's room and sit "one-on-one" with him, right next to his bed, to make sure none of these bad things can happen to him. It takes a little longer for me to explain why we should not give anticoagulants (blood thinners) to Mr. Warner, not even the low doses given routinely to almost all hospitalized patients today to prevent life-threatening blood clots in their legs and lungs. But, after I lay it out, Ms. Croft tilts back her head, whistles ominously, and says, *Got it. We'll take care of it right away*.

Urgently, I call down to the ED to speak with the staff who took care of Mr. Warner last night. I need to know more than what was scribbled in his chart. As I wait, holding on the phone, I'm wondering whether the ED guys know. Why did Mr. Warner come to the ED in the first place? Who brought him here? Who knows him? How long has he been sick? What do we know about his HIV disease—especially its impact on his immune system? Who is his doctor? *Where* is his doctor? What is his "baseline" mental status? Is his confusion new? Did anyone in the ED find the left-sided weakness and visual field deficit when they examined him? If not, why did they do the CT scan of his brain? All of these questions must be answered for me to fill in the blanks, help clarify whether I'm thinking straight.

But the ED guys can't answer my questions.

None of them knows Mr. Warner.

Like the nurses here on 10 Central, the ED staff changes over at 7:00 a.m. The doctors and nurses in the ED work long, hard, busy twelve-hour shifts and the 7:00 p.m. to 7:00 a.m. night shift has signed off. They've left the building. The oncoming day-shift staff have received their "hand-offs" for the patients in the ED now. But they don't know anything about Mr. Warner. He left the ED hours ago. He doesn't belong to the ED docs anymore.

He belongs to me.

So, for all I know right now, Mr. Warner is like Ms. Jackson, our bipolar homeless lady who wanders the fifth floor, ranting. It's like Mr. Warner has dropped down from another planet. We have no history, medical records, or friends to corroborate what he says. From the look of him, he isn't a homeless psychotic, but, right now, he might as well be.

I log on to a computer at the nurses' station. All tests done in the hospital, including those from the ED, are recorded there. According to the ED doc's written note, Mr. Warner's white blood count is high and there are red blood cells and white blood cells in his urine (an abnormal but nonspecific finding). But his other blood tests look good and the preliminary report of the CT scan, dictated at 1:12 a.m. by the radiology resident, is "normal for patient's age." I make a mental note of the uncertainty this raises. The "preliminary" report means that an attending radiologist, much more experienced than the radiology resident, hasn't read the CT scan yet. The "normal for age" interpretation raises the possibility that the scan isn't normal but that potentially important abnormalities have been attributed erroneously to "old age."

I will need to review the CT images myself this morning with an attending radiologist. In Mr. Warner's case, my working diagnosis—acute bacterial endocarditis with septic emboli to the brain—depends critically on the fact that his CT scan is normal. If it isn't normal—if the resident's preliminary interpretation is incorrect—then I'm back to square one.

Now I see in the computer that spinal fluid specimens were received in the laboratory at 2:57 a.m.; the results of the fluid analysis are still pending. Based on my own examination, I'd be surprised if the spinal fluid results will help us much, but at this point we're missing so much critical information about Mr. Warner that every piece of objective data is welcome. We should have the preliminary spinal fluid results very soon.

Finally, I look at the orders entered into the computer for Mr. Warner by Dr. Tina Johansen, the resident on my team who has been in the hospital all night and who admitted Mr. Warner. As usual, Tina has done the orders meticulously well. She has started several different antibiotic drugs simultaneously. This means Tina isn't sure what kind of infection Mr. Warner has—good for her, she's thinking independently, not passively accepting the diagnosis made by other doctors in the ED—but I can see from her antibiotic choices that she may not be thinking the same way I am.

We need to get our heads together about this. *Now.* If I'm right, we have no time to lose.

I page Tina on her beeper. She answers right away.

Sorry to interrupt, I say into the phone, but we'd better start rounding now. I'm worried about Mr. Warner. So let's see him first, up here on 10 Central, okay?

Tina's voice is crisp and clear, all business. You'd never know she'd been working hard, continuously and sleepless, for twenty-four hours straight. And you'd never know that she's not happy about my call. I'm interrupting her own rounds with the other members of our team, a process she (like all residents here) guards jealously, because this is the time when the residents see and talk about our patients without me, when they run the show themselves, sharing their opinions and teaching each other without feeling inhibited or intimidated by their attending physician. Resident rounds is an important part of their education—it won't be long before they finish training and assume the responsibilities of an attending physician like me—and it's a long-standing tradition here at Cornell. Knowing this, I interrupt residents' rounds no less apologetically than I interrupt nurses' change-of-shift meetings.

But medical care isn't about the doctors or the nurses.

Tina doesn't miss a beat.

We'll be right there, she says.

* * *

Hospital medicine is all about teamwork. This has always been true to some extent, but the need for teamwork has grown dramatically in recent years because hospitalized patients are "sicker and quicker" than ever before. They are sicker because medical progress has allowed patients to live longer with chronic illnesses (such as heart failure, cancer, and AIDS). Because many diagnostic procedures and treatments that once required hospitalization are now done routinely *outside* the hospital, the average patient admitted to hospitals today is older, suffers from more comorbidities (multiple chronic conditions), and receives more sophisticated inpatient treatment than patients hospitalized in the past.

Remarkably, these sicker patients are also "quicker"—many of them remain in hospital, on average, only half as long as (less sick) patients did years ago. This acceleration of inpatient care has happened because hospitals no longer are reimbursed for every day the patient stays in hospital; instead, hospitals now receive one lump sum based on each patient's principal diagnosis (regardless of how long the patient remains in hospital). So, hospitals try to minimize each patient's "length of stay," because shorter stays reduce the hospital's per-patient costs. Today, hospitals' profit margins are all about "patient throughput."

These two trends—older, sicker patients and hospitals' financial incentives to compress more care into less time—place a premium on efficient "24/7" inpatient care that is more intensive than ever before. Only *teams* of caregivers—working, of necessity, in shifts—can handle this around-the-clock responsibility well. (It is possible, but unproven, that this explains the "Friday-night curse"; even today, many hospitals are not staffed as well on weekends as on weekdays.)

In 2000, the Institute of Medicine reported that medical errors in hospitals caused almost as many annual deaths (98,000) in the United States as motor vehicle accidents (43,000), breast cancer (42,000), and AIDS (16,000) *combined*. Improved teamwork among doctors, nurses, and other hospital staff can mitigate many of these errors. Most important is clear communication of patient information and treatment goals among the many different caregivers who help "staff" patients around-the-clock throughout their hospital stay. This sounds easy but it's deceptively hard to do well. Patient hand-offs, for example, are notorious occasions of error. This is why nurses guard their change-of-shift meetings—and focus their efforts so closely—when transferring care of patients from one shift of nurses to the next.

Most doctors don't do hand-offs or work as a team nearly as well as nurses, because, until recently, we never had to learn how; unlike nurses, doctors didn't do shift work. Now we have a lot of catching up to do.

Today, only two of my team's regular seven members are in the hospital. The other five have the day off. The same will be true tomorrow, Sunday—but it will be a different two. Tina, by law, must leave the hospital no later than 10:00 a.m. today. (The legal maximum for residents is twenty-seven straight hours on duty.) Chris, not a regular member of our team, has been called in today to supervise Dan, an intern, because Brian, our team's regular senior resident, has today off. Leah, a physician assistant, also has been brought in as a pinch hitter because our regular PA (and our two medical students) don't work weekends. Leah will help to manage our team's twenty patients today while Chris and Dan are busy admitting new patients. Tomorrow, Dan will leave the hospital in the morning after working all night tonight; Tina will have Sunday off. Brian and Ashley (our other intern), both off today, will take over the team tomorrow—but only after Dan and I catch them up early tomorrow morning on all our new patients and everything else that will have happened in the thirty-six hours since Brian and Ashley went off duty Friday evening.

If you find this hard to follow, so do we. It's a challenge just keeping track of who will be here when—and who needs to "hand off" what to whom—to ensure that we take good care of our patients twenty-four hours a day.

Keeping track also of who's teaching whom—and who's learning what—is a whole other story. I pay attention to such things because, in addition to diagnosing and treating the patients in this teaching hospital, I'm expected to diagnose and treat the learners, too. This is especially challenging because my team consists of seven learners at six different levels of training—two residents, two interns, one physician assistant, and two medical students—each of whom deserves individual attention. Chris and Brian are senior (third-year) residents, both of whom will begin prestigious cardiology fellowships a few months from now. Their educational needs are different from those of Dan and Ashley, interns (first-year residents) who are new to clinical medicine, or Tina, a junior (second-year) resident who is somewhere in between. All of them are far more experienced clinically than my two medical students—one of whom is a third-year "clerk," the other a fourth-year "subintern"—and different from Leah, a physician assistant who has a lot of clinical experience but never went to medical school.

For generations, U.S. medical learners have taught each other: Senior residents teach junior residents, who in turn teach interns, and so on down the line. This tradition endures today, but it has become much more difficult to sustain (and evaluate), because only rarely is the whole team on the playing field together. More than ever before, the team needs a coach.

Jeez, Tina says.

Doe-eyed and pretty, smart as a whip, Tina has answers to all of my questions without my even asking. Three nights ago Mr. Warner had dinner with his niece and was his usual bright, witty self. The next day, he had a slight fever and didn't feel well. His niece called yesterday to inquire about him but no one answered the phone. Alarmed, she went to her uncle's apartment, where she found him confused and unkempt and called an ambulance. Mr. Warner has been HIV positive since 1995. He had told his niece as recently as last week that his antiretroviral medications were a "miracle" that had kept him "healthy as ever." We will need confirmation from his doctor, but this suggests that Mr. Warner's immune function has not been severely compromised by his chronic HIV infection. Equally important, we now know that his baseline mental status is normal—his confusion is new—and he's been ill for only a few days. Unfortunately for Mr. Warner, these facts support my own diagnostic suspicions.

Tina admits now she still isn't sure what's going on, which is why she took the time and trouble to do a spinal tap last night, even though she was busy with other patients and the ED docs didn't think the tap was necessary. Tina was worried about bacterial meningitis or viral encephalitis as well as sepsis from a kidney infection. To cover all these possibilities, she started several different antibiotic regimens simultaneously, pending further test results from the lab. She did all the right things, given the information she had.

But now she has new information.

We've just finished examining Mr. Warner together.

Jeez, Tina says again, biting her lip.

When we first gathered at Mr. Warner's bedside, he had resumed his peaceful, meditative pose. He remained this way—silent, motionless, eyes closed—even when Chris took down Mr. Warner's damp gown, put a stethoscope to his bare chest, and listened carefully to his heart. Only after we roused Mr. Warner to attention—we needed his cooperation to test his strength and vision again—did he actually meet his team of doctors. Then, he opened his eyes wide, looked around at all of us, and blinked hard.

Well, good evening, good evening! How nice to see you all! My, my, there are quite a few of you, aren't there? Was I expecting you? Oh, but that doesn't matter, does it? Do come in, let me get you all something nice to drink. Come in, come in . . .

Dan and Leah suppressed giggles. But Chris lifted an eyebrow when that one upgoing toe went up. His other eyebrow rose when Mr. Warner's left hand pronated, then drifted down, again. And when I threw my right cross at Mr. Warner's face and he didn't blink, Dan and Chris murmured *Whoa!* in unison.

This is all new to Tina. She hadn't seen any of it last night. But it doesn't take her long to put it together. She looks at me wide-eyed.

The neurological findings, she says, you think these are . . . ischemic? You think he's had a stroke . . . or maybe multiple strokes?

That's the most likely explanation, yes.

She considers this, then looks at Chris.

I wasn't impressed by the heart murmur, she says. Were you?

Yeah, Chris says. Actually, it sounds to me like two different murmurs: aortic stenosis and mitral regurgitation—not severe, probably, but real.

Now Tina and Chris examine Mr. Warner's hands and feet, inspecting his fingernails and the bottom of his toes. Then Tina looks at me again.

I don't see any peripheral signs of endocarditis, she says. Do you?

No.

Even so, Tina muses aloud, fever . . . heart murmurs . . . strokes . . . And here I am treating him for everything *except* endocarditis!

The several antibiotics Tina had ordered didn't cover the deadly staphylococcal infection that I was most worried about. Just as I hadn't known everything Tina knew about Mr. Warner's history, Tina hadn't seen everything I'd seen on his physical examination. As a result, in her mind's eye, Tina hadn't seen those lethal vegetations growing in Mr. Warner's heart—and now, maybe, in his brain.

But she's seeing them now. And she's kicking herself for not seeing them before.

Jeez, she says, shaking her head and looking sheepishly at me.

Don't get ahead of yourself, Tina. We don't know anything yet for sure.

We leave Mr. Warner with the nurse's aide sitting by his side. I'm hoping his confusion will lessen after we get his fever down. Maybe then we can explain some of this to him, too.

As we walk out to the nursing station, Tina turns to Chris.

Occam's Law, right? Tina says.

Could be, Chris answers.

Tina takes a seat in front of a computer terminal. She searches for incoming lab results. We can see now that there are forty white blood cells and twenty-five red blood cells in the fluid she removed during the spinal tap she performed last night. This is abnormal—normally, there aren't any cells seen in spinal fluid—but it's nonspecific, a finding compatible with Tina's diagnostic hypotheses (early meningitis or encephalitis) as well as my own. We talk briefly about this. We agree we must wait for additional tests before we can draw any firm conclusions.

Tina types urgent new orders into the computer, her fingers a blur. She amends her previous antibiotic orders to cover the deadly staphylococcus. She asks the nurses to give the new antibiotics STAT. She places an order to transfer Mr. Warner to an intermediate cardiac care unit, where we can monitor his heart more closely. She arranges an urgent Cardiology consultation, an ultrasound examination of his heart, and an MRI of his brain.

I'm impressed, and it's not Tina's typing skills that catch my eye. It's her honesty. Tina readily admitted that she must have missed Mr. Warner's neurological findings when she examined him last night. Such confessions are not easy to make in the competitive environment of a top teaching hospital—even when her sin is easily forgiven, as in this case. Mr. Warner's findings are subtle; I could easily have missed them myself. Equally impressive, Tina not only understood the implications of her mistake immediately, she also exhibited the single most difficult cognitive skill in medicine: the ability to change one's mind—to reconsider, or reject outright, one's previous conclusions when new facts render those conclusions less tenable. This sounds easy but it isn't. Some doctors learn it, then lose it. Many never learn it at all.

Tina finishes typing in her new orders. Staring at the monitor now, she wonders aloud why the nurses have held her order for heparin, the blood-thinner I asked the nurses not to give a short while ago.

I look at Chris. He's not sure. I explain.

Patients who have endocarditis-related stroke are much more likely to bleed into the brain than patients who have other kinds of stroke. If this is what's happening to Mr. Warner, we must do everything we can to minimize his risk.

If this is what's happening . . . Tina says.

Right. We don't know yet. The other possibilities you mentioned—sepsis, early meningitis, encephalitis—are definitely still in the game.

Chris gives Tina a thumbs-up.

Whew! Tina says. I'm glad I did *something* right!

You did fine. Mr. Warner's a tough one.

I look at my watch. It's 7:42. We've got a long way to go. We hustle down the corridor toward the elevators.

Leah nudges Tina as we walk.

What's Occam's Law? she asks.

William of Occam was a monk, or something like that, like hundreds of years ago, Tina says. He claimed that when you're trying to find the cause of a complex set of phenomena, the simplest explanation is usually the correct one.

Simplest? Leah asks.

Yeah, Tina says, not simplest like . . . easiest or . . . dumbest, but like . . . if one cause can explain *all* of the phenomena in question, then that one cause is more probable than multiple different causes operating at the same time.

O-kay, Leah says, unconvinced.

Like in this case, Tina continues. We're saying that one diagnosis—bacterial endocarditis—can explain *everything* we've found in Mr. Warner: his fever, heart murmurs, the neurological findings, the cells in his urine and spinal fluid, the CT scan. Occam's Law says it's more likely that Mr. Warner has this one diagnosis that can explain everything than that he has multiple diagnoses—a kidney infection *and* a stroke *and* heart murmurs—all unrelated but present simultaneously.

The elevator arrives, empty. We get on board, push the button for the fourteenth floor.

Leah looks at Tina.

So . . . this Occam's Law thing . . . it's always right?

Tina hesitates, then turns to me.

No, I say. Actually, in medicine it's often wrong. It tends to be right in young, previously healthy patients. In them, an illness characterized by many complex phenomena usually does follow Occam's Law. But elderly people who already have lots of different things wrong with them? Or people who have underlying conditions like AIDS that predispose them to many other diseases, too? Often those cases don't follow Occam's Law.

So . . . ? Leah says as we get off the elevator. In this case . . . ? I mean Mr. Warner is old. *And*, he's got HIV . . .

Yeah.

Hickam's Dictum, Chris says.

Leah rolls her eyes. Dickam's what? she says.

Hickam's Dictum, Chris repeats. Hickam was a doc at Duke ages ago, like in the sixties or seventies maybe . . . Uh, no offense, Dr. Reilly.

Everyone laughs.

Anyway, Chris continues, Hickam wasn't an Occam fan. So he came up with his own saying. It's . . . kind of . . . the flip side of Occam.

How's it go? Tina asks.

Chris makes rabbit ears with his fingers and intones, "The patient can have as many diseases . . ."

He pauses for the punch line, smiling.

". . . as he damn well pleases."

Tina guffaws, a big belly laugh.

Leah looks at me.

So . . . ? she asks.

We'll see, Leah. We'll see.

Chapter 2

CAUGHT IN THE MIDDLE

None of us is as smart as all of us.

—Japanese proverb

7:45 a.m.

The hospital's fourteenth floor is for rich people. This is New York, so let's be clear about rich: If you're willing to pay an *extra* sixteen hundred dollars per night, in addition to the astronomical hospital bill you (and your insurer) will receive anyway, the fourteenth floor is the place for you. In return, you receive magnificent views of the Manhattan skyline; a solicitous, manicured concierge at the front desk; a hushed, luxurious ambience; an enormous private room with an extra bed for family or friends; and a customized menu from a special kitchen whose chef will prepare whatever you want whenever and however you want it. Compared to some high-end Manhattan hotels, this is a pretty good deal, so some patients who can afford it want to stay even longer than their medical condition requires. For every one of those, though, there are many others whose presence on the fourteenth floor serves as a daily reminder that you can't take it with you.

Mr. Atkins is one of those. An architect in his early fifties, he was helicoptered in last night from a wealthy town on Connecticut's gold coast. For several years now he's been receiving various experimental treatments in Boston, at Sloan Kettering across the street, and here for a rare kind of pancreatic cancer. He hasn't been eating for the past few weeks and yesterday he became so weak he almost passed out. An oncologist here arranged his urgent transport to New York Presbyterian. When I saw him briefly earlier this morning, he was sleepy but his only complaint was discomfort in his right upper abdomen. I didn't spend much time with him then because, after I put my hands on the place where he said his belly hurt, I knew I would be spending a lot more time with him later today. In the place where his liver should be is a rock-hard lumpy mass the size of a basketball; it feels like there's more cancer in his liver than there is liver. Tina's admitting note in the computer shows that she saw Mr. Atkins around midnight and found the same things I found this morning. She wrote orders for pain medicine and left a message for the oncologist who had arranged his transfer here.

All of this sounded right to me, especially Tina's concluding remark in her admission note: "Not sure whether we have any further active treatment to offer this unfortunate patient. Will contact Oncology. Would strongly consider palliative care."

Smartly dressed attendants and attractive waitresses pass us in the oak-paneled corridor. Tina suggests that she not present Mr. Atkins's case at his bedside, as we did with Mr. Warner. Ordinarily, I prefer the bedside because most patients, when you ask them, want to hear what their doctors are saying about them. But I haven't spent enough time yet with Mr. Atkins to know what he knows or what he's expecting or what his hopes may be. So I defer to Tina's judgment about this and we gather together outside his room.

It takes Tina only a few minutes to tell the team about the inoperable metastatic neuroendocrine carcinoma of the pancreas; the many standard and experimental therapies Mr. Atkins has received; what Tina found last night on his physical examination and laboratory tests; and, finally, a summary of her own impressions and recommendations. She looks at me when she says that this rare type of pancreatic cancer sometimes has a better prognosis than the more common type but she doesn't know if there are any more experimental treatments still left to try.

He's still a young man, Tina concludes sadly. His kids are in grade school. So I hope Oncology has *something* to offer him, but . . . I don't know . . .

Chris asks Tina whether Mr. Atkins's cancer has caused any "paraneoplastic syndromes." It's a good question, because this rare kind of neoplasm arises in cells of the pancreas that normally make insulin and other hormones. Sometimes these wildly proliferating cancer cells continue to perform their normal functions; in such cases, they manufacture massive amounts of these hormones, which can cause the patient to have low blood sugar or high blood pressure or various digestive troubles that can be as difficult to treat as the cancer itself.

Despite her busy night, Tina has done her homework and reviewed all of Mr. Atkins's previous medical records, a big job. His blood and urine tests for every hormone associated with this type of cancer have been normal.

Chris has heard that this is often a poor prognostic sign. I've heard the same thing: When these types of cancer cells don't function well enough to manufacture their hormones, they tend to spend all their time and energy multiplying and metastasizing, not a good thing for the patient.

You may be right, Chris, but if you want to know this poor guy's prognosis, you don't need many fancy tests. You'll see what I mean when you take a look at him—and feel his belly.

Hmmph, Dan says.

Dan is an intern, a lanky, athletic, laconic guy very different from Chris, who is geeky, slightly built, and hyperkinetic. Chris is the senior resident but Dan is several years older. Before beginning his clinical training this year, Dan completed not only his M.D. degree but also a Ph.D. in molecular biology to prepare for his career as a cancer researcher. He's a scientist—a skeptic, a Doubting Thomas, by training. I'll make sure Dan feels Mr. Atkins's belly, too.

As we begin to enter Mr. Atkins's room, Julie, our team's other patient on the fourteenth floor, staggers drunkenly into the corridor from her own room two doors down. She grabs her IV pole with both hands, struggling to regain her balance, then turns 360 degrees to get her bearings before heading in our direction. Her constant companion, Gordon, is right behind her. Together, they move slowly toward us—Julie scowling and titubating, her face swollen and pasty gray, her eyes half shut; Gordon, movie-star handsome, buoyant despite his customized wheelchair, smiling his world-class, toothy grin. As they approach, Gordon raises a hand from his wheelchair and waves at us impishly.

Good morning, doctors! he says, his tone hushed and deferential yet brimming with delight. Gordon is the spitting image of Sidney Poitier in his prime, right down to his mellifluous speaking voice. He is so happy to see us. Life is grand, isn't it? he seems to say, his gaze lingering slightly longer on Tina and Leah, the two women in our group. Despite themselves, they melt a little. When he looks at me, it's hard to tell whether his smile is courteous and grateful—or cocky and in control.

Gordon's a piece of work. Julie's a mess. What I don't know yet is whether Julie's a mess *because* Gordon's a piece of work.

When Julie first arrived here three days ago she was barely conscious, worrisome enough that we considered putting her in the ICU. Now she has improved dramatically. This morning is the first time I've seen her standing. She's taller than I thought, nearly my height, surprising for an Asian woman. I wonder what Julie looks like when she's not all puffy, dried out, and groggy from myxedema, the life-threatening thyroid deficiency that landed her in the hospital. Again. It's the third time this has happened to her in the past eight months.

Why this is happening is a mystery. Prevention of myxedema in patients with thyroid deficiency requires nothing more than taking one pill a day to maintain complete normality. Not taking the thyroid pill can make you more than drunk and ugly; it can kill you. So how does this happen—not once, but three times? Julie and Gordon claim that they have solved the mystery. After consulting many specialists over the past several months, they found a "genius" endocrinologist who explained that Julie must not be able to absorb the thyroid pill from her stomach into her circulation. Theoretically, such selective malabsorption is possible, but there is only one reported case of this phenomenon in the entire world's medical literature and there's something about Gordon's shit-eating grin that makes me think Julie is not the second. When we hospitalized her, we tried to contact the genius endocrinologist but his telephone had been disconnected with no forwarding address. This did not inspire our confidence. Neither did the other specialists whom Julie and Gordon had consulted; when we called them, most of them just groaned and said, Best of luck with those two.

I've met many remarkable patients in my life, people who endure extraordinary disabilities yet seem genuinely happy and grateful to be alive. But Gordon gives me the creeps. He looks to be about thirty, at least a decade younger than Julie. I've asked him about his wheelchair in an offhanded way, not wanting to seem to pry. (I'm doctoring his girlfriend, not him, so it's really none of my business.) All he said was that he'd had an accident several years ago and injured his back. Several *years* ago. But sitting there, grinning in his wheelchair, Gordon's legs look beefy and strong, not wasted as one would expect of a chronic paraplegic. And I cannot ignore the fact that Gordon proudly claims to "supervise" Julie's medical care. Why she needs such supervision is unclear, but it is Gordon who makes sure that Julie takes her thyroid pill every day.

Now my team and I watch as they pass us in the corridor. (Yes, we'll be in to see you soon, Julie, we're seeing our other patients now.) The whole scene is bizarre: a wealthy cretinous woman and her handsome crippled consort, basking in the luxury of a hospital's VIP amenities while she recovers from a near-fatal illness that shouldn't have happened even once, much less three times. It pisses me off. Here we are, trying to help our patients get better—or, as we're about to do with Mr. Atkins, help them die in peace—while these two characters are jerking us around, wasting our time, using us. Worse, I'm the one who has to get to the bottom of it. Whatever is going on here, Julie's life is in danger. Whether I like it or not, she and Gordon are my problem now.

Farther down the hall, Julie totters next to Gordon, using her IV pole and his wheelchair to steady her gait. Gordon turns and looks back at us, watching. That grin again.

Have a wonderful day, doctors.

Medical care in the United States is a buyer's market. Not in the sense that it's cheap. Far from it. Medical care is far more expensive in the United States than anywhere else in the world. It's a buyer's market in the sense that most of us can get what we want when we want it. This might be a good thing if it were true for all of us (it isn't) and if all of us really needed what we want (we don't).

Persuasive research has shown that about one-third of all medical care in the United States is unnecessary, that is, wasteful, redundant, or ineffective, providing no net benefit to patients' health. Examples of this are everywhere. MRI scans costing thousands of dollars to evaluate trivial, self-limited symptoms. Expensive new drugs that work no better than cheaper old ones. Hospitalized patients who undergo the same battery of tests every single day even though these tests were normal yesterday and there is no reason to think they will be abnormal today or tomorrow. Frequent return visits to doctors' offices, scheduled not because patients need them but because doctors' schedules want filling. Outrageous administrative costs of countless different for-profit insurers. Having spent the past twenty years working in hospitals where most of the patients were poor and uninsured, I've seen too many people in the United States suffer or die because they couldn't get the care they needed—even as many others received care they didn't need at all. But, even if you've had no personal experience with these (sometimes tragic) inequities, it's important to know that inefficient, wasteful use of medical resources in the United States is hurting everyone, including you. Reducing unnecessary care would go a long way toward making medical care more available, and more affordable, to us all.

Part of the problem is the definition of "unnecessary." Are the fancy flat-screen televisions, oak paneling, and gourmet chefs here on the fourteenth floor of New York Presbyterian Hospital "necessary"? Wealthy people, who willingly pay the extra cost, seem to think so. But such hospital amenities are no longer relevant only to Wall Street tycoons and oil-rich sheikhs. Many U.S. hospitals now spend enormous sums to upgrade their "hotel" accommodations. Then they market these creature comforts directly to patients. Just as drug companies and medical device manufacturers gain market share by advertising their products directly to patients in the mass media, hospitals attract patients by promising a more comfortable "nonclinical experience" to their "guests." In fact, in a McKinsey study of this new business model, patients reported that, when choosing among hospitals, they considered the hospital's amenities twice as important as its reputation for high-quality medical care!

Don't get me wrong. Making sick patients more comfortable in the hospital is an admirable goal, but how much these amenities cost (and who pays for them) has become an increasingly important question. As we struggle to define the value of medical care, how will we measure its quality? Will we include patients' satisfaction with their "nonclinical experience" in the hospital? How about the "appointments" in doctors' offices? Are the chairs in the waiting room plush enough? Are the magazines up to snuff?

The generic question here is how to accommodate what patients want when what they want is largely a matter of personal preference *and* provides no known benefit to their health. This issue is not limited to hospital amenities. A much larger problem is the enormous amount of unnecessary medical care provided to patients because it reassures them, despite a lack of scientific evidence that it benefits them in any other way.

For example, do low-risk women under age fifty ever get breast cancer? Yes. Then performing annual mammograms for such women will save lives, yes? No. Do elderly men ever get prostate cancer? Yes. Then offering these men a PSA test (the prostate cancer blood test) will save lives, yes? No. Do adults with acute bronchitis (a chest cold) ever develop pneumonia? Yes. Then prescribing antibiotics for these patients will prevent pneumonia, yes? No. (Well, then, at least the antibiotics make the patient feel better faster, right? No.)

But try telling these folks that the mammogram, prostate test, or antibiotic is "unnecessary." (In fact, in some cases, it's worse than unnecessary, it's harmful.) A few patients listen. Most don't. Not surprisingly, many doctors have given up trying. That's probably why Julie and Gordon have been able to wheedle what they want from some of the doctors they've seen.

Educating patients about unnecessary medical care doesn't get much traction in the United States because it's essentially a conversation about cost-effectiveness, a subject about which most Americans (including doctors) know little and care less. People need what they need—and, in health care, our needs are largely conditioned by what Daniel Callahan calls "regnant social expectations." Individual patients and doctors don't deserve all of the blame for this mess. Often, unnecessary care reflects a local "culture" of medical practice that tacitly condones patients' excessive expectations and doctors' cost-inefficient behavior. Manhattan and Miami, for example, rank high on the scale of unnecessary care; Minneapolis and San Francisco do not. Just as all politics is local, so, too, is medical care. This phenomenon, exhaustively documented and deeply ingrained in regional medical cultures, illustrates how difficult it will be to reduce unnecessary care nationwide in our fragmented health care system.

Sadly, most of the research documenting wide variations in cost-effective medical care comes from studies of patients whose death is near. In some regions of the United States, terminal patients routinely receive futile treatments, remain in intensive care for weeks, or undergo "lifesaving" surgical procedures. Then, as expected, they die. "Unnecessary" doesn't begin to describe this kind of medicine; neither does "care." But, as many Americans know—including Julie and Gordon—you can buy it if you want it.

A small vestibule separates Mr. Atkins's room from the main corridor, another special amenity on this floor that enhances patients' privacy. As we open the door, twenty-foot-wide floor-to-ceiling windows frame the rising sun, its white winter light spilling across the river from Queens and Long Island to our east. The large guest bed by the window is empty. In the center of the room Mr. Atkins lies peacefully, his eyes closed, much as he looked when I met him earlier this morning. Now, though, his gaunt face and torso are bathed in brilliant sunlight. It's a stark, striking scene, beautiful in its way, a modern pietà *sans* Madonna.

We shield our eyes against the sun as we approach his bed. Leah moves to the window to draw the shades.

Tina touches his shoulder gently.

Good morning, Mr. Atkins, I'm Dr. Johansen, remember? We met last night . . .

He doesn't open his eyes. He doesn't move.

Mr. Atkins . . . ? Tina repeats.

Nothing.

Mr. Atkins . . . ?

I go to him and feel his pulse. It's strong and regular. His breathing looks normal. He is emaciated and pale, more noticeably now in the sunlight, but no different than earlier.

Mr. Atkins, I say loudly. I shake him at his shoulders.

Nothing.

I shout his name, louder still. I lift his lids with my fingers. His eyes loll, unseeing. Uh-oh.

I press my fist into his chest, hard.

Nothing.

Chris bolts from the room, yelling down the corridor for a nurse. Dan grabs a blood pressure cuff and wraps it around Mr. Atkins's arm. Tina tries again to arouse him by tugging hard on his ears. I check his IV; it's running slowly, normal saline dripping into his arm, no medications piggybacked into it.

Dan says, BP's okay, 120 over 70 . . .

Tina says, Jeez, he's comatose . . .

Okay, guys, let's . . .

Suddenly, a young woman crashes through the doorway, followed immediately by Chris and two nurses. Petite but surprisingly strong, the woman pushes Dan out of her way and throws herself bodily on top of Mr. Atkins.

Oh, my God, the woman cries out. Oh, my God! What have you done to him? What is happening here? Peter! Peter, talk to me! Oh, baby, please talk to me! Peter! Oh, baby!

Pummeled, now pounced upon, Mr. Atkins doesn't stir.

Mrs. Atkins . . . Tina begins.

His wife turns, looks up at me. Her blue eyes are bloodshot red, rimmed with tears.

Who *are* you? she asks, furious. What have you done to my husband? *What have you people done?*

The nurses go to her. They take her by her elbows, say something soothing, lift her off the bed. She protests, tries to fight them off.

She's a slim, slight woman but it takes all of the two nurses' strength to get her up.

Leave me alone! she yells. What are you doing? He's my husband! Peter! Peter! *He's my husband!*

Standing now, unrestrained, she is seething, spewing spit as she speaks.

He was fine when I left him! He was . . .

Mrs. Atkins, I'm Dr. Reilly, your husband's attending physician . . .

No, you're not! You're not our doctor! Our oncologist is . . .

I turn to Chris and Tina.

You guys take over here. Please come with me, Mrs. Atkins. These doctors have to take care of your husband now.

I motion to the nurses.

No, you don't! Who *are* you? Call Dr. Mortola immediately! I want . . .

One of the nurses and I move her into the adjoining vestibule. As the door closes behind us, I hear Tina saying, Okay, guys, let's move. Get me an amp of Narcan, Marcie, and let's check his finger-stick. Dan, let's get going on another IV . . .

Outside, in the vestibule, Mrs. Atkins is screaming at me through clenched teeth.

I . . . *told* . . . you! I . . . want . . . Mortola! And I want him now! I'll sue you for all you're worth, whoever you are . . .

Mrs. Atkins . . .

Hysterical now, she explodes.

They told us they would run more tests! They said there could be new treatments! There are always new treatments, I know that! He's young. He's in good shape. He eats right . . . or . . . he did . . .

Her voice slows now. Still furious, she's also exhausted.

. . . he did before . . . he has no appetite now . . . I make him smoothies, you know, he likes them . . . he and the kids like them . . . he and the kids . . . oh, God, the kids! He's . . . he's too young . . . oh, God, he's too young! Is he dying? Is that it? Is he dying?

Now she wails piteously, so distraught that her legs give way. She collapses into the nurse's arms, her sobs muffled against the nurse's gown.

Inside the room, I hear Chris say loudly: O2 sat is fine, his pupils aren't pinpoint, let's hold the Narcan for a minute, Marcie.

We sit Mrs. Atkins down in the lone chair in the vestibule. I crouch low so that my eyes are level with hers.

We don't know yet, Mrs. Atkins. I saw him a couple of hours ago and he seemed okay, he was sleepy but not like this . . .

As I speak, somewhere in my brain an idea is aborning. I can't see it yet and, whatever it is, it's drowned out by all the ruckus. But it's there, I can feel it there.

. . . he wasn't like this, he was able to tell me about the pain in his liver and losing all the weight . . .

Oh, God, she says, he's been suffering so . . . the pain and . . . and everything. He never complains . . . never . . . he didn't even want to . . . come back here . . . he just wanted to stay home . . . with the kids . . . oh, God, the kids . . .

She begins to sob uncontrollably. The nurse holds her closer.

Inside the room, I hear Tina shout: *Twenty-two? Did you say twenty-two? Oh, Jeez* . . .

That's it! That's it! I push through the door back into the room.

Mr. Atkins looks the same. Tina is standing on his left, her hand holding his IV line. Dan is connecting a bag of fluid to the second IV he's just placed in Mr. Atkins's right arm. Marcie, the nurse, is holding a small box used to measure patients' blood sugar at the bedside.

Chris hands Tina a big-barreled syringe the size of a beer can. Tina sticks the needle of the syringe into the IV line and pushes the entire contents of the barrel into Mr. Atkins's vein.

Mrs. Atkins barges back into the room. What are you doing? she says. *What are you doing?* she screams again, looking around the room at each of us.

It's a good question. Because, right now, we're not doing anything. We're all just standing there, looking at Mr. Atkins.

Waiting.

She pushes past Dan and Leah to her husband's side.

What are you people doing?

She looks down at her husband.

Is he dead? Oh, God, no, is he dead? Oh, God . . .

Mrs. Atkins, we're . . .

Oh, God, is he gone? He can't be gone . . .

She kneels by her husband's side, cradles his head gently in her hands, kisses him on his cheeks and forehead and mouth. Then she rests her head on his chest, sobbing.

We all stand there, watching.

A minute passes. It feels like a lot longer.

Then Mr. Atkins opens his eyes. He blinks a few times. He looks down, sees his wife's head on his chest. He puts his arms around her.

Startled, she jumps, thinking it's one of us.

Leave me alone! she growls, starting to rage again. How dare you . . . !

Then she looks into her husband's eyes. They're the same color as hers.

She gasps.

Hiya, hon, Mr. Atkins says softly, sleepily.

She yelps, then smothers him in kisses again.

Oh, my God! Peter . . . I thought you were . . . Oh, my God . . . Peter . . .

I look around the room.

Dan and Leah are grinning. Tina is frowning, mulling over something in her head. Chris confers with Marcie, the senior nurse.

Marcie asks the other nurse to get a new IV solution, one with concentrated glucose. She asks Mrs. Atkins, who is hugging and kissing her husband, to please let her have his hand so she can draw more blood.

Now what? she says angrily, turning to me. Can't you all just leave him alone? Haven't you done enough already?

Before I can answer, Tina steps forward.

Mrs. Atkins, she begins, let me . . .

I don't want to hear it! Just leave us alone . . .

Now Mr. Atkins sees Tina. Weakly, he waves at her.

Dr. Johansen, he says softly, his voice sleepy and warm. Hi, Dr. Johansen. Honey, this is Dr. Johansen, she's been very good to me . . .

Tina musters a smile.

Hi, Mr. Atkins, she says. Good morning, ma'am.

Mrs. Atkins smolders.

Undeterred, Tina introduces the team. When she comes to me, I step forward and ask Mr. Atkins if he remembers meeting me a few hours ago.

He looks at me doubtfully. I'm not sure, he says.

I glance at Tina. She looks puzzled, says nothing.

I tell Mr. Atkins that his blood sugar was dangerously low, so low that he was unconscious until Dr. Johansen and her team treated it and made him better. I tell him the nurse needs to stick his finger again to check his blood sugar.

Sure, sure, he says softly, offering his hand. He turns to Tina.

Thanks again, Dr. Johansen. You seem to be my guardian angel.

Tina's eyes fill.

Mrs. Atkins watches and listens but remains silent. She gets up from the bed to let Marcie draw blood. The second nurse re-enters the room with the new IV solution.

I tell Mr. Atkins that we'll all step out for a moment while the nurses do their work.

Sure, sure, he says. Thanks, doc . . . thank you all . . .

I motion to Mrs. Atkins to follow us out of the room. She looks at me, then at her husband.

I'll be *right* back, Peter, she says, more to me than to him.

Outside, in the vestibule, she isn't backing down.

What's going on here? she says to me. *Why* did his blood sugar get so low? He's never had that problem before. What have you done to him?

At this point, part of me wants to tell her to go to hell. But I've been here before. I don't know her, but I know where she's coming from, and I know it's not an easy place to be. I take a deep breath.

Mrs. Atkins, your husband's liver isn't functioning normally because of the cancer. On top of that, he hasn't been able to eat much lately. The combination of his sick liver and not eating is probably what made his blood sugar drop so low. We'll make sure it doesn't happen again. We want to be sure he's comfortable.

She considers this.

Well, he can't stay on an IV forever! she says, angry again. How do we get him to eat? Can't you give him something to stimulate his appetite? He can't go on like this!

No, he can't, I say.

She looks hard at me. Her bloodshot eyes well up again.

What does that mean? she says, fighting through the tears.

Mrs. Atkins, he's not eating—he has no appetite—because his liver is full of cancer.

She wipes her eyes and fires back at me.

They already told us the cancer has spread to the liver! We know that! That's why he's here! To treat the cancer!

We'll speak with the oncologists this morning, Mrs. Atkins. I'm sure they'll be seeing you and your husband soon. But I don't know if they'll have other treatments to offer him. I hope they do. But once the liver gets this sick, the treatment options are pretty limited . . .

Tina is nodding.

Mrs. Atkins looks around at all of us, each in turn. Leah's eyes are cast down to the floor. Dan can't look at her either. Chris hurries back into the room to check with the nurses. Tina and I exchange glances.

Mrs. Atkins, we need to be thinking about . . .

What? she says, combustible again. What? A liver transplant? You want to do a liver transplant? Fine! Whatever! Let's . . . get on with it . . . whatever it takes, she says, whatever he needs . . .

No, ma'am, he can't have a liver transplant. If the cancer were only in his liver and nowhere else in his body, he might be a candidate for a new liver. But, as you know, his cancer is in his pancreas and other organs, too. A liver transplant can't help him.

She steps close now and looks up at me, her eyes a foot from mine.

You're saying . . . You're saying . . .

He's very sick, Mrs. Atkins.

You're saying . . . he's . . .

We need to . . .

. . . dying, she says, matter-of-factly, her eyes dry now. She puts her hands on her hips defiantly.

You're saying he's dying, she says again.

Let's see how he does today, ma'am, and let's see what the oncologists think. They know more about this than I do.

Yes, she says coldly, I'm sure they do. I'm *sure* they do. What I want . . .

Her voice trails off. She begins to cry quietly. Tina comes to her, puts her arm around her.

What I want, she repeats, . . . What I *want* . . .

Mrs. Atkins, I know this has been very hard for you and your family . . .

Sobbing audibly now, she puts her head on Tina's shoulder. Tina closes her own eyes. They both look exhausted.

. . . we will do everything we can to help, Mrs. Atkins. But now we need to focus on what *he* wants, what your husband wants . . .

Slowly, she opens her eyes, lifts her head, turns to me.

Yes, she says, sniffling. You're right, we need to . . . we need . . .

We go back into the room. Mr. Atkins's knees are flexed. He's holding his right side. His wife goes to him, kneels by his bed, takes his hand. I grab a chair, sit close to them, our eyes level.

I point to his hand holding his side.

Are you having pain now, Mr. Atkins?

Yes.

We can help with that.

He closes his eyes. That would be good, he says.

I tell him the oncologists will see him this morning. I tell him we'll leave now for an hour or two to see our other patients but we can be here in a minute if he needs us. I tell him I'll be back after he has spoken with the oncologists so that we can discuss together what to do next.

If you can make this pain better, doc, I'd be grateful. But I don't want you to knock me out, okay? I want to be with Sarah . . . see my kids . . .

He turns to his wife. She takes a deep breath, then holds her hand against his cheek.

Whatever you say, sweetie . . . she says, her eyes wet but smiling. Whatever you say . . .

I get up to leave.

There are things to talk about, Mr. Atkins.

He looks me straight in the eye. Yes, he says.

Who is your regular doctor, sir? We can call him. Maybe you and Mrs. Atkins would like to discuss some of these things with him?

The question puzzles him. He looks at his wife.

You mean like a family doctor? she asks.

Yes.

There's no one like that, she says dismissively. Peter's doctors are all cancer specialists. Nothing but the best.

Okay. But, then, do you know any of the oncologists well? One doctor who knows *you* well? You mentioned Dr. Mortola . . .

We've met him only once, she says. He arranged the transport here last night. We've seen so many others. Here . . . Sloan Kettering . . . Boston . . . But there isn't any . . . one . . . regular one . . .

Okay. I understand. We'll talk more when I come back.

Mr. Atkins nods. Thanks, doc, he says.

His wife regards me silently as I leave.

How is this possible? How can it be that an intelligent, reasonable man with considerable financial resources and a loving family whose cancer has failed treatment at not one, but several, of the world's best hospitals finds himself in this situation? Near death, yet not knowing it? Assuming, despite multiple failures, that "there are always new treatments"? Unaware that heroic interventions like a liver transplant are not even conceivable in his case, much less feasible? And, throughout his long, wracking ordeal, not having a single doctor who knows him well, who is watching out for his best interests, who is talking to him about how he feels, what he needs, what he wants to do? How can it be—even in the best U.S. hospitals, the crown jewels of the "best health care system" in the world—that such an utter lack of communication is possible?

It happens every day. In fact, increasingly, it's predictable.

Part of the communication problem is doctors like me. "Hospitalists" who do the kind of clinical work I do now—we take care of patients *only* when they are in the hospital—today number in the tens of thousands. Most of us do the best we can in a difficult job. But what makes the job hard is not just the long hours, the frequent crises, the attendant risks of burnout or cynicism. In addition, what makes it hard is knowing that, from patients' perspective, my involvement in their care is a double-edged sword. I'm good at what I do, and most of the time, they're lucky to have me. But I'm not their doctor—the one who knew them *before* they came into the hospital, the one who will resume their care after they leave the hospital. And, when you're really sick, that's what you need: *your* doctor.

For older doctors like me, who remember the way it used to be, this is irritating not because the good old days were better—in many ways, they weren't—but because this drastic change in the way medicine is practiced has been precipitated by the medical profession's (and U.S. society's) preoccupation with money. In many parts of the United States, your "real" doctor—if you're lucky enough to have one—doesn't take care of you in the hospital because this has become a money-losing proposition (for both your doctor and the hospital). In the new economics of U.S. medical care, hospitalists are more cost-effective. In addition, fewer and fewer people have a "real" doctor anyway—one who takes care of you whenever and wherever you need it, through thick and thin, a doctor who knows you as a person. Why? Largely for the same reason: This kind of doctoring doesn't pay well. As a result, in many U.S. medical schools and teaching hospitals, physicians-in-training (most of whom amass enormous educational debts) are actively discouraged from, even ridiculed for, pursuing careers as primary care doctors.

The other part of the communication problem is you. All of us, really. Put yourself in Mr. Atkins's place. Wouldn't you do what he has done? Suppose you have everything to live for—and incurable cancer. Wouldn't you seek out the top specialists in the best hospitals? Take the treatments they recommend? Fight to get better, beat the odds, stay alive—for your own sake and your family's? I know I would. But if, after fighting the good fight, the writing is on the wall—if your cancer is galloping and you look like a concentration camp victim and you can't eat or get out of bed—what do you do? Voluminous research has shown that different people, when confronted with this existential crisis, make different choices. Ideally, then, doctors try to talk to their patients, explore their feelings and hopes, help them make the best decision for themselves and their family. But there's the rub: Not only do many doctors *not* do this, many patients *don't let them.*

Almost twenty years ago, researchers published results of the SUPPORT trial (The Study to Understand Prognoses and Preferences for Outcomes and Risks of Treatments), a landmark four-year study of more than nine thousand patients hospitalized for life-threatening illnesses at five top U.S. teaching hospitals. SUPPORT documented frequent disturbing failures in doctor-patient communication in hospital. In many cases, patients' preferences were not solicited by their doctors, their wishes not followed, their pain and suffering not relieved. Worse, despite $28 million in funding from the Robert Wood Johnson Foundation, intensive efforts to redress these shortcomings failed in every measurable way.

SUPPORT found that many people—doctors and patients alike—*don't want to talk* about failing treatments, dire prognoses, losing hope, dying. To try to overcome this reluctance, SUPPORT study staff met with each patient (and, in most cases, family members) an average of six times during their hospital stay. Specially trained nurses discussed the patient's prognosis, pain level, and likely outcome of resuscitation efforts (such as CPR). Yet, despite these substantial efforts to "support" patients, answer their questions, and encourage further discussions with their doctors, fewer than half of all SUPPORT patients (40 percent) actually then talked about these issues with their doctors. An equal proportion of SUPPORT patients (40 percent) not only did not discuss these issues, they actively *refused to discuss them*, despite the obvious severity of their illnesses. (One-half of all SUPPORT patients were dead six months later.) The remaining 20 percent of SUPPORT patients did not discuss these issues with their doctors but said they wanted to.

In one sense, results of the SUPPORT study are not surprising. William Saroyan's famous line resonates with most people: "Everybody has to die but I have always believed an exception would be made in my case." This is why SUPPORT investigator Joanne Lynn sometimes calls human beings "the temporarily immortal"; most of us so blithely take life for granted that we deny the inevitability of its end until it punches us in the face. In addition, some very sick patients don't want to talk about their prognosis or preferences, choosing instead to focus all of their physical energy on getting better and all of their mental energy on optimism and hope. (In fact, for a long time most doctors believed that such talk upset patients—and maybe even made them sicker. Before the SUPPORT study, doctors rarely spoke to *any* sick patients in hospital about dying.)

For these reasons, it is naïve to think that doctors can engage hospitalized patients in these uncomfortable discussions. But it is even more naïve to think that any doctor will do. If you were severely ill in hospital, would you want to discuss your most personal hopes and fears—literally, your life and death—with a doctor you just met? This aspect of the SUPPORT study received relatively little attention: Who were all those doctors with whom so many SUPPORT patients (40 percent) *refused* to talk? Were they doctors who knew the patients well? Did they have a personal relationship with these patients?

We don't know. SUPPORT researchers reported that they had relied on "the senior most available physician acknowledging responsibility for the patient's medical decisions" in hospital. Right now in the United States, that tends to be doctors like me. But the Atkinses, for example, don't know me from Adam and I don't know them. Today, all around the United States, doctors who've just met sick and dying patients in the hospital are struggling with this same problem. We're caught in the middle of an uncoordinated, depersonalized "system" of care that values subspecialist doctors (many of whom don't take responsibility for the "whole" patient over time) and cost-efficient hospitals (most of which eschew any responsibility for the patient's pre- or posthospital care). The patient is often lost in the shuffle. Despite the many important lessons learned from the SUPPORT study long ago, the situation in many hospitals today isn't getting much better.

At the nursing station on 14 South, we confer again with Marcie and try to reconstruct what happened to Mr. Atkins and why. She came on duty at 7:00 a.m. In the change-of-shift meeting, the night nurses told Marcie that Mr. Atkins was sleeping comfortably. She had no reason to think otherwise. We don't spend time now talking about how to make sure this doesn't happen again with another patient. There's a formal hospital process to get to the bottom of such things, do better next time. For now, we just talk about what we need to do for Mr. Atkins.

While we talk, Tina enters new orders into the computer. She looks discouraged.

You okay, Tina?

Mmm . . . I'm . . . I'm feeling kind of bad about what happened in there.

Why? You did great in there.

I should have thought of this, Tina says. I should have anticipated it. I could have prevented it.

He was okay when you saw him, Tina. His blood sugar was normal last night. You're not expected to be clairvoyant.

Yeah, Chris murmurs. Dan is looking over her shoulder at the computer screen.

Hey, look, he says. Oncology has seen him already. They've entered a note.

Huh, Tina says, clicking her mouse.

It's just a few lines, typed by Dr. Mortola, the senior oncologist, at 7:10 this morning. Tina reads it to us: "Fifty-three-year-old man with widely metastatic neuroendocrine pancreatic cancer refractory to all treatment admitted for reevaluation. Therapeutic options are limited. Patient currently unresponsive. Suspect brain metastases. Please obtain STAT MRI of the brain. Will return after MRI."

Chris whistles.

They all look at me.

You did good in there, guys.

Tina isn't satisfied with that.

Mortola didn't tell the nurses? she says.

I look at the time of the oncologist's note.

Nurses' change-of-shift, I say.

Oh, Jeez, Tina says.

But now I'm remembering the vague feeling I had about Mr. Atkins when he was unconscious a few minutes ago and I wasn't sure why until Tina and the others figured it out. When I saw him around five this morning, he had been pretty drowsy. Like the nurses, I had assumed he was just sleepy.

I tell Tina and the others that Dr. Mortola probably wasn't the only one who missed it. I tell them I'd bet anything Mr. Atkins's blood sugar was dangerously low when I saw him, too.

My team doesn't say anything, but they look uncomfortable. They're not accustomed to their attending physician admitting to serious mistakes. In fact, I'm pretty sure they don't want to hear it at all.

People get hurt in hospitals. This has been well known ever since a nurse named Florence Nightingale blew the whistle 150 years ago, and the problem hasn't gone away. In one year recently, 98,609 hospitalized patients *in New York State alone* suffered a serious injury (which prolonged their hospital stay or resulted in disability). One in seven of these hospital-acquired injuries was fatal. Extrapolated nationally, this number of iatrogenic (health care–related) deaths was the equivalent of three fatal jumbo-jet crashes every two days in the United States throughout the year. About one-third of these health care "crashes" are unavoidable. (Bad things happen to sick or dying people *because* they're sick or dying.) But the remaining two-thirds of these serious errors, caused by me and other people who work in hospitals, are preventable.

Shame on us? Yes and no.

The more we learn about medical error, the more daunting it seems. In one medical intensive care unit, for example, careful research documented an average of 1.7 errors *per day per patient*, of which 29 percent had the potential for serious or fatal injury. This sounds terrible until we realize that patients in this intensive care unit required, on average, 178 important actions daily, 99 percent of which were done timely and well. However, as Lucien Leape pointed out in his classic analysis of medical error, 99 percent proficiency in health care—even in medical intensive care units where the patients are complex, the work stressful, and crises unpredictable—isn't nearly good enough. Even if health care workers were ten times better than this—99.9 percent proficiency, an error rate of only one in one thousand—Leape noted that this would be the equivalent of two unsafe landings *every day* at Chicago's giant O'Hare Airport, or sixteen thousand pieces of mail lost *every hour* by the U.S. Post Office.

Clearly, then, other industries can teach the health care industry how to do better and there is good reason to be optimistic about this. Anesthesiologists, for example, have reduced deaths caused by anesthesia from 1 in 10,000 patients (0.01 percent) two decades ago to fewer than 1 in 200,000 patients (0.0005 percent) today. We have a long way to go before we reduce error this much in other areas of medical care, but we're learning.

Although individuals like me perform the actions that "make" the errors, the cause of most errors is more complicated than one individual's screwup. In effect, less-than-fail-proof systems fail to protect patients adequately from all-too-human errors. And, as anesthesiologists have done, these systems can be improved (in many cases, through computerization), "error-proofed" to reduce the impact of fallible people's (inevitable) missteps.

Traditionally, doctors have been "bred" to be perfect. Mistakes are considered unacceptable. Infallibility is the goal. This pursuit of perfection is admirable in one sense: It is in patients' best interests if their doctors strive relentlessly to get it right. But, in reality, this ambition is absurd: No one is perfect. And, in practice, setting the bar this high is downright harmful, because "perfect" doctors don't want to see their mistakes. As a result, we often don't see them or, when we do, we reconstruct the facts to explain them away. To paraphrase a famous quotation about history, doctors who deny their mistakes are doomed to repeat them.

People in denial often experience extreme emotional distress when the object of their denial reveals itself (to themselves and others) to be . . . undeniable. When this happens to doctors—and every one of us has made mistakes that hurt patients—many of us freak out. We feel ashamed, guilty, humiliated. We think everyone will think now that we're not good doctors (because good doctors don't make mistakes). We agonize, replay the event repeatedly in our mind, relive the horror of it. It becomes a kind of post-traumatic stress disorder for many of us: We become anxious and fearful, hesitant and defensive—not where you want your head to be if you work on the front lines of medical care. Professional perfectionism not only doesn't make a better system of care, it doesn't make better doctors, either.

Why, then, is Tina beating herself up about Mr. Atkins? If the medical profession has learned these important lessons—that all doctors are fallible, like everyone else; that most errors in medicine are systems flaws, not character flaws—then why is Tina feeling guilty, or thinking she *should* feel guilty? Because, as a matter of fact, most doctors have not accepted these new ways of thinking about error. Young doctors like Tina are taught and mentored by an older generation of doctors like me. And many of us dinosaurs, still in denial, continue to demand perfection—of ourselves and others. Cultures die hard.

But Tina's reaction is more complicated than simply feeling guilty. Tina knows that *someone* must take responsibility for the patient's welfare. Systems can't do this; only people can. And with personal responsibility comes personal accountability. Doctors take the credit when things go right. (That's what keeps most of us coming to work every day.) But we must also step up and take the blame when things go wrong. That's what Tina is doing, and I admire her for it.

Yet taking responsibility isn't enough. We also need to learn from what happened to Mr. Atkins, because it will happen again—to another patient—and maybe, by learning from this experience, we will do better the next time. It has long been a truism in medicine that doctors learn most from their mistakes (although most doctors don't tell this to their patients). But the essential first step in this process is to *want to know what really happened*, regardless of how it makes us feel.

Mr. Atkins suffered a potentially catastrophic adverse event. (Severe hypoglycemia, if unrecognized and untreated, causes permanent brain damage or death.) This event occurred after, not before, Mr. Atkins came to the hospital. Was it caused by medical error? Did we, the doctors and nurses entrusted with Mr. Atkins's care, commit a terrible mistake? The easy answer is No. Mr. Atkins's hypoglycemia was caused by his disease (liver cancer and resulting anorexia), not an error by his caregivers. As in one-third of all serious patient injuries in hospitals, medical error did not cause Mr. Atkins's problem.

But regardless of who or what *caused* his blood sugar to drop to dangerous levels, the relevant question is how his caregivers could have protected Mr. Atkins from the damaging effects of hypoglycemia. Could we have anticipated its occurrence—and prevented it? Could we have recognized it earlier—and treated it—before it hurt him? If the answer to either of these questions is Yes, then we must take responsibility for errors of *omission*—things we didn't do but should have done—even if we are not culpable of errors of *commission* in this particular case.

Yes, we could have anticipated the problem and prevented it from happening. And, failing this, we could have (and should have) recognized the problem earlier and minimized the harm it caused. We didn't do what we could have done to keep Mr. Atkins safe. Importantly, in this case "we" is not some disembodied "system" of care. We is all of us who cared for Mr. Atkins during his first twelve hours in the hospital. *Every one of us* committed errors.

In retrospect, Tina wishes that she had done one simple thing differently and ordered a sugar water (glucose) solution instead of the standard saltwater (saline) solution for Mr. Atkins's intravenous feeding. Then his blood sugar would not have fallen to such a low level. The nurse who carried out Tina's order last night also missed an opportunity to avert disaster by simply asking Tina whether, in Mr. Atkins's case, glucose would be a better choice of IV fluid. In hindsight, both of these actions seem obvious: Mr. Atkins was very sick, had lost a lot of weight, and hadn't eaten solid food in days. But that's the problem with "Monday-morning quarterbacking." Knowing the outcome of a past event influences one's perception of it; this "hindsight bias" distorts one's appraisal of what happened and why. If we hope to avert similar disasters in future patients, we may need to include a "stop order" (in the computerized order entry system) in the routine process of ordering IV solutions for patients. This would require the physician to consciously choose which of several intravenous solutions is best for this particular patient *before the computer will accept the order.* As with smart algorithms for diagnosing heart attacks, a smart system can protect patients from one doctor's—or one nurse's, or one team's—human error.

In the current vernacular of patient safety efforts, Tina's (and the nurse's) error is called a "slip" (as opposed to a "mistake"). Slips are glitches in "automatic" activities—routines performed largely without thinking about them—where unintended deviation from the routine (or, in this case, failure to deviate from the routine) causes an adverse event. Slips tend to happen when we don't pay sufficient attention to the "routine" task at hand, usually due to fatigue, stress, or distraction. Tina, for example, had been up all night taking care of sick, complex patients like Mr. Warner. She'd been bombarded with pages and phone calls and other distracting interruptions. Under these conditions, other doctors—including me—might have made more than just one slip. Better systems are the best way to protect against slips.

But the errors made this morning by myself and Dr. Mortola, the oncologist, were "mistakes," not slips. Mistakes are errors in conscious thinking due to lack of knowledge or misapplied knowledge or misinterpretation of the problem. This type of medical error is not so easy to fix with better systems. It's the kind that doctors, ever susceptible to denial, tend to "explain away." In my case, I misinterpreted the problem I encountered when I first met Mr. Atkins: He was very drowsy. I assumed that he was just sleepy, not a "problem" at all. This was a perfectly reasonable assumption at five o'clock in the morning, especially after Mr. Atkins had had an exhausting day and night (and several doses of strong pain medicine). In similar situations, my assumption would be correct 99.9 percent of the time. But that's not good enough. I was wrong: Mr. Atkins was drowsy because he had begun his gradual slide into hypoglycemic coma. *Why* was I wrong? Not, as I would prefer to think, because I was unlucky, the victim of a rare, unpredictable event (spontaneous hypoglycemia) masquerading as an unremarkable nonevent (normal sleepiness). No, I was wrong because I assumed that the most obvious explanation was the correct explanation. I was lazy. Not physically lazy. Mentally lazy. I "closed" the problem prematurely. I didn't ask myself: What else could this be?

Dr. Mortola was lazy, too. When he saw the patient an hour or two after I did, Mr. Atkins wasn't just drowsy, he was unresponsive. Comatose. Dr. Mortola *assumed* that Mr. Atkins's uncontrolled, widely disseminated cancer (which, he knew, would kill Mr. Atkins soon) had spread to his brain, and he recommended further testing (a brain MRI) to confirm this assumption. But, like me, he didn't ask: What *else* could this be? And, for the same reasons, he didn't make the effort to alert either the nurses (cocooned, at the time, in their change-of-shift hand-off huddle) or the residents (on rounds, seeing other sick patients, on other floors). One can argue that Dr. Mortola's mistake was more egregious than mine. (Coma is *always* a medical emergency, never to be confused with mere sleepiness.) Naturally, I like this idea because it makes my own mistake seem more forgivable by comparison. But we both made mistakes that could have killed Mr. Atkins. Indeed, Dr. Mortola couldn't have made his mistake if I hadn't made mine a couple of hours earlier.

Mistakes often reflect well-known "cognitive dispositions" and biases. In Mr. Atkins's case, "premature closure" was the main problem. But many other pitfalls like it—including attribution bias, availability bias, visceral bias, and "satisficing"—predispose doctors to make medical errors every day, wherever medicine is practiced. Knowing more about these potential sources of error can help doctors reduce mistakes. But even doctors who know a lot about these cognitive biases—as I did when I met Mr. Atkins—don't always recognize them and avoid their hazardous effects.

We're human. We make mistakes.

It's 8:15. I ask Leah to page Dr. Mortola to let him know what's going on. The rest of us hustle toward the elevators to go to the ED.

As we walk, Tina and I are side by side, the others trailing behind.

I'd like to be there when you talk to the Atkinses later, she says.

In saying so, Tina is asking permission to stay longer in the hospital today, beyond the legal twenty-seven-straight-hours maximum work shift for residents. Regulations allow exceptions to this rule but only in special circumstances. Talking to a patient about dying isn't one of them. Tina knows this.

Yeah, I know you would.

Tina doesn't push it. She's dog-tired. She's also five months pregnant. I'd like to put my arm around her shoulder, give her a hug, and tell her I'm proud of her, as if I were talking to my daughter, Caitlin, a young professional who's just had a baby of her own. But I can't do that. I'm Tina's teacher, not her father.

When you're back on Monday, Tina, I'll give you the blow by blow.

Tina grimaces.

Blow by blow? Jeez! Let's hope it doesn't come to *that*.

Chapter 3

A SAFE BET

All practical teachers know that education is a patient process of the mastery of details. . . . There is no royal road to
learning. . . . There is a proverb about the difficulty of seeing
the wood for the trees. . . . The problem of education is to
make the pupil see the wood by means of the trees.

—Alfred North Whitehead. *The Aims of Education* (1929)

8:18 a.m.

As we navigate the narrow intersecting hallways that connect the
various parts of the emergency department on the ground floor, a
rabbit warren comes to mind. We pass other teams, doctors scurrying
as we are from Area A or Area B (the older parts of the ED) past the
Pediatric ED to Area C (the new part of the ED) and back again,
hunting for our newly admitted patients, nibbling at their charts,
nosing behind their curtains, introducing ourselves to people we don't
know and who don't know us except for what they were told by the
ED docs last night or yesterday (or the day before): No, you can't go
home, you must stay in the hospital, the Medicine doctors will come
take care of you as soon as we can find you a bed upstairs. That's what
these folks want more than anything else, a real bed in a real room, a
little privacy, a chance to rest and gather themselves for whatever they
face next—which can't be good or they wouldn't be here. The ones
who can talk say: Okay, okay, just get me upstairs, will you, please?

New Yorkers who don't know from rabbit warrens would say it's more like a maze of subway tunnels down here. There's nothing natural about twenty-foot ceilings and long tight white-washed corridors that tee and turn at precise right angles, with mysterious unmarked gunmetal doors that appear unexpectedly here and there. Though I've negotiated this labyrinth for more than a year now, I still sometimes reach for the wrong door or take a wrong turn or get lost altogether and have to stop and retrace my steps.

The young doctors never seem to get lost down here, so I fall back a pace or two behind Tina, Chris, and the others and let them lead the way.

Mr. Tosca, our team's final new admission from last night, is in the old part of the ED. To reach him we hustle past Area C, the fancy new wing where patients lie in private, glass-enclosed cubicles around a central nurses' station, next door to their very own CT scanner. The new ED wing opened just a few months ago to accommodate the swelling crowds who come here day and night, testament to New York Presbyterian's reputation for excellence but also a reflection of national trends. More than 120 million Americans will make visits to a U.S. hospital emergency department this year. Sometimes it feels like most of them are waiting right here.

My cell phone rings as we pass Area C. This surprises me; cell phones typically die down here. Perhaps the fancy new ED wing, along with its flat-panel TVs, has better wireless coverage, too. Ordinarily, when my phone rings during rounds, I ignore it and deal with the message later. But this time it's my own mom and dad's phone number that flashes on my call screen. Ruth, one of two full-time, live-in health aides employed to care for my parents, is calling. I tell Tina and the others to go ahead and start on Mr. Tosca without me.

Both ninety-one years old and in failing health, Mom and Dad desperately want to stay in their own home. They're not wealthy and their home care arrangement is very expensive, but as long as their modest savings last, home is where they want to be. Dad, a retired physician, knows he won't be around much longer—he's bedridden with metastatic bladder cancer—but he hopes Mom will have more time. A former New York City school teacher, Mom has Alzheimer's disease but still says every day how much she loves the house on Shelter Island that she scrimped and saved to buy thirty-five years ago. Despite her advancing dementia, she sometimes remembers where she is. When she does, she smiles happily, looks out her window at the Great Peconic Bay, and says, Thank God I'm not in a nursing home.

Ruth apologizes for calling. She knows I'm on-service in the hospital this month and busy around the clock. But she also knows that I would want to know that Mom passed out, unconscious, just a few minutes ago. Mom is alert now, apparently unharmed, but Ruth has called an ambulance to transport her off-island by ferry across the bay to the tiny community hospital in Greenport. Shelter Island doesn't have a hospital; in fact, these days it doesn't have a doctor—and the doctors on the mainland don't make house calls on the island. Because Mom and Dad never leave the second floor of their house, much less the island, I have become my parents' doctor, by default. This is crazy, of course. Any physician will tell you that only a fool tries to doctor his own family, but this is a damned-if-you-do-damned-if-you-don't kind of deal. There's no one else. It's the main reason I'm here, why I left a job I loved in Chicago to come back to New York.

Ruth says Mom's pulse and blood pressure are normal now, but Mom has never passed out before and Ruth is right to do what she's done. Now she tells me the ambulance guys have just pulled up to the house. Before hanging up, I tell her I'll call the Greenport hospital emergency department to make sure they know about Mom's medical history when they see her.

Ordinarily, I would ruminate about this, because syncope—the medical term for transient loss of consciousness, or fainting—can be the sign of a serious, even life-threatening, condition. From long and sometimes painful experience, I know that it requires careful attention, especially when it happens to an elderly person. But there's nothing I can do about this right now. Shelter Island is a hundred miles away. And I can't do much good here if my head is out there with Mom.

So as I push through the big double doors into our bustling ED, I tune Mom out. I've been her son for more than sixty years, but I've been a doctor for almost forty of those years. You don't survive in my line of work unless you learn how to tune in one situation and tune out another quickly, as the need requires. I'm not sure this is a good way to be but it's in my bones, who I am.

I enter Area A in the old part of the ED, an open rectangular space about forty yards long and twenty yards wide. Its design is a relic of the past when emergency rooms looked like army barracks, rows of beds lined up along the walls. A long central nursing station divides the room down the middle. On one side of the room, patients lie on gurneys, each surrounded by a flimsy cotton curtain. On the opposite side, glass walls and sliding doors isolate patients from each other, providing a semblance of privacy. That's the intent, anyway. Today, like most days, the ED is hopping, sick people on stretchers in the corridors and everywhere else, too many to put behind curtains or glass doors. This ED is one of the few truly egalitarian places in Manhattan, a place where sniveling crack addicts from East Harlem and doubled-over undocumented Dominicans from Queens wait on gurneys alongside wide-eyed, terrified Park Avenue matrons. The hospital's board of trustees, whose members know more folks on Park Avenue than in Harlem, aren't thrilled about this situation, but, unlike the fourteenth floor upstairs, there's no special place in the emergency department for rich people.

If there were such a place, Mr. Tosca would be there. A seventy-year-old man with an expensive haircut and a surgically refined jaw line, he looks anxious as I approach. A pencil-thin, plastic oxygen tube stretches across both of his cheeks and into both nostrils. Tina and the rest of my team surround him, the curtain around his bed half open. Directly across the room, on the other side of the nurses' station, the cardiac arrest team is working frantically on a patient in a glass-enclosed cubicle. There, standing high above the crowd, a young intern rises and falls mechanically, like a derrick in an oil field, pumping the patient's heart. Wide-eyed, Mr. Tosca is watching.

I close the curtain behind me as I enter.

Mr. Tosca blinks. He takes a moment to collect himself. Then he bows courteously in my direction.

Dr. Reilly, he says.

Today—and, on average, every day—about 350,000 people will seek care in U.S. hospital emergency departments. In the past decade, this number has increased at a rate twice the rate of U.S. population growth, despite the fact that almost five hundred emergency departments (10 percent of all EDs in the United States) went out of business during this time. As a result, today's EDs are overcrowded, overburdened, and sometimes overwhelmed.

True emergencies comprise only a small proportion (about 10 percent) of all patient visits to U.S. emergency departments. Relatively few ED patients arrive by ambulance; more than 3 out of 4 walk in, unassisted. Most ED patients aren't sick enough to remain in the hospital. Nationally, about 6 of every 7 patients go home after their ED visits; only 1 in 50 needs intensive care or immediate surgery. These statistics highlight the daunting challenge EDs face—treating true emergencies skillfully while inundated by crowds of patients with less serious illnesses. No doubt EDs save lives and provide an essential "safety net" for all communities lucky enough to have one. But the U.S. health care system doesn't use EDs wisely or cost-effectively.

How did this happen? It wasn't so long ago that the "ER" was just that—an emergency *room*, one small space (even in very large hospitals) equipped to handle urgent accidents. (Emergency rooms were originally called "accident units.") In 1958, one large urban hospital, whose emergency room had treated an average of eight patients per twenty-four hours in the preceding decade, reported a sixfold increase in its daily number of ER visits, most of which didn't involve accidents or emergencies of any kind. The principal reasons for the dramatic increase in ER volume at this hospital (and scores of other hospitals surveyed nationwide) were the "inability of patients to reach physicians on nights, weekends, or holidays and the orientation of the public to the hospital as a place where one can receive aid at all times." That was fifty years ago.

Since then, this trend has accelerated. The "ER" has become the "ED"—one room has become an entire "department"—which, in many hospitals, is a sprawling, crowded, high-tech complex with its own radiology and laboratory facilities. Staffed twenty-four hours per day, equipped to handle everything from gunshot wounds and heart attacks to hangnails and sniffles, EDs today account for 11 percent of all outpatient visits in the United States, 28 percent of all acute care visits, and 50 percent of all hospital admissions.

Medical insurance or the lack of it explains some of this phenomenon. One of every six ED patients today is uninsured; these patients can't get care anywhere else. (ED care is the one health benefit to which all Americans have a legal right, regardless of their ability to pay.) In addition to these uninsured, one of every four ED patients is covered by Medicaid, the insurance program for the poor that reimburses care so poorly that most doctors can't afford to treat these patients. (Like the uninsured, many Medicaid patients become "frequent fliers" in the ED because they have nowhere else to go.) Patients with Medicare or commercial insurance account for the remainder (60 percent) of ED visits, yet most of these encounters address nonemergency problems, too, for reasons similar to those that prevailed fifty years ago. In a litigious society where patients demand skillful attention right now—and where doctors are either unavailable or unwilling to constrain those demands—easy access to the ED is the path of least resistance. If you build it, they will come.

Many EDs are swamped today also because hospital capacity has shrunk for patients who really are emergencies. In many hospitals, inpatient beds are full, unavailable to patients who are seriously ill (the 10 percent of ED patients who can't go home). Then, when there's no room at the inn, these sick people wait—in the ED, for hours, sometimes for *days*.

This situation is more than inconvenient, it's dangerous. Most EDs are not equipped or staffed to care for the sickest of the sick beyond their initial triage and stabilization. This higher level of care is what the inpatient hospital is for. When staff and space in the ED are consumed with sick patients waiting for inpatient beds, both the sick and the not-so-sick people in the ED suffer. The "bed crunch" has a domino effect. Crowding, long waits, and lack of privacy affect everyone.

The solution to this problem would seem obvious: If there's no room at the inn, we need a bigger inn, right? And, in fact, there are 25 percent fewer hospital beds in the United States today than twenty years ago (about 900,000 versus 1.2 million), despite a growing U.S. population and many more elderly, infirm patients. But during this same twenty-year period, the average *duration* of patients' hospital stays has also declined about 25 percent (from seven days to five days), the result of hospitals' efforts to cut costs, increase efficiency, and improve profit margins. Under these stressful conditions—and because inpatients today are older and sicker than ever—delays and bottlenecks are inevitable. Increasingly, sick patients wait in the ED because getting patients out of the hospital—so that others can get in—is anything but simple.

Part of the problem is finding somewhere to send them. Homeless hospitalized patients are just the tip of this iceberg (although sending a sick person "home" to a cardboard tent under a bridge always gives one pause). More prevalent is the challenge presented by patients who have homes but can't go there. In New York State, for example, only two-thirds of hospital inpatients over age sixty-five are discharged to their homes (579,000 of 889,000 in 2006); the remainder go to institutions, such as nursing homes and "acute rehabilitation" facilities. This is increasingly problematic because, as U.S. society ages, there is a growing shortage of such institutions (and inadequate funding for more). Furthermore, about one-third of hospitalized patients who *can* go home (175,000 of 579,000 in 2006 in New York) require additional "ancillary" services—physical therapy, dietary counseling, assistance with transportation or insurance—to assist them after they leave the hospital. Formerly provided (during longer stays) in hospital, these services must now be provided elsewhere. All hospitals now employ social workers to oversee this "discharge planning" process and advocate for patients' needs.

Even for patients who *can* go directly home from the hospital and who *don't* need many ancillary services, the hospital discharge process is complex. Every patient (and, often, their family members) must be instructed about which medications to take after discharge, how to take them, and which previously prescribed medications to discontinue. (Despite intensive efforts to improve this "medication reconciliation" process, posthospitalization surveys show that as many as 70 percent of all patients discharged from hospital don't know which medications to take!) In addition, all patients discharged from hospital must be educated about their medical condition, how it was treated in hospital, and what to expect in the future. Detailed "discharge summaries" about patients' hospitalization must be written (and made available to the patients and their outpatient caregivers). Timely follow-up appointments also must be arranged, not infrequently with several specialists as well as a primary care physician (if the patient has one).

Most important, efforts to "transition" care from the inpatient to the outpatient setting are more cumbersome today than in the past because the doctors who care for patients in the hospital ("hospitalists") are not the same doctors who will care for these patients after they leave the hospital. Many hospitals are trying hard to improve these "transitions of care" because poor discharge planning can result in patients' being *readmitted* to the hospital unnecessarily and new government regulations will deny payment to hospitals for these readmissions. (Hospitals, whether for-profit or not-for-profit, are businesses; to understand them, follow the money.)

Despite these intensive efforts, the process of hospital discharge remains fraught with unpredictability and last-minute glitches. Most patients don't leave the hospital until late in the day, thus delaying availability of their vacated room, which must be cleaned meticulously before a newly admitted patient can use it. (Hospitals aren't hotels; they can't charge guests for an extra day if they stay past checkout time.) Other patients, despite the best-laid discharge plans, don't leave even then: Unexpectedly, they may take a turn for the worse or, at the last minute, simply refuse to leave.

As this complex dance plays itself out on a hospital's inpatient wards, patients in the ED wait. And, as they wait, their doctors often must make uneasy decisions. *Must* this patient stay in the hospital? Might it be safe to send him home? *How much* does this patient "need" to be in hospital? Different doctors understand and answer these questions in different ways. Ultimately, these differences are the main reason why managing "throughput" in busy hospitals is so hard to do well.

Mr. Tosca regards us warily. Above his head, a cardiac monitor bleeps his heart beats, tinny plinking sounds. An IV line runs into his arm. To his right, behind a curtain, we hear a surgeon telling someone, *Hang on now, hang on, just a little longer, we're almost done.* To his left, an unseen person snores loudly, the stuttering exhalations a mix of wheezes and moans. I tune it out. I suspect Mr. Tosca can't.

Tina says she's just finishing her presentation to the team.

Mr. Tosca turns to me.

Dr. Reilly, I thought . . .

I hold up a finger, interrupting him.

Mr. Tosca, let's see what Dr. Johansen thinks first, okay?

He turns to Tina, bows his head deferentially, and murmurs, But yes, of course.

I can almost hear him saying this in the same courtly way to a countess requesting a tour of his Tuscan villa: But yes, of cawss. Mr. Tosca's accent is Noo Yawk continental—a mix, he told me earlier this morning, of Milan and Manhattan. His demeanor is polite but formal. Surrounded by the suffering masses here in the ED, his aristocratic mien and manner seem surreal, as if we've all just walked into a Fellini film.

In summary, Tina says to us all, Mr. Tosca is a seventy-year-old man with Type 2 diabetes who came to the ED last night after experiencing chest pain, palpitations, and shortness of breath at home. When he arrived, his symptoms had begun to resolve and his physical examination and electrocardiogram were normal. A CT scan of his chest was negative, no evidence of pulmonary emboli. Overnight, a repeat electrocardiogram and two sets of troponins drawn four hours apart ruled out myocardial infarction. The ED has admitted him to us with a diagnosis of acute coronary syndrome. We've started him on aspirin and IV heparin. We've held the clopidogrel and beta-blockers for now. The plan is to admit him, observe him over the weekend, get Cardiology involved if his symptoms recur but otherwise stress him on Monday, and then decide whether he'll need a cath.

I know these things already, because I saw Mr. Tosca a couple of hours ago and read Tina's admitting note, which summarized her impressions and plan. But the other members of my team have just met Mr. Tosca and they're hearing all this for the first time.

So you think this is unstable angina? I ask Tina.

Most likely, she says. I don't get any history of prior angina or coronary disease. But a man of his age with diabetes and a story like this? We have to assume it's an acute coronary syndrome until proven otherwise.

Okay.

Tina nods, seems satisfied. Unlike her other two overnight admissions, Mr. Warner and Mr. Atkins, this is an easy one.

We talk briefly about the spectrum of "acute coronary syndromes." These range from acute myocardial infarction—a life-threatening heart attack—to unstable angina, a less severe precursor of myocardial infarction (MI) whose timely recognition and treatment can prevent serious heart damage before it occurs. Tina is on top of all this: She has analyzed Mr. Tosca's history, physical exam, and electrocardiograms and concluded that his unstable angina falls into the "intermediate risk" category. This means that his short-term risk of MI or death is neither "high" nor "low" but somewhere in between. Given this assessment, Tina and the ED docs have chosen the correct initial treatment, a combination of blood-thinning drugs proven to improve outcomes in patients with this condition.

Mr. Tosca listens carefully to what we say. He's tired. He's been here in the ED all night and hasn't slept much. But when he hears us talk about short-term risks of MI and death, he scowls and begins to protest.

Dr. Reilly, you said . . .

I put my finger to my lips.

Yes, I know, Mr. Tosca. All will become clear in a few minutes. I'm sorry if we've upset you. Would you prefer that we talk outside, without you?

Certainly not! he says emphatically. It is *my* heart, yes?

A few more minutes, then, all right?

Tina squints. She and the others still haven't gotten used to the idea that I see their new, overnight admissions before they "present" them to me. (This practice is countercultural at Cornell and most other large teaching hospitals.) She doesn't know yet what Mr. Tosca and I talked about earlier.

Dan and Chris and Tina are holding copies of Mr. Tosca's electrocardiograms (ECGs), the paper tracings that depict the electrical currents and rhythm of his heart.

Everybody agree about those ECGs? I ask.

They all nod.

Cold normal, Chris says, the two done here in the ED and the one the ambulance guys did at his home. No Q waves or ST changes to suggest infarction or ischemia.

No signs of heart failure on his physical exam, right?

Right, Tina says.

No recurrence of symptoms since he's been here? No more chest pain or palpitations or shortness of breath?

No, Tina says. He's been fine.

She puts her hand lightly on Mr. Tosca's shoulder and leans toward him.

You're doing just fine, sir, she says.

He lies back against his pillow. But his eyes dart from Tina to me and back again.

I turn to Tina.

So everything depends on his story, doesn't it? His physical exam and his tests look good. So we're basing our decision *entirely* on the history. Unlike the two admissions we've just seen upstairs—neither of them could tell us much of anything—in Mr. Tosca's case, what he tells us is *all* we've to go on. True?

True, Tina says.

Mr. Tosca, Dr. Johansen has brought our whole team with her this morning. Maybe they can help us with your problem. Can you tell them what happened to you last night?

Certainly, doctors. I am sitting in my apartment with my wife. I begin to feel . . . discomfort here. (*He puts his hand over his heart.*)

Mmm, heaviness . . . tightness, maybe, but very strong . . . and I am having trouble to catch my breathing . . . my heart, it is pounding hard like it will jump out of my body, *Boom-ba-boom-ba-boom* . . . and I feel very bad . . . *very* bad, like I will die.

Dan tilts back on his heels, purses his lips. He's impressed.

Chris, our future cardiologist, asks, How long did this last, sir?

Last night? Mr. Tosca says. Mmm . . . twenty minutes, thirty? Mmm, maybe longer . . . I am still feeling this way when I am coming to the hospital.

Chris points to the electrocardiogram papers.

And when the ambulance people did this first cardiogram at your home, Mr. Tosca? You were feeling sick then?

Oh, yes, doctor. I am very bad. The ambulance people, they say the cardiogram doesn't show a heart attack. They say . . . they must take me to hospital . . . to make sure . . . do more tests.

Uh-huh. And when you got here? You were better?

Aah . . . I am a little better, yes, doctor. But my heart, it is still going *Boom-ba-boom* and I am not catching my breathing. The doctors do this test again. *(He points to the electrocardiograms.)* They say it is good. I am glad for this. Soon I am feeling better. But they say I need more tests. When Dr. Johansen tells me that my tests are all coming good, I am very happy.

Chris holds up the third electrocardiogram and scans it again quickly.

And this last one, sir? This says it was done at . . . 4:45 this morning. How did you feel then?

I am fine, doctor. No problem.

Chris turns to Tina.

So. No dynamic ECG changes. That's good.

Tina nods. Mr. Tosca nods, too.

No previous episodes, right? Chris asks Tina.

Tina consults her notes, then touches Mr. Tosca's shoulder lightly again.

Sir, I believe you told me that you had had similar symptoms the night before also, is that right? Not as severe as last night but something like it?

Yes, Dr. Johansen. Mmm . . . when I am speaking to Dr. Reilly this morning? I am remembering . . . I have this same feeling every night this week.

Tina closes one eye.

Every night? she says.

Yes, doctor.

Tina bites her lip.

Hmm, Chris says. Exertional symptoms? he asks Tina.

Tina is struggling now, trying to make sense of what Mr. Tosca just said.

No, she says. He hasn't had any symptoms when he walks or does physical exercise.

Unnerved, Tina looks to Mr. Tosca for confirmation.

Yes, this is so, Dr. Johansen. I have no problem doing the physical things. Knock on the wood, yes?

Hmm, Chris says again.

Suddenly, the patient behind the curtain to our left is moaning more than he's snoring. Moaning *loudly*. I can't tune this out. I pull the curtain back to check on him. The guy barely fits on two gurneys pushed together; he weighs six hundred pounds if he weighs an ounce. He looks like hell but two nurses are tending to him, adjusting his breathing mask and drawing blood.

I pull the curtain closed, turn back to Mr. Tosca.

His eyes are wide. He licks his lips. He doesn't speak.

Mr. Tosca, can you tell the doctors what kinds of physical activity you've been doing recently?

Certainly, doctor. Ah, how to begin? My son-in-law, he is renovating a penthouse on Seventy-fourth Street, you know? This is very expensive, I think maybe too expensive, this house. So I am helping him, you know? Every day we go to the Home Depot on Fifty-eighth Street and we pick up the supplies we need and we bring them back to the house and we do the work.

You do this in a car or a truck or what?

Oh, no, doctor, like I told you, we walk.

So every day for the past week you have been carrying supplies from Fifty-eighth Street to Seventy-fourth Street?

Yes, doctor.

What kind of supplies?

Lumber. Sometimes other things.

Lumber? How heavy?

I don't know, fifty, maybe sixty kilos. This is not a problem for me, doctor.

Tina's shoulders slump.

And when you are doing this, Mr. Tosca, carrying these heavy supplies and walking all that way, do you ever feel the chest discomfort or shortness of breath or *Boom-ba-boom* in your heart?

No, Dr. Reilly.

Tina and Chris exchange glances.

Let's be sure about this, Mr. Tosca. For the past week, you've been doing heavy manual labor all day, every day, without any problem at all. But in the evening of those same days, *every* evening, you have experienced these symptoms at home, resting, not doing anything in particular. Is this correct?

Yes, doctor.

Tina shakes her head.

That doesn't make sense, she says.

No, I agree, it doesn't make sense, does it?

Indignant, Mr. Tosca says, But I am sure about this, Dr. Reilly.

Yes, I know, Mr. Tosca. We're not saying that *you* don't make sense. *You* make perfect sense. What doesn't make sense is what *we* think.

Ahh.

Let me explain. Heart pains typically happen during physical exertion, because that's when the heart must pump harder and faster. If the heart can't get enough blood and oxygen to do this harder work, then the physical exertion causes the heart muscle to hurt.

Mr. Tosca nods vigorously.

I understand, doctor. So . . . this is not my problem, yes?

An unseen voice suddenly yells out from behind the curtain and across the room: *No, no, no! A pericardial needle, for Chrissakes! Come on! Come on! We're losin' this guy!*

Then we hear voices Sh-shing, feet shuffling. A heavy glass door slams shut.

Mr. Tosca closes his eyes. We both pretend we didn't hear this.

So, what do you think, Tina?

Last night I was worried that he'd ruptured a plaque.

Right.

But if his symptoms started a week ago—and given what we've just heard—then I don't think that's right. I don't think he has unstable angina.

Yeah. So what do we do now? The ED guys want to admit him to the hospital. Do you?

Tina pauses, looks at Mr. Tosca.

Yes, she says. From what he's just told us, I agree he's very low risk for any serious cardiac event. *Very* low risk, like less than one percent. So, from that perspective, sending him home seems like a safe bet.

Mr. Tosca nods appreciatively.

But . . . Tina says, shaking her head.

But?

But if this isn't unstable angina, then what is it? *Something* is happening that's pretty scary for Mr. Tosca. If I do your mother-father test, Dr. Reilly, I'm thinking let's keep him, work him up, find out what's going on . . .

A puzzled look crosses Mr. Tosca's face but I don't interrupt Tina to explain to him the "mother-father test." (When discussing uncertain clinical decisions with physicians-in-training, I sometimes ask them what they would do if the patient were their own mother or father. Their answer is enlightening sometimes.)

. . . so, if Mr. Tosca were my dad, Dr. Reilly, I'd admit him to the hospital, take no chances.

I look at Mr. Tosca.

He doesn't seem puzzled now. He can't take his eyes off Tina. It's like he's seeing her for the first time.

The elephant in the room—in this case, the emergency room—is the reality that all clinical decisions in medicine are probabilistic. *Every* clinical decision is uncertain, its outcome unsure. Many patients don't know this.

It is not a small matter. Patients like Mr. Tosca are not hard to find. At this very moment, more than eight thousand Americans are being evaluated for a possible heart attack in U.S. emergency departments. Chest pain is the single most common reason adults seek care in EDs, accounting for about six million annual visits. Large EDs admit a new chest pain patient, on average, *every hour* over the course of a typical twenty-four-hour period, every day. Ironically, this deluge of such patients in hospital emergency departments reflects a remarkable public health triumph. Public awareness of coronary heart disease—long the leading killer of Americans, including several U.S. presidents—has grown to a point where most adults today know that chest pain may be a sign of an impending "coronary" (a myo-cardial infarction, or heart attack). This awareness, combined with scientific and clinical advances in treatment, has reduced mortality from coronary heart disease by more than half in the past generation, an extraordinary accomplishment.

This achievement, however, has come at a high cost, because the great majority of people who come to EDs worried about chest pain have nothing wrong with their heart. And yet, most of these patients—whose pains are caused by minor problems like indigestion or a strained chest muscle—are kept in the ED for twelve hours or more, undergoing repeated tests on their heart. Because these tests are often inconclusive, many of these patients are then admitted to the hospital for even more sophisticated (and expensive) cardiac test-ing. In other words, our well-intentioned (and successful) effort to combat coronary heart disease spends substantial medical resources on patients who don't need them. Many experts believe that this is the price we must pay to continue "winning the war" against coro-nary heart disease (which, despite great progress, remains the leading cause of death in the United States).

But, as with other wars, inevitable questions arise about whether the price we pay is too high. Consider, for example, a large (fifty-bed) ED that treats twenty chest pain patients per day. These pa-tients will stay in the ED, on average, for at least twelve hours. This means that, on average, at least 20 percent (ten of fifty) of all beds in that ED are *solely* devoted to chest pain patients. This would be a smart investment if most of these patients were having heart attacks, but they're not. Very few of them have any heart problem at all.

Why, then, do we do this? As recently as ten years ago, between 1 and 4 percent of all patients who actually *were having* heart attacks were "missed" in the emergency department and mistakenly sent home. Nationwide, this meant that thousands of heart attacks were being missed annually in U.S. EDs. Not surprisingly, missed MIs became the single most costly cause of medical malpractice lawsuits filed against physicians working in EDs. As a result, doctors became extremely risk-averse when treating ED patients with chest pain.

This is why, today, the tail wags the elephant. The "tail of the curve"—the very small percentage of heart attacks that are hard to diagnose, easy to miss—drives our elephant of a health care system to strive *never to miss a single one*. Consider an ED where, on average, 10 percent of all patients presenting with chest pain will have a proven heart attack. (This "MI rate" varies widely among different EDs.) Now assume that the best evidence-based diagnostic protocol (including evaluation by a physician and performance of serial tests over a twelve-hour period in the ED) will miss 2 percent of these heart attacks. If this ED evaluates a total of 2,000 chest pain patients per year (10 percent, or 200, of whom are having heart attacks), then it will miss 4 heart attacks (2 percent of the 200) per year. But the only way to avoid these 4 "misses" is to perform additional diagnostic tests in *all* of the chest pain patients. Remarkably, this is exactly what we do, usually by keeping these patients in the ED (or in specialized "ED chest pain units") until they can undergo more sophisticated testing. To avoid missing 4 heart attacks in a year, then, we perform additional, expensive cardiac testing on 1,804 patients! (Clearly, this practice does not alleviate the problem of overcrowding in emergency departments.)

Hospitals and some doctors (especially the ones who perform the expensive heart tests) tend to applaud this practice because they profit from it financially. Most (insured) patients applaud, too, because they end up feeling reassured about their heart—and it doesn't cost them a dime. Even the insurance companies tend to buy the elephant act because it's less expensive than what we used to do—"observe" the patient in the hospital for two to three days. (For decades, "rule out MI" was the most common admitting diagnosis in U.S. hospitals.) But it's hard not to conclude that we are wasting precious resources (ED and hospital beds, doctors' and nurses' time, billions of dollars) by overreacting to this very important public health problem.

There may a better way, but it depends on how you feel about probability and risk, the two things that bedevil all medical decisions.

For example, Tina has concluded that Mr. Tosca has less than a 1-in-100 chance of having a bad outcome if she sends him home from the ED. To her credit, Tina is quoting the best scientific research about the probability that a patient like Mr. Tosca will suffer any serious cardiac complication over the next few days (which, if such a complication did occur, would have justified his being admitted to the hospital). This research shows that patients like Mr. Tosca—whose vital signs, physical examination, and ECGs are normal and whose history is not typical for a heart attack—are "very low risk" for one of these bad outcomes. Specifically, the probability that a patient like Mr. Tosca will suffer a serious cardiac complication requiring urgent hospital treatment is about 1 in 200.

Remember: There is no way to predict a *zero* probability of such a complication. *Absolute certainty is not achievable.* Mr. Tosca's 1-in-200 chance of a serious complication—or, in other words, 199-to-1 odds *in his favor* that he will do fine—is "as good as it gets" when predicting outcomes for ED patients with chest pain. When advised of this fact, some very low-risk patients (and their doctors) will say, Well, I don't want to be the *one* who has the bad outcome! (Such people, if given the choice, typically don't want to leave the ED; they want additional cardiac tests.) Other patients, however, consider a 1-in-200 chance so remote that it's not even worth their thinking about. (Given the choice, these people typically want to go home without further testing.) But, in most EDs today, patients are not informed about these odds and risks. Nor are they given a choice. Instead, the "standard of care" in U.S. emergency departments is to do further testing on *all* such "very low-risk" patients despite the fact that 199 out of 200 don't need it.

Or do they? "Need" is a tricky thing. Put yourself in Mr. Tosca's place. If you were told today that you have 1 chance in 200 of having a life-threatening cardiac emergency some time in the next three days, would you want to be admitted to a hospital now and undergo testing and monitoring of your heart to mitigate that risk? (This is not an idle "What if?" Given the high prevalence of this problem in the U.S. population, there's a pretty good chance you will have to make this decision yourself someday.) In part, your answer to this question will depend on how much you fear the possibility of having a cardiac emergency. (If you're one hundred years old and have terminal cancer, for example, you might not fear this possibility so much.)

But your answer will also depend on how you "feel" about the 0.5 percent (1-in-200) probability itself. Psychological research about decision-making has shown that people vary not only in how much they fear particular outcomes of a decision, we also vary in how we "weight" the probabilities of those outcomes. Many of us do this in an irrational way: We treat small probabilities as if they're much larger than they really (mathematically) are. This phenomenon explains why taking effortful steps to circumvent a tiny risk (such as 1-in-200) appeals to many people. For them, that tiny risk doesn't "feel" tiny at all.

Such "irrationality" affects doctors, too. My clinical decisions "feel" different—and, sometimes, I decide differently—when emotion complicates the calculus. When the patient is my mother or father, for example.

Mr. Tosca listens patiently while we briefly review the possibilities. If it's not an impending heart attack—this is now very unlikely—then what is causing Mr. Tosca's symptoms? He doesn't say anything when we use words like tachyarrhythmia, hypertrophic cardiomyopathy, or pheochromocytoma. It's all Greek to him. But he bristles visibly when we talk about cocaine.

Tina sees this. She pats him gently on the shoulder and winks.

Mr. Tosca, we're just talking, trying to learn.

Still, he looks at her sternly, then at me.

Dr. Johansen, Dr. Reilly, I do *not* do the cocaine.

Yes, sir, we know, sir, Tina says soothingly. (The ED docs have already tested Mr. Tosca's urine for cocaine and other drugs.)

Soon, however, our team runs out of other ideas. I push them. Think, guys. His story is the key. The answer is in Mr. Tosca's story.

But . . . Tina says. We've already . . .

Not that story, Tina. Mr. Tosca's story is that he came to this country from Italy as a young man. He started with nothing. He worked hard. Now he owns *La Tosca*—do you know it?—very exclusive, one of Manhattan's finest restaurants, very fancy.

Mr. Tosca makes an appreciative bow in my direction.

Now Mr. Tosca is helping his son-in-law to do the same. In fact, recently he helped his son-in-law buy his own restaurant here on the Upper East Side. It's going well but maybe, Mr. Tosca thinks, maybe not well enough for his daughter and son-in-law to buy a multimillion-dollar penthouse on Seventy-fourth Street. So, he is doing everything he can to help them, including help with the penthouse renovations himself. But he's worried about this. He thinks maybe his kids are taking too many chances, overspending, moving too fast. He says he worries about this a lot these days.

Mr. Tosca looks down at his hands. He purses his lips pensively and nods.

This is so, doctor, he says.

And so, I continue, for the past week, after spending every day working with his son-in-law in his expensive new penthouse, Mr. Tosca comes home, has dinner with his wife, and thinks about these things. And that's when he develops his symptoms: the chest discomfort, the feeling of air hunger, the palpitations.

Chris isn't buying this idea. Neither is Tina.

Okay, Tina says, I see where you're going, Dr. Reilly. But . . . at this point . . . you can't *prove* that these episodes are anxiety attacks any more than I can prove that they're caused by coronary disease or . . . or a pheo, for that matter. Our job is to *know*, isn't it? Not just make our best guess . . .

Yes.

So?

It's in your hands.

Uh . . . well, okay, thanks for your confidence, Dr. Reilly . . . but, like I've been saying, I think we should admit him to the hospital.

No, I mean it's *in your hands*. Chris and Dan's hands, too.

They look at each other's hands. They're all holding Mr. Tosca's ECGs.

His electrocardiograms are all normal, Tina says. We've already . . .

They're all the same.

Uh . . . right . . . normal, same . . . same difference, right?

Not exactly. It all depends on what you're looking *for*.

O-kay . . .

We've looked at the ECGs to see if they show any signs of cardiac ischemia, right? That's why the ECGs were done in the first place. True?

True.

Let's look at them again. But now let's ask a different question. We're trying to make sense of Mr. Tosca's *story*, right? Well, those ECGs are objective pieces of information obtained *during* his story.

Yeah . . . ?

Look at the first one. It was done at Mr. Tosca's home when he felt so bad he thought he was dying—his heart going *Boom-ba-boom* and all that. Where's the *Boom-ba-boom* on this ECG? Now look at the second one. It was done here in the ED, when Mr. Tosca was having the same symptoms. Again, do you see any *Boom-ba-boom* on that ECG? And these first two ECGs are identical to the third one. When that one was done, how was Mr. Tosca? He tells us he felt fine.

Tina's frown is incredulous. She leans forward and speaks softly to Mr. Tosca.

Sir, you are sure about this?

Yes, doctor, I am sure. When Dr. Reilly shows me these papers, earlier this morning, I am surprised, too.

Tina turns to me.

You're saying . . . Mr. Tosca was feeling these things . . . his heart racing and all that . . . but it wasn't really happening?

Not exactly. Mr. Tosca *experienced* the feelings he told us about. He certainly didn't make them up.

Then . . . ?

Chris is studying the ECGs carefully, comparing each to the others.

Very cool, he says. I've heard of this but never . . . *Very* cool.

This? Tina says. What's *this?*

Chris holds up the ECGs.

They say this is what you see sometimes with anxiety attacks . . . panic attacks. The patient *perceives* symptoms like a rapid heartbeat even though there's no objective sign of it when it's happening. There's some kind of disconnect in these anxiety disorders between what the patient *feels* subjectively and what's *actually* happening objectively.

Tina considers this.

How is that possible? she asks.

Hah! Mr. Tosca interjects. Exactly, Dr. Johansen! This is what I say! This is my question, too!

Tina looks at me skeptically.

So . . . ?

I look at Mr. Tosca. He turns to Tina.

Dr. Johansen, Dr. Reilly tells me that if he knows the answer to this question, he will not be here . . .

Her patience fading, Tina rolls her hands in a forward spinning motion.

Mr. Tosca chuckles and continues.

. . . Dr. Reilly said if he knows the answer to this question he will be in Stockholm . . .

Chris begins to laugh.

. . . receiving the Nobel Prize for Medicine.

Mr. Tosca beams. Dan grins. Tina smirks.

The residents have all seen patients with serious cardiac arrhythmias. That's what Chris and Tina and Dan are trained to worry about when a patient complains of palpitations, Mr. Tosca's *Boom-ba-boom-ba-boom*. But, working in hospitals, residents see patients who are just the tip of the iceberg—the "sickest" tip. Even Chris, a budding cardiologist, is surprised when I tell them that the single most common cause of palpitations in the general population is panic attacks, not heart diseases.

We talk about this briefly. How panic disorders often present with physical symptoms even when the patient is not consciously aware of feeling panicky or anxious. How, as in Mr. Tosca's case, the key to diagnosis is the recognition of discordance between what the patient reports and what doctors actually observe (or know to be physiologically possible).

It all sounds neat and tidy in the telling of it. In fact, somatization is a mystery. Medical science doesn't understand it at all.

Somatization is the medical term for "the propensity to experience and report somatic (bodily) symptoms that have no pathophysiological explanation, to misattribute them to disease, and to seek medical attention for them." It is extraordinarily common. No physical cause can be found to explain patients' physical symptoms in 25 to 50 percent *of all patient visits* to doctors; psychosocial factors play the major role in prompting these visits. Somatization is also highly democratic: It affects people of all ages, personality types, cultures, and intellectual levels. Medical students, for example, when first learning about symptoms and signs of human disease, often become convinced that they have one or more of the diseases they are studying. Older people, as they endure the sickness and death of their loved ones, sometimes develop "sympathetic" symptoms themselves (not unlike some husbands who, in sympathy with their pregnant wives, experience their own morning sickness).

For many patients, somatization is extremely disabling, a source of great suffering. ("Somatoform disorders" comprise a whole spectrum of debilitating conditions.) Sadly, it has become a mode of communication, a way people express distress in our "medicalized" secular society. Lacking confessors or confidants, many people today take their worries and anxieties to a doctor, complaining only of headaches or fatigue or other vague physical symptoms. Many doctors fail to recognize these symptoms as an expression of psychological distress, the patient's ticket into the doctor's office. When the doctor misses this connection, the patient's "real" problem remains unaddressed.

No one knows how somatization "works" biologically, the physical mechanisms whereby psychological tension causes headaches or anxiety causes rapid breathing. Especially mysterious is the subconscious nature of the process. Tension headache sufferers, for example, often deny any "tension" in their lives. This makes the doctor's job doubly difficult. Convincing a patient that physical symptoms are due *entirely* to psychological distress is hard enough; doing so when the patient adamantly denies any psychological distress or mood disturbance is an even taller order.

We also don't understand the flip side of somatization: how some patients with obvious, advanced, symptomatic diseases (like cancer or AIDS) can deny what they see in the mirror, repress what they feel in their bones, or delay seeking medical help until it's too late. How the brain achieves these mysterious "disconnections" between the conscious "soma" (body) and the subconscious "psyche" (mind) is one of the great scientific unknowns.

An extreme example of mind-body interaction is panic attacks, defined as a discrete period (developing abruptly and peaking within ten minutes of onset) of intense discomfort or fear characterized by four or more of thirteen common symptoms: palpitations, sweating, trembling, shortness of breath, choking, chest pain, abdominal distress, dizziness, feelings of unreality or "depersonalization" (feeling detached from oneself), fear of losing control or going crazy, fear of dying, numbness or tingling sensations, and chills or hot flushes. In some patients, the "psychic" symptoms (such as fear or depersonalization) predominate and diagnosis of panic attack usually is easy. But, in most patients, it is the "somatic" symptoms of panic that bring them to doctors, often in emergency rooms. This is not an overreaction; it makes perfect sense. Mr. Tosca's panic symptoms, for example—chest pain, shortness of breath, and palpitations—are the classic symptoms of a heart attack. If this ever happened to me, I'd call an ambulance, too.

Remarkably, doctors tend to trivialize the suffering of patients with panic attacks—and somatization in general. When it becomes clear that the patient is not having a heart attack—it's "only" a panic attack—many doctors lose interest or, worse, blame the patient for wasting their time. (I did this myself many times before I learned better.) These dismissive attitudes and behaviors have deep roots in the medical profession: They go to the core of *what medicine is for.* For many doctors, the purpose of medicine is to cure disease. For these "curing" doctors, if you don't have a definable disease—panic attacks are not a disease—then you've come to the wrong place. But, for other doctors, the purpose of medicine is the same today as it has been for centuries: to relieve human suffering—*sometimes* by curing disease (when we can) but *always* by empathizing with, understanding, and trying to comfort the sufferer.

Doctors' dismissive attitudes toward patients with "psychosomatic" illness are not only unhelpful, they are harmful. Patients with panic attacks, for example, don't just go away after they've been told that their chest pain or palpitations or choking "is all in your head." They suffer. They get worse. They somatize more, not less. They make more visits to doctors and emergency rooms, undergo more tests, spend more of our precious health care resources. The less well they are understood, the more hypochondriacal (and angry) they become. These patients get sicker the more doctors tell them they're not sick.

Occasionally, as in Mr. Tosca's case, the doctor (and patient) gets lucky: Unassailable, objective evidence confirms that what the patient feels, although "real," is *purely* subjective. Knowing this—and knowing that the single most common cause of heart palpitations in the general population is a panic attack, not a heart attack—made it easy to diagnose Mr. Tosca. Often, though, it's anything but easy, because the "hidden reasons" that patients visit medical doctors—emotional distress, psychiatric disorders, loneliness, fear, a need for reassurance or understanding—are hidden from the patient as well as the doctor.

The clue to diagnosing somatization is the doctor's own intuitive feeling that the patient's motivation for seeking medical help is unclear or seems odd. Sometimes, the genesis of this intuition is commonsensical. For example, in Mr. Tosca's case, the obvious question was: Why did he come to the ED *last night*? Why not the night before, or the night before that? After all, he's had these episodes *every* night for a week. But, in other cases, the doctor's suspicion of somatization seems to come out of nowhere. The doctor has recognized some clue, but its recognition remains subconscious. It's just a feeling. How this occurs is a mystery, like somatization itself.

So what can we do for Mr. Tosca? I ask my team. How can we help him?

Chris, Tina, and Dan don't know much about this subject—they're training to be internists, not psychiatrists—but they mention several classes of drugs used for anxiety and panic disorders and some behavioral treatments they've heard about.

Interested? I ask Mr. Tosca.

No, doctor, he says emphatically. These things are not for me. Like we talked before, Dr. Reilly, I need to . . . accept my . . . situation . . . what makes me feel this way . . . I . . . I must talk to my family . . .

I look at Dan, then Tina. So, what do you think Mr. Tosca needs now? How can we help him? His cardiologist checks his heart every year. His endocrinologist checks his diabetes. His ophthalmologist checks his eyes. His podiatrist checks his feet. And yet . . . here he is . . . spending all night in a crazy emergency room having an anxiety attack . . .

Tina and Dan know where I'm going with this, because we seem to talk about this same thing almost every day. So many of the patients we see here have an "-ologist" for this and an "-ologist" for that, multiple subspecialists each taking care of his or her own piece of the person. But when we ask these folks the question I asked the Atkinses upstairs, most of them look at us like we're speaking a foreign language.

He needs a doctor, Tina answers.

Mr. Tosca looks at me. He doesn't repeat now what he had said to me a few hours earlier. Then, he had said, Will *you* be my doctor, Dr. Reilly? There was a time when I would have answered him, Yes, flattered to be asked. But that was then. Now, I never say Yes. I tell them that I do a lot of administrative work in my job here, that I get to see patients only during occasional month-long stretches like this one, and even then, I see patients only in the hospital. I never explain further. I don't tell them about Fred and Martha, my patients from years ago, or how I got this way. I turn to Tina.

Yes, I agree. Mr. Tosca needs a doctor.

Tina looks whipped. She's exhausted from being up all night and thinks she should have done better with Mr. Tosca. She expects a lot of herself, even though she's been out of med school for only a little more than a year.

But I won't need to reassure Tina again, as I did upstairs. Mr. Tosca turns to Tina and makes a courtly bow.

Dr. Johansen, will *you* be my doctor?

And, just like that, Tina isn't tired at all. She looks like a young girl who's just been asked to the prom.

It would be an honor, Mr. Tosca. Thank you.

He bows again. Thank *you*, he says.

We make the necessary arrangements at the nursing station: discharge orders, a follow-up appointment with Tina in the clinic next week, an address where Mr. Tosca can send his medical records. Before we go, Tina steps back behind the curtain and gives Mr. Tosca her pager number so he can reach her if he needs to. Then she asks him if he'd like her to call his wife at home.

She's probably worried about you, Tina says.

Oh, no, Dr. Johansen. Tina and I exchange puzzled looks.

My wife, he explains, we have been married for forty-five years. She knows me better than anyone.

Yes . . . ? Tina says.

He shrugs his shoulders, smiles, and throws up his hands.

How can I say? My wife, she is no doctor . . . but . . . she tells me every day this week . . . this is all in my head!

We laugh.

I'd like to meet her, Tina says.

And so you shall, Mr. Tosca says warmly. So you shall.

We say good-bye. I look at my watch. It's 8:40. It's taken us an hour and a half just to see Tina's three new overnight admissions. We have all of our other patients to see before Tina leaves at ten.

On our way out, Tom, one of the ED docs, overhears that we are sending Mr. Tosca home. He doesn't know Mr. Tosca. But Tom took his hand-offs this morning when the ED shifts changed at 7:00 a.m., so he knows that Mr. Tosca is an elderly man with diabetes being admitted to the Cardiology floor with an acute coronary syndrome. I explain briefly what's happened, what we think.

Even so, Tom says, pretty gutsy to send him home. An old guy with diabetes . . . ?

I've had hundreds of conversations with ED docs in the past about patients like Mr. Tosca, so I know "gutsy" isn't what Tom really means. He means "dumb."

Why not keep him, work him up, make sure you're right? Tom says.

Because it won't help him. Plus, it's a waste of another ten thousand bucks.

Tom shrugs.

Plus, we need the beds. Where we gonna put all these people? I say to Tom, looking around at the dozens of bodies lying here on ED gurneys.

Tom shrugs again. Not my problem, he says.

Tom's right, of course. It's not his job to make sure that our hospital has enough beds for every patient who comes here. Tom's job is to do what he thinks is best for every patient he sees. But this gets tricky when Tom's opinion about what's best for one patient conflicts with what may be best for other patients. Tom knows this, but he doesn't talk about it. It's the elephant in the room.

Instead, Tom tilts his head toward the glass-enclosed resuscitation room. There, ED nurses and technicians are cleaning up the mess after their unsuccessful cardiac arrest effort. The patient lies there on his gurney, a tube sticking up out of his throat, waiting to be wheeled down to the morgue.

See that guy there? Tom says. He was in some other ED yesterday. We don't know the details yet but his wife says they sent him home. They told her he was okay.

Tom shakes his head. He nods in Mr. Tosca's direction, then looks at me.

So, this guy? What's his name, Tosca?

Yeah.

So, what if you're wrong?

Chapter 4

WHAT'S THE PLAN?

The simple view is that medicine exists to fight death and disease, and that is, of course, its most basic task. Death is the enemy. But the enemy has superior forces. Eventually, it wins. And, in a war that you cannot win, you don't want a general who fights to the point of total annihilation. You don't want Custer. You want Robert E. Lee, someone who knew how to fight for territory when he could and how to surrender when he couldn't, someone who understood that the damage is greater if all you do is fight to the bitter end.

—Atul Gawande, "Letting Go" (*The New Yorker*, 2010)

9:50 a.m.

Mr. Mukaj doesn't look like a guy caught between a rock and a hard place. Right now, he's caught between two beautiful young women lying in bed with him. One languishes on her side facing away from us, her head at his feet. Honey-blond hair cascades down her back, the curves of her body tapering to long bare legs stretched out atop the sheets. Mr. Mukaj, propped on pillows like a pharaoh at court, caresses her feet absentmindedly as he laughs at whatever the other woman is whispering to him. This one, auburn-haired and stunning, is under the covers with him, her body spooned against his from behind, her lips nibbling, murmuring in his ear. His eyes are closed, his expression rapturous. Mr. Mukaj is in heaven.

It's no easy trick to simulate heaven on the tenth floor of New York Presbyterian Hospital. This floor is filled mainly with people referred here for treatment of refractory leukemia and bone marrow transplants, not a group prone to rapture. Mr. Mukaj doesn't have leukemia but you'd think he did from the gruesome paraphernalia around his bed. Six gallon-size plastic bags of fluid dangle from poles above his head. An even bigger bag, nearly filled with several liters of his blood-red urine, hangs below his bedrail. An electric pump attached to his IV line propels morphine into his vein. As his right hand strokes the blond woman's ankle, his left hand fondles the red button he taps whenever he wants a bigger dose of painkiller.

His auburn-haired granddaughter smiles when she sees us, welcoming us with a silent wink, a dazzling come-hither look impossible to refuse. She doesn't move or disturb her Papa's reverie. Her blond cousin turns her head, looks over her shoulder at us, and nods a happy hello.

Chris and Leah, pinch-hitting on our team today, haven't seen Mr. Mukaj and his harem before. Chris's eyes widen as we enter the room. It looks like a *Saturday Night Live* sketch about hospital amenities.

Tina speaks softly, almost a whisper, to the granddaughter. Good morning, Magdalena, she says.

Dr. Johansen, Magdalena murmurs into her grandfather's ear.

Mr. Mukaj stirs now, opening his eyes.

Aahh, he says, seeing Tina, his speech slurred but sensuous, Zee luffly doaktoor Yo-hahn-sen, how happy to see you.

He reaches for her hand, as if inviting her to join his threesome. Tina gently pats his arm, humoring him. She likes Mr. Mukaj. We all like him. He's a charming guy even when he's not high on morphine, a "good" patient with bad problems. We're all hoping we can help.

It won't be easy. He's been here for almost two weeks now. He'd had groin pain for some time, even back home in Croatia, but ignored it until, while visiting his granddaughter here in New York, his urine turned blood red. After a while he couldn't pee at all and his bladder began to hurt so bad he had to come to the ED. It didn't take us long to drain his bladder with a catheter through his penis to relieve his pain. Nor did it take long to find the grapefruit-size bladder cancer causing his bleeding and urinary obstruction. A CT scan showed the reason for his groin pain—the cancer has spread through his pelvis and into his right hip bone—which means we can't cure the cancer no matter what we try.

That's the rock: Mr. Mukaj's metastatic bladder cancer. The hard place is his heart. We discovered this quickly, too, if not in the most elegant way. On the first day, Dan was doing a simple rectal examination with his finger (to make sure all that blood was coming from Mr. Mukaj's bladder, not from his rectum, too) when Mr. Mukaj experienced crushing chest pain that lasted until we were able to get enough morphine into him to relieve it. His electrocardiograms and blood tests showed that he was having a heart attack—not the "major" kind that needs a heart operation immediately but the "minor" kind that means he is on the brink of having the big one any time now. Whether precipitated by the discomfort of Dan's rectal examination or, more likely, the stress of everything else that was happening to him, Mr. Mukaj's heart attack meant three things. One, his heart could kill him before his cancer does. Two, we can't treat his cancer until we treat his heart. And three, it will be a long time before the other interns stop ribbing Dan about his rectal examination technique.

Two weeks later, we haven't made much progress. We've had to keep Mr. Mukaj in bed because his cancerous hip looks ominous on the X-rays, maybe ready to fracture if it bears any weight. He's bleeding a lot from his bladder, so much that he's needed blood transfusions to keep up with it. On several occasions, the bleeding has been so heavy that blood clots formed inside his bladder and obstructed the catheter in his penis, causing excruciating pain in his belly (and dangerously stressing his heart). The cardiologists can't operate on his heart because doing so would require the use of powerful blood-thinners, which could make his bladder bleeding even worse. Conversely, the urologists can't operate on his bladder to stop the bleeding because the stress of surgery on his heart might kill him. For the same reason, the orthopedists can't pin his hip to prevent it from crumbling.

So, we're biding our time. For the past week, we've been "irrigating" his bladder—running liters of saline into his bladder through the urinary catheter, then letting the bloody fluid drain out into the catheter bag before repeating the process all over again. Called continuous bladder irrigation, this procedure dilutes the blood in his bladder to prevent it from clotting and obstructing his urinary catheter. The urologists say sometimes the irrigation slows the bleeding, too, but this hasn't happened yet. Despite our efforts, his catheter has clotted twice in the last three days. The only good thing is that Mr. Mukaj has had no further heart episodes. If he's lucky, as each day passes his heart will heal a little from the heart attack two weeks ago. If he's unlucky, he'll have the big one before we can prevent it.

Mr. Mukaj doesn't look like a man living with a death sentence. He could easily pass for ten years younger than his seventy-two years. A full head of thick, dark hair frames his ruggedly handsome Serbian face. The morphine makes him loopy but he's a brilliant guy, an emeritus professor of political philosophy who speaks six languages. His home in Croatia, on the Adriatic coast near Albania, is in what his granddaughter describes as "the most awesome picture-perfect-postcard town you ever saw." She told us proudly that he is the elected mayor of his town, an honor he himself pooh-poohed by explaining that his large extended family accounts for half of the town's voting population.

But he makes no bones about the fact that that is where he wants to be. He wants to go home.

Last week, this raised the option of finessing both the rock and the hard place: We could do nothing about his cancer or his heart and simply arrange his discharge home. Mr. Mukaj himself took to this idea eagerly. The sooner, the better, he said, which also made the hospital's social workers perk up. Mr. Mukaj's medical insurance will cover everything in Greece, Italy, or France but little, if anything, here in the United States. He doesn't have much money. So, neither New York Presbyterian Hospital nor any of the doctors here will be reimbursed for the hundreds of thousands of dollars his care will cost. It would be far less expensive for the hospital to foot the bill for his transportation back home, even if it meant paying for a special medical transport plane to fly him direct to Dubrovnik.

But now we know we can't do that. Because now we know what he wants. We enlisted the help of a Serbian interpreter who also speaks Italian and Greek. (When the morphine kicks in, Mr. Mukaj sometimes alternates among several languages.) After explaining the pros and cons of his going home, I said, It's a hard decision, Mr. Mukaj. Only you can make it. But perhaps I can help if you can answer a question for me.

Yes, doak-toor?

Knowing all these details about your medical condition, what is the most important thing you want right now?

My question puzzled him. He asked the interpreter to repeat it.

Ah! he said. I want . . . to be young . . . and healthy.

Yeah. Me, too.

He was not amused. He harrumphed and flicked his fingers at me.

Okay, okay, I understand.

He thought for a moment, then spoke again.

Do you know my country, doak-toor?

No. I would like to visit someday.

You must. You must come to my village. I will tell my people about you.

Thank you.

How can I explain, doak-toor? Every day in my village, in the afternoon, I walk from my house to the . . . how do you call it . . . the piazza? . . . the town square, yes? . . . It is a short walk. Mine is a small town . . . I go to the piazza to sit, in the sun . . . We are on a high hill, my village. On the coast. We look out to the sea. The gulls there, they ride the breeze—the wind is good, they don't need to work their wings, you know? It is like this for the people, too. Life is good in my village. I watch the men play . . . Mmm, the boule? . . . the boccie, you know it? . . . We drink some wine, we talk about the football . . . these are my cousins, my friends . . . We have known each other all our lives. When the sun begins to go into the water, the women come out of their houses, too. They walk in the piazza. They look out to the sea. The men tease them, make the eyes at them, you know? The women, they laugh . . .

As he spoke, the Serbian interpreter modulated her own voice.

A tired-looking, middle-aged woman who had seemed hurried and peremptory at first, she began to translate his words more slowly, almost reverently. She didn't turn to me now as she spoke. She looked only at him, repeating his words like a chant or a prayer, talking to him, not to me.

. . . and the young ones, they are watching, you know? And sometimes they will sit with me there in the piazza and we will talk . . . family, love, life, you know, doak-toor? . . . And then we light the lamps when the stars come out . . . someday you will come and see the night, the sky, in my country . . . We talk and laugh and drink the wine and then we walk back to our houses for the supper time and then . . . tomorrow . . .

His voice trailed off. He looked down at his hands, remembering. The interpreter seemed to hold her breath.

It took only a few more minutes to answer my question. What was important to Mr. Mukaj wasn't just to *be* back home. He wanted to *walk*. He didn't care if he dropped dead from another heart attack. Or if he gradually bled to death from his bladder. In the time I have left, he said, I want to be with my people. I want to walk from my house—like a man—to the piazza. And I want to walk back to my house when the night comes.

Then, he said with a shrug, we will see if the morning will come.

So, there it was. Our job is to help him walk. We can't just ship him home.

Dan and Tina quickly explain the situation to Chris. He needs to know these things because he will be Dan's supervising senior resident in the hospital today. It's a lot to digest but Chris, after asking a few questions, gets the picture. He shoots me a look that seems to say, Wow! This, too? Mr. Mukaj is the final patient on our team rounds this morning and, yes, he's complicated, but Chris sees he's just the icing on the cake. Most of our other patients are every bit as tough.

Dare I ask? Chris says. What's the plan?

Dan chuckles. Chris is making a little joke. He's asking the same question I've asked the team repeatedly this morning, about each of our other patients.

Just before coming up to 10 South to see Mr. Mukaj, we had left another patient, Mona Lisa, down on 8 West. Talk about complicated. Out loud I use her real name, Ms. Rhodik, but in my mind I call her Mona Lisa. It's her eyes. They don't move—they don't even blink—but somehow they follow you around the room. It's spooky. Ms. Rhodik's looking at you, no doubt about that, but we don't know what she sees. Or hears. Or wants. And that's the question: How can we do right by her—how can we make a plan—if we don't know what she wants?

I know what her family wants. But what they want is bananas.

Ms. Rhodik is seventy-five years old. She's Russian. That's the only language she speaks—if she speaks at all. Her family says she speaks to them sometimes and maybe she does but, during the week I've known her, I've never seen or heard it. On a few occasions, I've stood outside her door, listening surreptitiously when I know she has visitors, trying to confirm what her family says about her speaking sometimes. But, as best I can tell so far, she's mute. I don't know what to think about the fact that her sons tell me otherwise. Her white-haired husband is worried, diffident, and speaks not a word of English. He visits and holds her hand, in silence, every day. She stares, straight ahead, mute. Even with a Russian interpreter present, her husband simply shakes his head and says to me, Please, doctor, talk to my sons. Ms. Rhodik has breast cancer, the bad kind, progressively metastatic despite multiple rounds of treatment. The oncologists say there's nothing more they can do. Ms. Rhodik was transferred to our team last week from the intensive care unit, where she'd been treated for aspiration pneumonia. It's the third time this has happened in the past four months. Each time the pneumonia has been worse than the previous one; this time she almost died. She's better now, but her family members—three sons and their wives—have been insisting that we feed her by mouth, despite her history and the fact that our swallowing specialists have documented repeatedly that, whenever she tries to eat or drink, she aspirates into her windpipe. Her gag reflex and cough are just too weak to protect her airway. Sometimes we have to snake a tube down her throat and suction her vigorously just to prevent her from drowning in her own saliva. Feeding her is out of the question.

Still, one of her sons (or one of their wives) calls every night to badger the nurses and our resident to feed Mona Lisa some "real food." Every night, they insist that food is all Ms. Rhodik has left to enjoy in life, why deny her? Her sons say she has had a "mental disorder" for her entire adult life. It's called something else in Kiev but it sounds like schizophrenia to us (and to the psychiatrists we've consulted here). She's taken large doses of antipsychotic drugs for years. Now, because she can't swallow, we must administer these drugs intravenously, along with her nutritional supplementation and the antibiotics for her pneumonia. To get her off IVs, she will need a feeding tube inserted into her stomach. Her family refuses to grant permission for this. If they persist in refusing, the only alternatives are to keep her in the hospital indefinitely or discharge her home, where, her family readily admits, they will feed her whatever she likes. (They know what she likes. They say she tells them so.) This is what the family did after her two previous hospitalizations for aspiration pneumonia; each time, within days of going home, she became deathly ill again.

We have told her sons—in her presence, in her room, just in case she's listening—that her swallowing weakness might be reversible. We have proposed that we try the feeding tube, transfer her to a rehabilitation facility where she can receive further nutrition and intensive physical therapy for her weakness and her swallowing dysfunction. After several weeks, she might improve enough to achieve what her family says is her own personal goal: to be at home, surrounded by her grandchildren, able to eat and drink. We have also recommended that hospice become involved now—to help Ms. Rhodik in the rehab facility and, if she improves, at home thereafter.

But her family says no. They are adamant. They want us to remove her IV, feed her food by mouth, and see what happens. If she develops pneumonia again, for a fourth time, okay, they say, then maybe we will reconsider.

We can't do this. We know it will hurt her, maybe kill her.

Hearing this, her eldest son responds, with a Russian accent and Tolstoyan rectitude, *How can you know this, doctor? The future is unknowable, is it not?* He's a smart guy, not at all naïve about medical care. (He works in a hospital himself.) Yet when I explain his mother's situation in detail, he simply says, *You know, you are a good negotiator, doctor*. He seems to think we're doing some kind of horse trade here: We give this, you give that, maybe we make a deal.

When we rounded this morning, one of Mona Lisa's daughters-in-law was in her room. This was the one, Tina told us, who had called her three times during the night. This morning, she wanted to argue more about Tina's refusal to feed Ms. Rhodik. I am a physical therapist, she said, I am an expert about these things. She said she *knows* Ms. Rhodik can swallow. She said this triumphantly, smugly, as if maybe she had just proved it to herself. Hearing this, I tried to see if Ms. Rhodik had any food in her mouth. But this Mona Lisa doesn't smile, much less open her mouth, so I didn't push it. The daughter-in-law smirked, as if she had just won something. I reminded her that we have arranged a family conference at noon today. (Saturday is the only day we can get all three sons and their father together.) I encouraged the daughter-in-law to attend. She smirked again, said nothing.

Watching all this on rounds, Chris had chewed on his cheek. As we left Ms. Rhodik's room, Tina gave him a see-what-I-mean? kind of look. Chris turned to me.

Don't worry, Chris, I'll do the meeting with the family. I've asked the Palliative Care guys to come in, too. Noon, here in the conference room, but only if you have time.

Chris looked relieved. Thanks, he said. Then, only half kidding, he added, Maybe you should ask the guy next door to talk to them, too.

The guy next door is going home today. Sort of. Home now for Mr. Gunther is Bethesda, Maryland, where he moved from New York nine months ago to live near the National Institutes of Health. Almost forty years ago, at age twenty-eight, Mr. Gunther had been cured of advanced Hodgkin's Disease by NIH doctors who were experimenting with new kinds of chemotherapy for his then-deadly type of lymphatic cancer. (Mr. Gunther was one of the first; today, 90 percent of Hodgkin's patients are cured.) But now he has a rare kind of leukemia, probably caused by his chemotherapy long ago. Last week, while visiting New York, he developed a high fever and shaking chills; he wanted to return immediately to Bethesda but the NIH docs wisely advised him to come here first. We found that he had

WHAT'S THE PLAN? 101

CLABSI (central line–associated bloodstream infection), blood poisoning caused by bacterial contamination of the intravenous catheter in his neck used to infuse chemotherapy drugs and blood products. After a few days of antibiotics here, he feels much better but he's anxious to get back to the NIH. He knows his central line catheter may need to be removed—it's the "permanent" kind of catheter whose insertion or removal requires a surgical procedure—but he wants this decision to be taken with the doctors who know him best. We've spoken with the NIH docs, who've graciously agreed to transfer him to their hospital today even though it's a weekend. We've tanked Mr. Gunther up with large doses of intravenous antibiotics to cover him during the long drive to Maryland.

On rounds this morning, I shook his hand and wished him luck.

Thanks, doc, he said, I'll need it . . .

He made a lopsided half-smile. He knows his chances of winning the lottery twice aren't good. He knows that, almost certainly, his leukemia will kill him. But he has the resources to fight it. And, God knows, he has the will.

. . . but . . . who knows, eh, doc? Maybe Pascal cashed in, too?

I laughed. This was our little joke.

I hope so, Mr. Gunther. I hope he did.

After we left him, on our way to see Mona Lisa, Chris stopped in the corridor and asked what Mr. Gunther meant. I hadn't told the team about an exchange that Mr. Gunther and I had the night before last. Then, Mr. Gunther made clear his wish to return to NIH as soon as possible. He thanked me for what we had done here, praised the hospital for the excellent care he had received, reassured me that his desire to leave was no reflection on us. I told him I would do the same thing if I were in his position. He has a long-standing, trusting relationship with one of his NIH doctors, and that's a big plus. Still, I probed a little. I said Mr. Gunther's story was a remarkable one. I asked him how he felt about it. Did he feel cursed? Blessed? Both?

He thought about this for a moment before answering, then said he'd never believed in God or an afterlife, not even when he thought he was dying young, years ago. So, for me, Mr. Gunther said, this life is all there is. I'll go anywhere, do anything to keep breathing.

I've made more money than I can spend and I'll gladly pay it all just to watch the sun come up again tomorrow, see my wife's lovely face. I'll do whatever it takes to beat this thing.

He paused. He could see that I was unconvinced. He asked me if I knew Pascal's wager.

Pascal, the seventeenth-century French philosopher and mathematician (who died at age thirty-nine), had made a famous "bet" that God exists. It's impossible to know for sure, Pascal had reasoned, but the smart bettor should go with God. Why? Because if you bet that God exists and you're wrong, you lose relatively little. But if you bet against Him and you're wrong, you lose everything. Even if we think that the probability of God's existence is infinitesimally small, Pascal argued, we should still bet on Him because, if we're right, our reward will be infinitely great.

It's like that for me, Mr. Gunther said. Life means everything to me. Its value, for me, is infinite. So it doesn't matter how high the odds are stacked against me. I'll do anything to stay alive. Anything.

I didn't mention what I knew about rebuttals to Pascal. The important thing was that Mr. Gunther knew what he wanted. And, God knows, he knew better than anyone what he was up against. That's why Chris, after hearing about Pascal, was only half kidding when he suggested that Mr. Gunther advise Mona Lisa's family. Mr. Gunther's plan was a long shot but it made sense. What Mona Lisa's family wants makes no sense at all. I was not looking forward to our family conference at noon.

Now, in Mr. Mukaj's room, his beautiful granddaughter puts her hand on her Papa's chest.

Monday is his heart operation, right? she says cheerfully.

Yes. That's the plan.

Wonderful, she says.

She gives her Papa a gentle hug and says, This will protect his heart for the cancer operations, right?

Mr. Mukaj, floating somewhere in his morphine haze, hears her voice, opens his eyes. He seems surprised to see me.

Ah, doak-toor! Hello, doak-toor! Thank you! You are protecting me, yes? You are protecting me! I am thanking you!

Yes, Mr. Mukaj, we will protect you.

It's a simple plan. The cardiologists will operate on Monday, try to open his coronary arteries to prevent another heart attack. If this goes well, then we will see whether the blood-thinning drugs used to protect his heart will make his bladder cancer bleed even more. If so, we will stop the blood-thinners. In the aftermath of his heart procedure, this could cause a fatal heart attack but . . . maybe not, he might get lucky. Then, if we can't control the bladder bleeding even after stopping the blood-thinners, the urologists will surgically remove his entire bladder. It's a big operation. It won't cure his cancer—nothing will—but, if he survives, at least it will stop the bleeding. Then, if he's still alive after the heart procedure and the bladder operation, the orthopedic surgeons can pin his hip to prevent his cancerous bone from fracturing when he gets out of bed. If he makes it through that final operation, too, then maybe he'll walk again, if he can handle the weeks of physical therapy to follow.

A lot of ifs and maybes, but that's the plan. Everyone has agreed to give it a go, even though the odds are against him and none of the doctors will get paid a dime for any of it. It makes sense to try, knowing what Mr. Mukaj wants.

For me, this case has been a hard one because, whenever I see Mr. Mukaj, I see my own father. Except for his heart, which is relatively healthy, Dad has *exactly* the same condition as Mr. Mukaj—a big bleeding bladder cancer with a painful metastasis in his right hip. Dad's plan is to do nothing. He's twenty years older than Mr. Mukaj and blind from macular degeneration. (The only good thing about this is that he can't see all that bloody urine draining out of his own catheter.) His hip hurts but he's used to worse pain than that. For several years now, he has suffered from postherpetic neuralgia, which, whenever it strikes, makes him double over in agony and grit his teeth. He doesn't like people to see this. None of the drugs help; they just make him confused. Still, somehow—I don't know how—Dad is able to laugh and enjoy visits from his children and grandchildren. His plan is to stay at home with Mom—confined to his bed, unable to ambulate or even sit up, listening to talk radio—and just wait for the end.

Now Mr. Mukaj's granddaughter hugs him again.

I will protect you, too, Papa, she says, tickling him.

He laughs, deliriously carefree.

Then, suddenly, he is groaning, deep piteous moans. He presses both fists into his lower abdomen, against his bladder. The girls leap up from his bed.

Oh, shit! Dan says.

In a flash, Dan grabs a large plastic basin from the floor and puts it beneath the urine collection bag, which, swollen tense with liters of bloody fluid, seems ready to explode. Mr. Mukaj is grimacing so hard now that his whole body shakes, his face twisted with pain. Dan opens the spigot on the urine bag. With a gush, bloody urine splashes into the basin with such force that it splatters the floor red. As the bladder bag begins to empty and deflate, Mr. Mukaj stops shaking, then begins whimpering with relief.

Oh! he says. Oh!

And then, just like that, he is smiling again.

Ah! he says happily, I am feeling good now! Thank you, doak-toor! I am feeling good!

Dan mutters something and leaves the room to find a nurse. Continuous bladder irrigation is a very demanding nursing task. The big drainage bag needs to be emptied every twenty or thirty minutes around the clock. If it isn't emptied on time, the bag fills, the fluid backs up into the bladder, distending it so much it hurts like hell. We may need to move Mr. Mukaj to an intensive care unit just to make sure a nurse can be with him all the time. I explain this to his granddaughter.

Yes, of course, of course, she says, we want you to do everything you can. Everything.

When patients (and their families) say they want doctors to do "everything," it's tempting to assume they mean what they say: I want you to use every available means at your disposal to save (or prolong) my life. The will to live is hardwired into the human genome; when faced with life-threatening illness, of course we want our doctors to do everything to beat it. This is a no-brainer. Dying is the worst thing that can happen to you, right?

Some of us, like Mr. Gunther, think so. But others aren't so sure. For them, the key question is: *compared to what?*

There are few sorrier sights in medicine than watching human beings—or what remains of them—tethered to life-support machines with no hope of recovery, victims of untold suffering, all because no one ever bothered to ask them what they meant when they said they wanted "everything." Too late, these folks (and their families) discover a not-so-closely guarded secret: Some fates are worse than death. If you surveyed U.S. hospitals and nursing homes today, you would find thousands of patients who, if they could still think and talk, would tell you they'd rather be dead.

Knowing this, some doctors take the time and trouble to ask what patients really mean. For some patients "Do everything" really means "Don't give up on me" or "Do everything you, as my doctor, think can help me." For other patients, it means they're scared, or they don't understand how sick they are, or they don't want to hurt loved ones who can't "let go." But, whatever it means for each person, the request to "do everything" cannot be understood (and respected) unless the doctor explores that person's own unique goals as the end of life approaches.

Tim Quill, an internist and palliative care expert at the University of Rochester, recommends that doctors begin to explore what patients want by asking them a simple question, the same question I asked Mr. Mukaj: Given what you have learned about your medical condition, what is most important to you? Quill's research has shown that, when answering this question, most patients who are faced with terminal illness don't focus on curing their disease (typically because they already know that cure is not an option). Instead, about three of every four such patients focus on quality of life, especially relief of pain and suffering (which may be psychological or spiritual as well as physical). But every patient is different. Each of us has his own feelings about the "trade-off" between prolonging life and the suffering this may entail. How much discomfort are you willing to endure to live longer? How much longevity are you willing to sacrifice to live better? There are no right or wrong answers to these questions. The only certainty is that you can't answer them reliably for anyone but yourself.

Mr. Gunther, the man returning to the NIH today for his leukemia treatment, wants every treatment that has any possible potential to prolong his life even a small amount, no matter how much suffering this causes. This is an extreme position, which requires questioning and clarification by his doctors, but Mr. Gunther knows whereof he speaks: He has already beaten one "terminal" illness, and it cost him a lot more than a pound of flesh to do it. Like Job, he's been down in the belly of the beast and, remarkably, he's willing to go down there again. When Mr. Gunther says he wants everything, he knows what it means and he means what he says.

In contrast, although Mr. Mukaj wants "everything," too, his goal is different from Mr. Gunther's. Mr. Mukaj wants to live out whatever time he has left the *way* he wants to live it. For him it's *all about* quality, not quantity, of life. He wants to go home and walk "like a man" even if it kills him. He wants to die with his boots on. This kind of decision is not unusual; many people choose quality over quantity of life and, for some of us, remaining physically active is the most important thing. What makes Mr. Mukaj unusual, like Mr. Gunther, is how clearly he has thought this through, how well he knows what's important *to him*, regardless of what others (including his doctors) may think. Mr. Mukaj's "everything" is very different from Mr. Gunther's but they both know what they want and why.

Many of us don't know what we want. When the question is posed hypothetically, most people say they want "everything" done to prolong their life, but when crunch time comes—when the hypothetical crisis becomes real—many of us change our minds. My father, for example, began his fight against cancer with an attitude similar to Mr. Gunther's. Dad wanted everything done that had a reasonable chance of prolonging his life even if it caused him suffering. Given his other burdens—Dad is very old, blind, suffers from chronic pain, and his dear wife of sixty-five years is demented—*any* increase in suffering was a lot to bear. Still, he traveled to Chicago for his first cancer operation. A few years later, he traveled to New York for two more operations. But when it became clear that Dad would lose his fight, despite everything the best of modern medicine could give him, his priorities shifted. His "everything" changed—from Mr. Gunther's priority to prolong life at any cost to Mr. Mukaj's quest for "quality time."

This trajectory is the road many of us will travel when we confront terminal illness. In the beginning, our hope of winning makes the suffering bearable. In the end, when we know we won't win, the same suffering becomes intolerable. The important point here is that what we want evolves over time. Ask a patient what "everything" means today and you may well get a different answer tomorrow. That's why it's so important that the patient have at least one doctor who *knows* her, who follows her over time.

Of course, understanding what the patient wants is only the first step. It is essential also to make sure that what the patient wants makes sense *for her*. I don't doubt that a patient like Mona Lisa, as death nears, *might* prefer the pleasures of eating and drinking to a slightly longer life devoid of those pleasures. But this preference, if true to Mona Lisa's own wishes, is inconsistent with her family's insistence on "doing everything" to keep her alive. Achieving both goals is impossible; pursuing both can only *harm* Ms. Rhodik, not help her.

Patients who want everything are everywhere, and their numbers are growing. But balancing the hopes and fears of patients and families, negotiating potential benefits and harms of treatment, finding ways to honor patients' values even as tough, pragmatic decisions must be made are not tasks that doctors can accomplish with pills or scalpels. It's all about listening, finding out who the patient is, what's important to her. The process must start there.

Most of the sad stories happen when this process doesn't start until it's too late. That's how all those folks wind up comatose in nursing homes and intensive care units, fogged with drugs and flogged by machines, not a prayer of getting better. It's a living hell—and the only hyperbole in that phrase is the "living" part.

10:50 a.m.

Standing in the vestibule outside Mr. Atkins's VIP room on 14 South, I'm struggling. There's a right way to do this. But first I have to get my own act together. I've just spoken to Mortola and the Oncology team. They told me what they told Mr. Atkins's wife—and what she told them. She's pissed. So I know this won't go well even if I'm on my game. But I'm not on my game, not yet anyway. Because I'm pissed, too. And that's not where you want your head to be at a time like this. You don't want distractions.

I don't want to be thinking about Mr. Warner, our delirious old guy with HIV and probable endocarditis, who just was wheeled into the elevator to go down to MRI. I'm worried about him. (Will the MRI show that he's bleeding in his brain?) But I have to tune him out. Right now, to do right by the Atkinses, I have to tune out Mr. Warner and Mona Lisa and her crazy family and Mom at the hospital on Long Island and Dad at home and Mr. Mukaj's heart and bloody urine bags. I have to put them all out of my head.

But that's not enough, because what I'm pissed about is Julie and Gordon. If I can't tune them out, I might just barge in here and make a mess of it with the Atkinses.

Gordon had been waiting for me in the 14 South corridor as I approached Mr. Atkins's room. It's hard to say no to a guy in a wheelchair, even one as creepily obsequious as Gordon. It'll just take a minute, doc, do you mind? Then the shit-eating grin again.

When I entered her room, Julie muted the TV. She had brought her own luxurious comforter, plush pillows, and silk bedclothes from home. Propped up in her bed, she looked like an Asian empress at the Beverly Hills Hotel.

I wonder, Julie said, her myxedematous voice croaking like a frog, I wonder . . . if you would be so kind . . . as to do me a small . . . favor, doctor?

I glanced at Gordon. That grin.

Julie said she needed a "leave of absence" from the hospital to take care of some very important business. It's a family emergency, Julie said, nodding, as if this explained everything. She wanted to continue her hospitalization indefinitely—as long as it takes to cure me, she said—but she wanted to leave the hospital Monday morning and return Monday evening.

Gordon regarded me with a soulful, supplicant look as fake as a three-dollar bill. They're in this together, whatever it is.

I'm sorry to hear that, Julie. What kind of emergency?

She lowered her eyes, tried to mimic Gordon's puppy dog look.

It's personal, doctor. Very personal. I can't talk about it.

I told them "leaves of absence" are against hospital policy. It can't be done. It's a legal thing. I told Julie she can be discharged on Monday—my team was planning to do this anyway—but then she would no longer be the hospital's responsibility. Or mine.

Julie began to whimper and whine. Her swollen lips quivering, she protested the "inhumanity" of such a policy.

Doctor, her life is in danger, Gordon pleaded. If Julie doesn't get her thyroid medicine in the IV, she could die. You wouldn't want that on your conscience, would you, doctor? Surely you can make an exception and override the hospital policy?

Julie nodded, looked hopefully at me.

I repeated what I'd already said.

Julie began to weep, loudly. I can't do that, she said.

Gordon rolled his wheelchair to her side, took her hand in both of his. He murmured soothing things.

Whatever they're up to, they're good. But I don't want to know what they're up to. It's none of my business and that's what pisses me off: They've made it my business. In the midst of all this—all these sick patients, like Mr. Atkins, struggling to handle the bad hands they've been dealt—I have to deal with these two?

Monday morning, Julie. Discharge from the hospital. Got it?

I didn't wait for her answer. I glanced again at Gordon as I left. He was grinning again.

Have a good day, doctor, he said soothingly, as I closed the door behind me.

So now, as I stand outside the Atkinses' room, just down the corridor from Julie's, I know I should wait. Cool off.

But I don't wait. I knock, walk in.

He's awake. She's sitting on his left, near the window, her hand on his shoulder. The room is flooded with bright sunlight.

Yes, Mr. Atkins says, I remember you.

They both watch me as I go to the windows. The sun is high. In the wake of the storm, it's a pristine blue-sky day. Far below, its banks piled high with snow, the big river rolls south. There, in the distance, beyond the great bridges, the sea is shining. It could take your breath away.

But now is not the time to marvel at how beautiful the world can be. I draw down the window shades. The big plasma TV on the wall is tuned to satellite radio, something classical, soothing. I switch it off. The sudden silence echoes in the room.

They watch me as I take the phone off its hook on the bedside table. I unplug the intercom to the nursing station, close the door after dragging in a chair from the vestibule. I sit down close to the bed on his right side, my eyes now level with his. I reach through the buttons of my white coat, remove my pager and cell phone, turn them off, put them on the bedside table. I ask Ms. Atkins to do the same.

She starts to protest but catches herself. She reaches into her handbag and silences her phone.

Thank you.

She nods, glowering. Her husband closes his eyes for a moment, then looks at me.

The oncologists were here, he says.

Yes.

Hmmph, his wife says.

I've spoken with them in some detail, Mr. Atkins. I'm sorry I couldn't be here when they were speaking to you. Maybe you could tell me what you took away from what they said?

Hmmph! his wife says again. Took away? That's the right word for it, all right.

Hon . . . he says, shaking his head.

I look from her to him and back again.

Mr. and Ms. Atkins, we've just met. You don't know me. But, as you can see, I'm not a young man. I've been doing this kind of work for a long time now. I think I have at least some sense of how hard this must be for you both. I wish for your sake things were different. But we need to talk about things the way they are.

They stare at me. Neither speaks.

So, please, folks, bear with me for just a minute. Mr. Atkins, now that you've spoken with the oncologists, can you tell me what you understand about your present medical condition?

Understand? his wife says indignantly. *Understand?* Oh, please! Do we *understand?* Who do you think has been living with this . . . ?

It's okay, hon . . .

. . . for all these months and years? *Do we understand?*

. . . it's okay, hon . . .

I don't respond. I just wait. A minute, maybe. It feels like a month.

Mr. Atkins breaks the silence.

They tell me there's nothing more they can do, he says in a soft voice. They say I've had all the treatments. Mortola said he checked with Sloan Kettering and M.D. Anderson and the others. There's nothing left, nothing else . . .

Yeah, we'll see about that! his wife interjects. She takes her cell phone out of her bag. I've got calls in right now, she says, to the people in Boston and the people at Mayo! We'll see about that!

Ms. Atkins, of course you can do whatever . . .

Honey, her husband says softly. Honey . . .

You bet I can! she says to me angrily. We're gonna . . .

Sarah, Mr. Atkins says quietly, Sarah . . .

. . . talk to the people at Dana Farber and we're gonna put him on a plane and we're gonna . . .

Suddenly Mr. Atkins yells at the top of his voice.

Sarah! Sarah!

Startled, we both look at him. His eyes are closed now. He seems to be concentrating with all his might. He's breathing hard and fast. The effort of shouting out two words has taken every bit of his strength.

Oh! his wife says. Peter, what . . . ?

He takes another deep breath. He opens his eyes, looks at her.

Sarah, he says, his voice breathless, soft again.

Yes, Peter? What . . . ?

I'm sorry, he says. Honey, I'm sorry.

What . . . ?

I . . . I can't do it, Sarah . . . Can't do it . . . anymore . . . I'm . . . I'm done, Sarah.

He closes his eyes, sunken in their sockets. He breathes in.

She watches him. He doesn't breathe out. He doesn't move at all. Frightened, she starts, looks at me.

Then he exhales. He opens his eyes, looks at his wife. You don't need to be a doctor to know. He's a dead man, waiting. It could happen any time.

Okay, she says to him, her eyes filling.

Okay, she says again. She gulps audibly, then holds his head lovingly in both her hands. Okay, she says.

There's a lot to do. Papers to sign and witness and put in his medical record. Decisions to be made, not just about CPR and mechanical ventilators and intensive care units, but about how awake he wants to be, who can visit, what to tell the kids. Neither of them asks about time but I know they're wondering. I suggest that we get his pain under control, let him rest a little, see how the afternoon goes. I'll be back in an hour or two, I tell them, we'll see how things are looking then.

They get the picture. We're not talking weeks here. We're talking days, maybe hours.

Through it all, she is astonishing. She has every right to be angry. This isn't the way it's supposed to be. But she turns on a dime, instantly seeing that it's all about him now. Not her. Not the kids. She sees it doesn't make sense to be mad at me, a stranger. I'm just the messenger. She tells me she's sorry for how she behaved.

Don't be, I tell her, I hope my wife does the same for me.

I leave the shades drawn on the big picture windows. The sunlight filtering through is pale but warm. His eyes are closed as I leave. So are hers.

This isn't the way it's supposed to be. Preparing for the end needs time. It's just not right to put people through this all at once. In fact, it's downright cruel, especially when kids are involved. But I didn't have any choice. I needed to know what to do—today, or tonight, or tomorrow. Because, make no mistake, Mr. Atkins will become unconscious again. He'll stop breathing. He'll have a cardiac arrest. And when he does, I need to know what to *do*.

But you don't begin this process by talking about what to do. You begin by talking about what the patient understands—and what's important to him now. Not what's important to the doctor. What's important to the patient. You want to know his concerns, his family's concerns, about what lies ahead. Does he understand what lies ahead, and how far ahead it lies? Does he have questions about his condition, his prognosis? Does he want numbers? Median survival statistics? It doesn't hurt to say that clinical prognostication is far from an exact science. Even when you're deathly ill, no one can tell you with any certainty when you're going to die. Some patients find some comfort in that.

You want to ask the patient who he wants to make decisions on his behalf if, as events evolve, he can't make decisions for himself. Things change. God knows, things change. There's just no way to anticipate and discuss every possible complication or new situation that might arise between now and when the end comes. This means that the patient must designate a "surrogate," an end-of-life decision-maker entrusted to do what the patient *would want* to do. This surrogate responsibility is a big deal; asking a friend or loved one to take it on is asking a lot. After the patient's death, surrogate decision-makers often feel guilty, regretful, depressed. (Did I do the right thing? Did I do what he would have wanted?) It's not a job for everyone.

Most important, it takes time. It's all about the nitty-gritty. The details.

The doctor will say: I can relieve your pain with strong pain medicine but there's a chance that this could slow your breathing. There's even a small chance that the pain medicine could cause you to *stop* breathing, hasten your death. Is this okay with you? Is relieving your pain "worth" this risk?

In Mr. Atkins's case, as in so many others, there was more, much more: I can prevent another episode of hypoglycemic coma by giving you sugar water in your IV. Or, if you prefer, we can insert a tube into your stomach and give you sugar that way. Do you want the IV? Do you want the stomach tube? Do you want neither?

What would you say? Do you want to stay in the hospital to die? Or would you rather die at home? Which do you think would be easier for your wife? How about your kids?

What would you say? If you become too sick to speak for yourself, what do you want your surrogate to say?

More than twenty years have passed since the U.S. Congress enacted the Federal Patient Self-Determination Act in response to growing concerns about the importance of end-of-life planning. This law requires that all states recognize advance directives of two different types: 1) "instructional" directives whereby patients stipulate their specific wishes about life-prolonging interventions (such as CPR) when terminally ill; and 2) "proxy" directives whereby patients designate a person their "health care proxy" to make treatment decisions on their behalf if they become incapacitated and unable to decide for themselves. All health care facilities that receive reimbursement from Medicare or Medicaid—including hospitals, nursing homes, home health care agencies, and HMOs—must provide patients with information about such advance directives and document in each patient's medical record any directives the patient has completed. This same information must be provided to all recipients of Social Security or Medicare.

The purpose of this law is to give all patients the information and legal authority they need to make decisions, based on what's important to *them*, about which medical treatments they want (and don't want) when they become seriously ill. The law's purpose is *not* to save money by minimizing health care costs at the end of life. Nor is it intended to simplify end-of-life decision-making for doctors. Quite the opposite, the law is intended to encourage personal reflection, discussion, and planning about end-of-life care before one's health care crisis occurs, before death is imminent, before the patient can no longer speak for himself.

So: How well is this law working?

Mr. Atkins, who has received care at some of the best medical centers in the world, hasn't done any of these things. Have you? Have you had discussions with your own doctor about these issues? Have you identified a health care proxy and given that person legal authority to speak on your behalf in the event you become incapacitated? Have you discussed with your health care proxy what's important to you? How you want to spend your time when death nears? What role, if any, you want your family members to play when these decisions must be made?

If, like Mr. Atkins, you haven't done any of these things, you aren't alone. Most Americans haven't done them either.

Some people aren't convinced it's necessary. If you're a healthy twenty-year-old, this attitude is understandable. (However, keep in mind that Karen Ann Quinlan, the woman whose decade-long tragedy trumpeted the need for advance directive legislation in the first place, became "vegetative" at age twenty-one.) If you're older, you probably think you can wait to decide these things until the need arises. But the one major research study that has examined this question found that, among people above age sixty who died during a subsequent six-year period, *more than two-thirds* had become incapacitated and unable to make end-of-life decisions for themselves when the need arose. Someone else (in many cases, a family member unprepared for this task) had to make these decisions for them.

Even if you think that having an advance directive is a good idea, it's not always easy to make one. Many patients can't predict what specific treatments they would want in a future, hypothetical medical crisis. (This is one reason some doctors don't encourage patients to complete "instructional" advance directives.) In many states, advance directive forms are written in legalistic language at or above twelfth-grade reading level, which means that many Americans can't understand them, especially elderly people who need them most. In addition, many advance directive forms have not been translated into non-English languages. Many states restrict who may legally serve as your health care proxy. (Each state has a different law; some allow only relatives to serve in this capacity—not domestic or same-sex partners, or close friends.) Patients who are homeless, migratory, or socially isolated may want their doctor or social worker to represent them, lacking other suitable candidates, but, in many states, health care providers are disallowed from serving as their patient's surrogate.

The obstacles don't end there. Even if you have completed an advance directive, it is useless in most states unless *the written form itself* is available to the doctors attending you in a medical crisis. When you're delirious or unconscious in an ambulance or emergency room, your carefully considered (signed, witnessed, and notarized) advance directive form can't help you when it's stashed away in your safe deposit box. (Verbal directives, even from duly appointed surrogates, are disallowed in many states.) Worse, many individuals who are duly designated health care surrogates simply don't know what the patient would want in a particular clinical situation. (Unfortunately, some surrogates then choose what *they themselves* would want in this situation—not what the patient would want.) Finally, doctors don't always honor advance directives when the crisis occurs, because they question the directive's validity. For example, the doctor on the scene—who may not know you at all—may be unconvinced that you really understood the implications of your directive when applied in this particular clinical situation. Or, the doctor may be challenged by one of your family members who, although *not* your legally designated surrogate, disputes the intent or content of your directive.

Despite a gradual increase in public awareness of advance directives (and some impressive local successes in their use), the current generation of advance directives is unlikely to optimize end-of-life planning. An alternative, new approach deemphasizes reliance on written documents that stipulate the *content* of end-of-life care. (Do you want a feeding tube? A breathing machine? CPR?) Instead, this new approach focuses on preparing the patient's chosen surrogate, *together with the patient's doctor*, to make decisions the patient would approve. The merit of this approach lies in its focus on the *process*, not the outcome, of end-of-life decision-making. It assumes that if, over time, you develop a trusting, informed relationship with your doctor *and* your health care proxy, you can be confident that the two of them *together* will decide well for you when and if the need arises.

The Achilles' heel of this new approach is that the requisite "personal" relationship between patients and their doctors is now difficult to develop and sustain. In many communities today, such meaningful doctor-patient relationships are dying. They must be resuscitated if we're serious about helping more Americans die a "good" death.

Laws won't fix this, but good public policy can help. Government and private insurers pay thousands of dollars per day to keep a moribund person "alive" in an intensive care unit, long after there is any hope of the patient's meaningful recovery. And yet these same insurers refuse to reimburse doctors for spending time to talk to patients (and their surrogates) about end-of-life care. Key federal lawmakers have blocked such reimbursement by stirring up fears about "death panels" hell-bent on killing patients to save money. This obstructionism is worse than wrong; it is the height of cynicism. Many of these "public servants" admit, behind closed doors, that their resistance in this matter is "not personal, it's just politics." Let them tell that to Mr. Atkins.

And his wife. And their kids.

1:10 p.m.

For my meeting with Mona Lisa's crazy family, we've gathered in a small conference room on 5 West. Her three sons and their wives sit together on a sofa and chairs, their arms folded defensively across their chests, their solidarity and intransigence unmistakable.

We go at it for more than an hour. I and my two colleagues—Nancy, a palliative care nurse, and Felix, a senior geriatrics fellow—have tried to answer their questions, understand their peculiar perspective, deflect their bizarre suggestions, and clarify what we can and cannot do. Yes, we will do whatever we can to minimize her suffering and maximize her comfort. No, this does not mean we can feed her shrimp risotto and peach cobbler, her favorites, because that would put her back in the ICU gagging on a breathing tube. Mona Lisa's family seems genuinely to care for her but it's taken an hour just to get them to understand that it's *her* comfort and suffering we're talking about here, not theirs. Right now, they haven't accepted anything we've said. But at least now they've all heard it, together, in front of witnesses. It's a start.

Ordinarily, when I've been on-service in hospital, day and night for weeks on end, my pager's vibration reminds me of the drill in the dentist's office when I was a kid, before novocaine became popular. Right now, though, I'm grateful for the buzz. Chris has sent a text message that reads: "2 new Area C—1? home—1? CT Surg."

This means that he's seeing two new admissions in Area C of the emergency department, one of whom maybe we can send home (like Mr. Tosca earlier today). But the other one, Chris thinks, may need a cardiothoracic (CT) surgeon. I'm no heart surgeon but that's the one that gets me out of my chair.

Before I leave, I summarize for Mona Lisa's family the bottom line about where we go from here. First, we cannot deal with six different surrogate decision-makers, each one saying and requesting different things. One of them, and only one, must be designated by Ms. Rhodik's husband as her sole spokesperson. Second, I make clear to them what I will do if the family continues to refuse our recommendation to transfer Ms. Rhodik to an excellent rehabilitation facility where, after intensive physical therapy, she *might* regain her ability to eat and drink. If they insist on taking her home again—where, I am sure, she would develop aspiration pneumonia for the fourth time—then I will have no choice but to involve the hospital's Ethics Committee and legal staff. And, if they simply refuse to decide anything, passively forcing me to keep Ms. Rhodik in hospital indefinitely (where she cannot get the intensive physical therapy she needs), I will do the same. I tell them I've had to involve the lawyers and the Ethics Committee only twice before in my entire forty-year career in medicine. But I won't hesitate to do it now.

If you refuse what we know is the only responsible way to try to help your mother, then you will be hurting her. *You* will be hurting her. And that we cannot allow.

When I said this for the first time about thirty minutes ago, it caused an uproar. When I said it for the second time ten minutes later, their petulant harrumphs and snide whispers ricocheted around the room. When I say it again now, all six of them glare silently, glad to see me go.

Down in the ED, Chris and Dan are in Bay 12 examining Ms. Dubois, an eighty-nine-year-old woman with a prosthetic heart valve. A portable ultrasound machine, the size and shape of a microwave oven, sits next to them on a cart with wheels. Jim, a Cardiology fellow, is positioning a small microphone on Ms. Dubois's chest, moving it here and there. Metallic clicks and mechanical whooshes echo from her heart, reverberating around the room. There, Jim is saying to Chris and Dan as I enter, there it is.

Whew, Chris says, they weren't kiddin'. That thing's huge.

From its ultrasound appearance alone, Jim can't be sure what the mass in Ms. Dubois's heart is. It could be a tumor but most likely it's a giant clot. Ms. Dubois has been taking blood-thinner medication for decades to prevent such a clot. Recently she was moved into a new nursing home where they screwed up her medications; for the past six weeks, she's been receiving only half as much blood-thinner as she needs. When the nursing home staff discovered their error, they obtained an echocardiogram, freaked out when they saw what we're looking at right now, and shipped her over here.

Ms. Dubois has Alzheimer's disease. She knows her name but that's about all. Luckily, she's peaceful, not at all agitated by the sudden change in her surroundings or the hubbub around her now. Hearing the dissonant plinks and hisses of her heart on the echo machine, she says to no one in particular, Can you change the channel, please? I don't think I like this show.

Jim, the Cardiology fellow, suggests that we consult the surgeons. Whatever it is, Jim says, maybe we should get it out of there . . .

Ms. Dubois farts, loudly. She doesn't apologize or seem to notice. She's picking at the little blue flowers printed on her jonnie, trying to gather them into a bouquet. Her head is shaking, involuntarily. She farts again.

Then again . . . Jim says, nodding sympathetically at me and Chris.

Chris hustles away to try to reach her family, a son in Miami.

Looking at Ms. Dubois, I can't help thinking about Mom. The docs at the hospital in Greenport told me an hour ago that she was doing okay after they'd given her drugs to calm her down and lower her blood pressure. But if Mom really did pass out at home, and if her pulse really was only twenty-eight beats per minute at the time, she may need a pacemaker for her heart. Would Mom want that? (Would Ms. Dubois want heart surgery?) Before Mom began losing her marbles, she always said she didn't want breathing machines or CPR or "any of that lifesaving stuff." But a pacemaker? We never talked about a pacemaker. I'm Mom's surrogate, her legally designated health care proxy, but I'm not sure what she would want.

Now Dan tells me he's just been paged to go up to the fifth floor to help the nurses deal with Ms. Tate, our patient with bad sickle cell disease who is protesting her discharge from the hospital. Dan asks me to see Ms. Finch, his other new admission here in the ED, without him. He and Chris have already seen her; they know what they would do but they don't have the authority to do it. Briefly, Dan tells me Ms. Finch's story, then heads upstairs.

I review Ms. Finch's medical chart before meeting her. She's sixty years old with a remote history of breast cancer. According to the ED doc's note, she "passed out" at home this morning. (Reading this, Mom pops into my head again. I tune her out.) Ms. Finch's vital signs, physical examination, and laboratory tests look fine but the scribbled note concludes: "See Dr. Rosenthal's recommendations. Admit to Medicine." Dr. Rosenthal, a private cardiologist, has typed a three-page consultation note into the electronic medical record, having been asked to see Ms. Finch here in the ED this morning by Dr. Nye, her private internist, who is away for the weekend. Dr. Rosenthal has concluded that Ms. Finch must be admitted to the cardiac floor and undergo a series of tests to find out what made her faint. His evaluation reads like something an excellent senior resident would write: He lists every cause of syncope (fainting) known to modern medicine, asks that tests be done to evaluate every one of these possibilities, no matter how rare or remote, and suggests additional consultations from Neurology, Oncology, Radiology, Electrophysiology, and Physical Therapy. Little or none of this work will get done today or tomorrow, Sunday. Implementing all of Rosenthal's suggestions likely will require Ms. Finch to remain in hospital for about a week. In one sense, Rosenthal has made my job easy. All I have to do is write in the chart, "Agree with Dr. Rosenthal."

But I can't do that. Ms. Finch, as I soon discover, is a lovely lady in excellent health whose only problem is that she is very sad. Her husband died two weeks ago—here, in this hospital—and she hasn't been eating or sleeping well since. This morning, when she got out of bed after another night of tossing and turning, she felt a little dizzy ("like

I *might* pass out") but quickly felt better after forcing herself to eat something. Her daughter insisted on calling Dr. Nye. His answering service instructed them to come to the ED and then contacted Dr. Rosenthal (who doesn't know Ms. Finch but is covering Dr. Nye for the weekend). Ms. Finch didn't want to come to the hospital; it's the last place she wants to be, so soon after her husband's death.

Despite her visible grief, Ms. Finch manages a wan, grateful smile when I tell her she can call her daughter to take her home. She has just told me that she has "never passed out in my life, including today." She has a "wonderful" psychologist who has been helping her through her husband's terminal illness. It's been hard, she says, but they tell me it takes time. Ms. Finch's main concern now seems to be that she doesn't want to "disappoint" Dr. Rosenthal, who, she says, "seems very nice." I tell her I'll take care of Dr. Rosenthal. She smiles gratefully again, shakes my hand, says good-bye.

I page Rosenthal and sit down to enter my own note into the computer. Officially, Ms. Finch has already been "admitted" to the hospital under my care so my note must be extremely detailed, explaining why Ms. Finch does *not* need hospitalization or any of the tests or consultations Dr. Rosenthal has recommended. As I'm finishing my note twenty minutes later, Rosenthal answers my page. He doesn't know me, asks who I am, then listens to what I say, interrupting me several times to remark, "I strongly disagree." He can't justify his disagreements except to say that he saw a patient "just like her" many years ago who turned out to have a brain tumor that was missed. It was his first personal experience with being sued for malpractice, and, he says ponderously as he hangs up the phone, *You can't be too careful, you know, you can never be too careful.* I think about Mom, about Fred and Martha, long ago, what I've learned about being careful.

Rosenthal's words echoing in my head, I leave the ED to go up to the fifth floor to help Dan with Ms. Tate. She's trouble. Dan will need all the help he can get.

As I exit the elevator on 5, Mr. Jefferson is waiting to get on. He's our guy with advanced HIV disease and chronic hepatitis who, on rounds this morning, had clapped his hands and jumped out of bed when we told him he could go. Forty-eight hours ago in the ED, he looked like he might die, but what initially looked like septic shock turned out to be nothing more than severe dehydration from acute gastroenteritis and this morning on rounds he looked like a rose. Before boogeying into the bathroom, he high-fived us all and said, No offense, docs, but I hope I don't see any of you again real soon. Now, at the elevator, Mr. Jefferson smiles broadly when he sees me and says the same thing again. But, as the doors shoosh closed around him, he winks and says, Thanks, doc.

This is not what Ms. Tate is saying to Dan or the head nurse on 5 Central as I enter her room. A good-looking woman of indeterminate age, Ms. Tate is in their face, haranguing them in a loud, hectoring voice. They stand silently around her bed, absorbing the incoming artillery. You call yourself a doctor? she says to Dan. How can you send me out when I'm still painin' so bad? You supposed to help me, man!

Then she sees me.

Aw, shit! she says, and shuts up, hunkering down in her bed.

Ms. Tate's a pro. She knows how hospitals work, especially on weekends. She figured that I, the senior guy, would have gone home by now. She was sure she could squeeze another day out of Dan, an inexperienced intern, despite what we had told her on team rounds this morning. Ms. Tate hasn't had it easy; lifelong, sickle cell disease is no picnic. She came in two days ago unable to move her shoulder. The slightest motion was excruciating. This can be serious in a sickler—joint destruction caused by infection or sludging of the sickled blood cells—so we gave her lots of strong pain medicine while we and the orthopedic guys figured out what was wrong. Ms. Tate thanked the Lord and told us how wonderful we all were until we discovered that there was nothing wrong with her shoulder and she was just jerking us around. Yesterday we had given her one more night to think again about our offers to help her—methadone, an addiction program, counseling, social services, the works—but she's been down that road before. When we stuck to our guns this morning and refused to give her more drugs, she knew it was over.

Y'all may be hot-shit doctors, she said, but you don't know nothin' 'bout me.

She's right about that last part. But there is no family or friend we can call in to talk to her, try to help. I'm pretty sure she'll wind up in some other hospital's ED before nightfall and get what she wants—but there's nothing I can do about it.

The afternoon passes. Visitors stream in and out of the rooms and corridors. There are families to see, questions to answer, a new admission from the ED. It's one thing after another—randomly, it seems—bouncing from one story to the next. Mr. Gunther, headed for the NIH, leaves with his wife. She gives me a long look as they head toward the elevator. I wish her well; living with Pascal's wager can't be easy. Mr. Kinney, a dapper corporate attorney, is also getting out of here after a rough two weeks. His pancreas is totally destroyed, replaced by puddles of necrotic fluid, yet he refuses to accept the fact that his fondness for single-malt scotch is the reason why. His wife gives me a long look, too, then they're gone. Jim, the Cardiology fellow, shows me the echocardiogram he just did on Mr. Warner, our guy with HIV. Nothing there, Jim says, no vegetation, no sign of endocarditis. We consider what this means, make a plan. Up on 10 Central, Mr. Mukaj's bladder irrigation backs up painfully again but there's nowhere else we can put him, no empty beds in the ICU or Step-Down Unit, no place where he can have his own nurse with him all the time. We bounce this around, too, decide to try this, then that, we'll see. Mr. Harris, our patient with Marfan syndrome, a plastic aorta, and a septic hip joint, spikes a fever again. Not good. We make a plan. And so it goes, on into the evening. On days like this, doctoring feels like pinball: nonstop random events—intercepted here, altered there, prolonged or postponed by this or that, the bells and boinks sounding all around—and sometimes you can't be sure whether you're the guy pushing the buttons, manipulating the levers, and bumping the machine, or whether you're *inside* the machine, whether you're the pinball itself.

In the evening, a small crowd has gathered in the plush atrium at the far end of the VIP corridor on 14 South. People stand around, looking out the huge picture windows at Manhattan, sparkling in the dark. The Fifty-ninth Street Bridge is lit up like Coney Island. Other people sit in small groups, talking in hushed tones. A few mill about, alone, unsure how or where to look. Veteran staff on 14 South will tell you that most Saturday nights here don't look like this, the patients and their visitors typically cloistered away in their private penthouse hospital suites. It's different when there's a death watch.

Outside Mr. Atkins's room, a young girl sits on the carpeted floor in the corridor, her back to the wall. An older woman stands nearby, talking quietly on a cell phone. The girl is coltish, prepubescent, eleven or twelve. Her blond hair tumbles and sways, half hiding her face. Her pink polka-dotted fingernails pick aimlessly at her jeans. She doesn't notice my approach.

What can this poor kid be thinking? I wonder as I approach her father's room. But it's not my place to ask, so I don't.

This is my fifth visit to Mr. Atkins today. Nancy, the palliative care nurse who helped me with Mona Lisa, was here with me two hours ago to make sure his morphine pump was doing its job. The pain was better, he said. He talked a little, about his kids, how he wanted to go home to his house on the beach. I know the Connecticut town where he lives. I asked him where his house is. When he told me, I said that's the prettiest place I've ever seen and he knew I wasn't just saying so, because it's the prettiest place he's ever seen, too. I said something about how his town has changed from the way it was when I was young and he said he would have liked to see it back then and he asked me about my kids, too. He didn't ask about time or what to expect when and I couldn't tell whether he wanted to know. So I said, Let's see how it goes today and tonight, and he nodded and said, Okay, I understand, and I think he probably did. His wife was very quiet, even when we talked about the kids. Nancy came back to speak with her some more after I left.

Now I'm back again just to check, make sure we're doing what we said, see if they have new questions. For most folks going through this, it's an awful lot to get your head around. After all these years, I've found that it's not a bad idea to stop in—be around—as often as you can.

I open the door a crack, peer inside. Mr. Atkins is lying flat, asleep, his breathing regular and unlabored. His wife is dozing, too, in a chair, her legs drawn up to her chest. One fist is clenched below her chin. In the big window, across the river, the city lights blink softly in the night. I don't go in.

Out in the corridor, a young boy is hopping on one foot, balancing a chocolate ice cream cone in one hand, trying to get his sister's attention. He's seven or eight. Like his sister, he's a beautiful kid, blond hair, blue eyes, with a smidge of chocolate on the tip of his nose. He looks up at me as I close the door.

Are you my dad's doctor? he asks, hopping.

Uh-huh.

He stops hopping. He tilts his head to his shoulder, his ear now facing the floor. He's looking at me sideways.

Is my dad getting better?

His sister, sitting on the floor, looks up at me.

Your dad's feeling better now, yes. He's sleeping.

The boy untilts his head, looks at me straight on. Then he begins to nod, confidently, like he's heard this before.

Yeah, he says, then skips down the corridor toward the crowd.

His sister is looking at me.

Hi.

Hi, she says, and looks down again, her blond hair swinging.

I stand there for a minute.

She doesn't look up again.

I stop down on the fourth floor to check on Mr. Warner. We've moved him so we can monitor his heart. He looks a little better. His temperature is down. He seems less confused, but, perhaps as a result, he's more anxious. Oh, he says nervously, when I tell him that he's in the hospital. Why? he asks.

I try to explain briefly what we know, why he'll be here for weeks (if he's lucky). But he drifts off again, not understanding.

Am I going home now? he asks.

On 5 North, I run into Dan and we quickly run our list of patients. We've been able to get four folks discharged today, not including Ms. Finch and Mr. Tosca, whom we sent home directly from the ED. Our team started the morning with nineteen patients and now we have only sixteen, including our new lady with the heart clot and another new admission downstairs. Dan knows that this means he may be in for a long night. He's "vulnerable" to get three or four more admissions between now and tomorrow morning. He's thinking ahead, cleaning up his charts, finishing his notes, getting ready.

Chris appears. You saw Warner's stuff? he asks Dan.

His echocardiogram was normal.

Yeah, but all three of his blood cultures are growing gram-positive cocci in clusters, probably *Staph*.

Hmmph, Dan says.

Did you see his brain MRI? Chris asks.

No, not yet.

Two enhancing lesions, exactly where we talked about. One in the right frontal lobe, the other right occipital.

Dan whistles.

Bleeding? I ask.

Yeah, Chris says. Both strokes look hemorrhagic.

So, his echocardiogram? Dan says.

False negative, Chris shrugs. The guy's got endocarditis with septic emboli to the brain, echo or no echo.

Chris turns to me. I'll let the surgeons know.

Okay, good. But the surgeons won't touch him, Chris. Not now anyway. Not with fresh blood in his head.

Sheesh, Chris says, nodding. Then he chews on his cheek.

He's all ours, guys. Keep a close eye on him. Call if I can help.

My office is a short way down the hall. It's small and cramped, not like the one I had in Chicago. People here are still figuring out where to put me. I take off my white coat, hang it on a hook. I open the electronic medical record in my desktop computer and settle in to write my patients' chart notes. If I don't do this, no one gets paid. Not including the two notes I wrote earlier to send Mr. Tosca and Ms. Finch home from the ED, I have nineteen more to do. I'm pretty fast at this, so it will probably take me less than three hours. I look at my watch. It's 7:20 p.m. If I'm lucky, I'm out of here by ten. Not bad for a Saturday.

Most doctors in the U.S. are reimbursed by (private or government) insurers based on the doctor's documentation in the patient's medical record of the specific type and complexity of service provided. For this reason, doctors pay careful attention to their "payer mix" (which type of insurance their patients have) and the accuracy of their documentation (which is audited periodically by external reviewers).

This "fee-for-service" reimbursement system has been criticized for a long time, and for good reasons. One problem is that it pays doctors' fees for services whether those services help the patient or not. Ms. Finch, the recently widowed woman in the ED, needed a little hopeful consolation, not a lot of hospital consultations. But if Dr. Rosenthal, who didn't know Ms. Finch, had had his way, many doctors (and the hospital) would have been reimbursed handsomely for doing things Ms. Finch didn't need. Another problem with the fee-for-service payment system is that it rewards technological procedures (surgery, CT scans, laboratory tests) much more than "cognitive" services (talking to and examining patients, diagnosing what's wrong with them, giving them advice, following them over time). There are cogent arguments favoring both sides of this "procedural versus cognitive" reimbursement debate, but most objective observers believe that the current system disproportionately rewards procedural services.

My employer (Cornell's medical school, which pays me a salary) will collect about $1,800 for the clinical services I've provided to my twenty-one patients today, an average of about $85 per patient. This total includes $240 for Mr. Warner (a newly admitted, complicated patient with "good" private insurance); $75 for Mr. Gunther (from Medicare); $37 for Ms. Rhodik (from Medicaid); and no reimbursement for Mr. Mukaj (who is uninsured). In contrast to my reimbursement rate (about $100 per hour on a day that began in the hospital at 5:00 a.m. and will end after 10:00 p.m.), the radiologist who reads Mr. Warner's CT scan and MRI pictures today will receive about $500 for these services (which will take about thirty minutes of his time). If Mr. Mukaj were insured, the cardiologist's fee for his (two-hour) heart procedure would be about $1,300. These "proceduralists" are highly skilled and provide outstanding, sometimes lifesaving service to patients. But should their (hourly) reimbursement rates be *six to ten times* higher than mine?

Make no mistake: The average worker in the United States would be thrilled to earn salaries paid to "cognitive" doctors like me. Annual incomes of hospitalists and primary care physicians average about $150,000 to $200,000 before taxes. (This represents about half of the revenue we collect for our services: The other half pays for medical malpractice premiums, practice expenses, and fringe benefits—especially health care.) But this level of remuneration places "cognitive" doctors at the bottom of the health care reimbursement food chain. U.S. medical students today, burdened with staggering educational debts, spurn these careers en masse, aspiring instead to become radiologists, ophthalmologists, dermatologists, or other specialists at the top of the food chain (who, in general, don't work eighteen-hour Saturdays). This trend is problematic because nations whose health care systems perform better and cost less than that of the United States have many more cognitive than procedural physicians. Why? Because, in order to provide high-quality medical care, *someone must take care of the patients*—not just their CT scans or their cataracts or their Botox injections.

How will this needed change in the composition of the U.S. physician workforce come about? No one seems to have a good answer to this question.

There was a time when the question itself was unimportant. A time when, believe it or not, most doctors didn't do medicine for the money. But it's a business now. Sometimes, a crazy business.

10:05 p.m.

I'm done. I sign my notes, log off the computer, check in with Dan.

Quiet, he says, at least for now.

Before I leave, I pick up the phone, call Dad on Shelter Island. He's been waiting to hear about Mom.

I tell him what the docs in Greenport just told me. Mom had been doing okay after they medicated her to calm her down. But a little while ago, she had a seven-second pause on her heart monitor. Her heart didn't beat at all for seven seconds straight.

Dad says, Wait a minute, Bren, I've gotta fix this damn hearing aid.

Along with everything else, Dad's losing his hearing. I wait, then tell him again.

Seven seconds? he says. Seven seconds?

Yeah.

Mmm, he says.

Dad's a retired cardiologist. I can almost hear his wheels turning, figuring the angles, slowly. He still has all of his marbles but he's very weak, every day a struggle now.

They put in a wire? Dad asks. (A wire is a pacemaker.)

No.

Why not?

I tell Dad about the two drugs they gave Mom in the ED to calm her down and control her blood pressure. Both drugs can cause a heart pause like Mom's, called heart block. If that's the problem, the heart block will just go away as the drugs clear out of her system. So the truth is we don't know yet whether Mom needs a pacemaker. It's equally possible that she just needs to be left alone.

I tell Dad this.

Yeah, he says doubtfully. But . . . seven seconds, Bren.

Yeah, I know.

It's a stretch to blame seven full seconds of no heartbeat on a drug. I tell Dad the plan is to see how Mom does overnight. I tell him that the cardiologist in Greenport is prepared to put in a pacemaker if the problem shows itself again. That is, if I give the cardiologist the go-ahead, which I haven't done yet. I don't tell Dad this last part.

Okay, Dad says, you're the doctor.

I don't remind him that I'm the son, too. And that the son shouldn't be the doctor. We ring off. As I put on my winter coat, glance at the picture of Amelia Earhart on my desk, and head down the hall, I can't say that I tune out Mom and Dad. Maybe that's why, when I get to the elevator bank, I push the Up button by mistake.

Quickly, I push Down. Now both buttons are lit. When the elevator arrives, it's going Up.

I get on and push 14.

The lobby on 14 South is empty now. The concierge is snoozing at his desk. Lights are dimmed everywhere, even at the nursing station. I look down the long corridor past Mr. Atkins's room. The crowd and the kids are gone. I approach his room, open the door slightly, peek in. He's asleep, the button for the morphine pump in his hand. His wife is sitting in her chair, looking out the big window. She hears the door, turns to me. I make a movement with my chin toward him. She makes a little shrug, nods approvingly. She doesn't speak or get up. I hold her gaze for a moment, then back out, close the door.

Blinking lights catch my eye at the far end of the corridor. Something is moving there, crossing in front of the big atrium windows. I walk there.

It's Julie. She's pacing, back and forth. Outside, the skyline and the big bridge glitter in the dark. I don't see Gordon. I've never seen Julie without Gordon.

At first, she doesn't recognize me without my white doctor coat. Workin' late, she says.

You, too.

Yeah, well . . . things on my mind.

Mmm.

It's a court case, she says. That's the personal thing I wouldn't tell you about earlier today. I have to be in court on Monday.

Uh-huh.

Divorce.

Ah.

I can't go, Dr. Reilly. I'm too sick.

Mmm. Can't your lawyer tell the judge? Get a postponement?

He tried that. Yesterday. The judge refused.

Oh?

Yeah, he's already postponed it twice before . . . June . . . then October . . . My husband's an asshole. So the judge won't postpone again.

Julie's hand trembles as she speaks. She's obviously distraught. And now I get it. I'm a little slow about such things but finally I get it. That's when she was in the hospital before. In June, and then again in October. Each time, like this time, nearly dead because her thyroid level was so low.

You can't do this all of a sudden. It takes time for the thyroid level to drop so low. You have to go without your thyroid pill for several weeks before you get this bad. You have to plan it.

I'm not a cop. I don't think that way. So I'm not thinking about Gordon's grin or the fact that he's the one who gives Julie her pills every day. I'm not smart enough, in the moment, to ask the obvious question: So whose plan is it? Julie's? Or Gordon's? Is she the mastermind? Or is she the victim? If I were smarter, I would have wondered about that.

As it turns out, Julie answers these questions without my asking. All I do is what I'm trained to do in these situations: keep the patient talking, see what comes out.

This must be hard for you, Julie. Divorce . . . it's a hard thing.

Her lip quivers. Her eyes gleam, wet now.

Yeah.

I'm sorry. It must be a very emotional time for you.

At this, Julie snorts, a deep guttural sucking sound, half guffaw, half jeer. She's laughing at me.

Emotional? she says derisively. *Emotional?*

She doesn't scream. She doesn't spit. She speaks with the cold, calm fury of a hit man.

I'll tell you what's fuckin' emotional. How 'bout fifty million fuckin' bucks? Eh, doctor? Would you call that *emotional?*

She looks at me like I'm a baboon. Then she turns her back, waves her hand dismissively, and walks away.

I almost sprint to the elevator. I don't want to know who gets Julie's fifty million bucks. Or whether Gordon really needs his wheelchair.

I just gotta get outta here.

Part II

THEN

Primary care . . . provides person-focused (not disease-oriented) care over time . . . and coordinates or integrates care provided elsewhere or by others. . . . The long-term relationship that characterizes primary care will be difficult to sustain if either party is uncomfortable with their encounters. Because many problems that patients bring to primary care physicians are of uncertain cause or prognosis, the relationship must be strong enough to tolerate ambiguity.

—Barbara Starfield, *Primary Care* (1998)

Chapter 5

AN END

What we call the beginning is often the end
And to make an end is to make a beginning.
The end is where we start from.

—T. S. Eliot, "Little Gidding" (1942)

Hanover, New Hampshire. February 1985

It was still dark outside our bedroom window when the phone rang.
Calls before dawn were always bad news, but ours was a doctor's
house, so we got a lot of them. Typically, it was someone else's bad
news, not our own, but this didn't make it any easier for Janice, my
wife. All those calls meant that bad things were happening to lots of
folks out there, decent folks like us, bad things they didn't deserve
and usually didn't see coming. And, if that's the way it is, then our
turn will come, too, right? So, is this the one? Is this call for us?

Janice sprang out of bed as if she'd been bitten.

Yes? she said anxiously into the receiver, her voice gruff with sleep
but suddenly wide awake. She listened for a minute, then exhaled
deeply.

No, she said. No . . . wait a minute . . . wait a minute . . .

Who is it?

Your girlfriend.

Which one?

Janice handed me the phone.

Remember, she said sternly, you're on vacation.

It was warm outside when I went to my car. That detail sticks in my memory now, twenty-five years later—that and the sound of Martha's voice on the phone. *Please come! Please, Brendan! Now! Please! You must come now!* She wasn't shouting. Martha wasn't a shouter, not even that day, but her whisper was so plaintive, so urgent—so fierce!—I knew I had to go. Martha hadn't asked for much in the years we'd been together. And she never begged for anything. But that's what I heard that morning, even more in her voice than her words: She was begging me. *Please! Come now! Please!*

Snow lay hip-high in the yard and along the road. First light had barely begun to crawl up over the eastern hills—just the gray, not the glimmer—but already, even before sunup, it was warm. I could smell the thaw, hear it trickle. The Volvo's tires had frozen flat in the driveway every night since Christmas, but I pulled out easily onto Wheelock Street. A pair of bluebirds tweeted in the bare lilac hedges.

Every year, for a day or two, this sudden reprieve in the dead of winter sent the temperature climbing into the fifties. It was always a surprise. And when it came, the whole town felt lucky, jubilant. During our thirteen winters here in Hanover, where I worked at Dartmouth's medical center, there had been entire months when the mercury never rose above zero, day or night. During those stretches, even the native New Hampshire folks took notice. (*Been some nippy out there, ayuh?*) But most people here endured the long winter without complaint. Beyond the skiing and Dartmouth's winter carnival and the fine snow sculptures on the college green, there would be ample compensation for the cold. Here in the north country, spring was triumphal, summer idyllic, and autumn so glorious you almost didn't care that winter was just around the bend again. Like most everybody else, Janice and I felt lucky to live here, especially on a day like today.

It was a Tuesday. I had taken the week off—it was the kids' winter school break—and we were all going skiing that day. When I hung up the phone and jumped out of bed to go see Martha, I told Janice, Don't worry, this won't take long, we'll make the skiway before the first lift.

Janice didn't say anything. She just gave me one of those looks: Again? *They* come first again?

Martha was eighty. So was her husband, Fred. They had been calling a lot these past few weeks, but we had worked it out, talked it through. We had a plan. But this was a new wrinkle. Martha was so distraught she couldn't even say what was wrong. *Please! Please come!* was all I could get out of her. I had been Martha's doctor for ten years. I liked her, admired her. I couldn't ask the on-call guy to handle this. He didn't know Fred and Martha. I did. I knew I could help, whatever this was.

Yet Janice had every right to be pissed about this. It was a different story when I was on call. Then, typically one weekday night per week and one weekend per month, my going would make sense. It was my job. Most of the time I could handle things on the phone—someone's minor illness that could wait until morning or a discussion with one of the Dartmouth medical residents about an inpatient on the hospital service. But if it sounded serious and uncertain, if it meant going to the hospital or someone's house even in the middle of the night, that's what you did, it came with the territory.

Janice accepted this. She knew all about responsibility and hard work. She was raising BJ and Caitie without a lot of help from me, despite having a busy full-time job herself. In her "spare time," she had just completed a graduate degree from Dartmouth. But there are limits, Janice said, there must be *boundaries*.

We argued about this and, as I drove down Wheelock Street that morning, I worked through these arguments again. Talking about it—boundaries and all that—is one thing. But what do you *do*? Some doctors say, *I'm sorry, I'm on vacation today, Dr. So-and-so is on call, you don't know him but he's very good.* Is that what you do? Martha and Fred were people I cared about. It didn't make any sense to ask another doctor to get involved.

A short way down the hill, I approached the old mansion on the corner of Jackson Road. Reflexively, I ducked, almost hiding under my dashboard as I passed. It was six in the morning and still dark outside but you never knew with Babs. She could appear out of nowhere, always when I least expected her, and start shrieking for attention.

Babs and her husband, Clark, a wealthy couple from New York, had moved into the mansion a couple of years ago. Soon after they arrived, they were invited to a dinner party hosted by a medical professor at Dartmouth, who was constantly courting wealthy donors to support his research. I lived just down the street. The professor apologized when he called me, said he didn't know if I was on call that night, but one of his dinner guests was having a stroke—or something, he wasn't sure what it was—and asked could I just come over and take a look at her?

As it happened, I was on call that night and, after asking a few questions, I had a pretty good notion what this "stroke" might be. It's peculiar, the professor had said, it's just her face that's paralyzed but it came on all of a sudden. During dessert, actually. The rest of her seems all right, she has no hemiparesis or headache or anything else. It's a bit . . . embarrassing, you know? I've got a house full of people here . . .

When I arrived a few minutes later, Babs had been secluded in the den with her husband, apart from the other dinner guests. In her forties, fashionably thin in the New York way, Babs would have been attractive had her meticulously cosmeticized face not been so grotesquely contorted. Everything on the left side of her face—her eye and mouth, even her nose—was straining desperately to occupy the right side of her face instead. Her tongue was stuck hard inside her right cheek, making a bulge like a huge wad of chewing tobacco, but the spit dripping down her chin was clear, not brown. Her lips and tongue could barely move at all, her speech was garbled, nearly incomprehensible. The rest of her looked all right but she was miserable, frantic, and she mumbled something about being too young to have a stroke. I tied a tourniquet tight around her arm, slapped the crook of her elbow to find a vein and shot her up with a slug of IV Benadryl from my little black bag. I wasn't sure myself how long it would take, so we laid her down on the couch and put a pillow under her head, but within less than a minute Babs was sitting up, exclaiming, Oh, Gawd, oh, Gawd, thank you, Gawd, her diction precise, her tongue untied, her face symmetrical and astonished. I hung around only long enough to make sure she wouldn't need more Benadryl and to explain that her problem was the medication she had taken earlier in the day. She had called her doctor in New York because she had an upset stomach, and he had phoned in a prescription for an antinausea drug, Compazine, which was well known to cause (rare) dystonic drug reactions like this one. After I left, Babs became the life of the party, which itself became a great fund-raising success. Apparently, Babs's dramatic "cure" became a perfect prop in the professor's after-dinner spiel about the importance of supporting medical research.

But no good deed goes unpunished. From that night onward, whenever Babs spotted me around town—in the supermarket, at the skiway, wherever—she would shriek and make a huge fuss. *There's my doctor! Dr. Reilly! He's my doctor!* she would shout, *He's my doctor!* as if everyone, now gawking at us in the vegetable aisle, would really want to know this.

Babs became a recurring reminder of one of the things I disliked about being a primary care doctor in a small town: the loss of anonymity. The townspeople here all knew me. Or at least they liked to think so. After all, I knew their secrets and their sins. For some of them, I was as much confessor as doctor. True, I didn't discourage patients from phoning me at home, as Janice thought I should. My patients knew they could reach me if they thought it was important. Most of them were respectful of my time and apologetic about bothering my family at home. It just didn't feel right to me to abandon them to the guy on call—someone who didn't know them, hadn't followed them for years, hadn't seen them in the hospital and at home, a stranger who didn't know all that they and their families had been through. Even if the on-call guy took the time and trouble to read through their stacks of medical records, he couldn't possibly do what I could do. Yeah, Janice would counter when I made this argument, do the other guys do the same for you?

The truth was that some did, but some didn't. So, for a long time, these "unnecessary" intrusions into our personal life had upset Janice. She began to understand my side of the story only after I told her about Laura Henderson. As I neared the bottom of the hill on Wheelock, I realized that Laura hadn't called for some time now. I hoped this was a good sign.

Laura didn't call often, but it was always late at night and always she was crying, saying she really couldn't talk to anyone but me. Laura lived alone in northern Vermont now, her six kids grown up and moved away. She didn't know me well—I had been her husband's doctor, not hers. She had friends, but she couldn't confide in them, not about this. And she had forbidden me to discuss it with anyone. Ever.

So I was the only one she had. I was the only one who knew.

Two years before, Saul Henderson had been referred to me at Dartmouth by his own internist up north, who knew Saul was seriously ill but couldn't figure out why. A charming, charismatic headmaster at a prestigious New England prep school, Saul's months of fever and weight loss had baffled his doctors. He'd had all the tests and empiric treatments they could think of, but he kept going downhill. After I put him in the hospital at Dartmouth it took us a while to figure it out, too, but a new virus had just been identified in Bethesda and Paris, so we asked the NIH people to do their new blood test for HIV—it wasn't approved yet for general use—because no other diagnosis made sense. This one didn't make sense either until Saul finally told me about his business trips to New York and visits to the bathhouses in Greenwich Village.

When the blood test came back positive, Laura couldn't believe it, not even after I insisted that Saul tell her about New York. She refused to be tested herself—This is not possible, she said—and they both instructed me to tell no one. This wasn't easy. Back then, HIV was rare in small-town America, but Christopher, the Hendersons' eldest son, was a savvy young guy who asked to meet with me privately more than once.

Talk to your mom and dad, Chris. That was all I could say.

We kept Saul in the hospital until he died about a month later. Under the circumstances—the bleeding, the diarrhea, how combative and confused he became toward the end—there was no way we could send him home to die, no way to protect his family and friends from infection. When the autopsy confirmed the diagnosis, Laura couldn't continue to deny it to me, but she'd never been able to tell anyone else.

After Saul died, Laura's entire adult life made no sense to her. They had married young, raised a large loving family. They had been happy, she said.

Do you understand what I'm saying, Dr. Reilly? We were *happy*.

Now, two years later, it still didn't make any sense to her. So, on some lonely nights when she'd had a few drinks, Laura would pick up the phone and call the only person who could know why she was crying.

One night when Laura called I had just gotten home from the hospital. It was late. I wasn't on call but I had missed dinner and hadn't seen the kids before they'd gone to bed. When I got off the phone with Laura, Janice hit the roof. So I broke my promise to Laura and told someone else about Saul.

I can't say it made everything better. But after Janice heard the story, she seemed less begrudging about the phone calls—Laura's and some of the others, too.

This business about boundaries isn't as simple as it sounds.

My headlights flashed past Kingsford Road, where Janice and I and the kids had lived when I first met Martha ten years before. Even then, at age seventy, Martha was striking, a dead ringer for the actress Jessica Tandy and every bit as vital, witty, and wry. Since I'd known her, she'd been lucky, her arthritis slowly getting worse but the rest of her remarkably well preserved despite her rheumatic heart. Fred, Martha's husband, had been even luckier. He'd never had any serious medical problems at all. Fred took no pills, had never had surgery, and, with his spry youthful demeanor and full head of white hair, he looked like a poster child for healthy aging. I had been his doctor for about a year now—I took him on after his own doctor retired—and, except for the fainting spell that brought him to me in the first place, he hadn't needed my help at all.

The phone calls had started a few weeks ago. Always at night. The first time it was Martha who called. She apologized, said Fred needed to talk to me. Then she listened in on the extension as Fred rambled on about this or that, coherent but oddly tangential. It wasn't clear what was on his mind. When I asked how I could help, Fred paused, then said, That's a good question, that's a very good question. But that was as far as I could get.

A few nights after that first call, Fred made the call himself. I could hear Martha tsk-tsking in the background and exclaiming in a loud exasperated whisper: *Fred! Leave the poor man alone!*

I was wondering, Brendan . . . do you know much about angels?

Angels?

Yes, you know, cherubim and seraphim, all that . . .

Uh, no. Not much. Why?

Well, I've been thinking about haloes . . .

Haloes . . . ?

Yeah, you know, the light around the angels' heads . . .

Uh-huh . . . ?

Well, I think maybe the shape and intensity of the light . . .

Click-click. Martha's persnickety voice came over the extension line.

Fred? For Pete's sake, Fred! It's the middle of the night!

Oh . . . well now, you see, Brendan, that's interesting, too, don't you think? I mean . . .

Fred, leave the poor man alone! Hang up the phone!

Well, I just . . .

For Pete's sake! Brendan, I'm sorry. Fred! Hang up the phone!

The whole thing was bizarre. As far as I knew, this was completely out of character for Fred. So I brought him in and checked him out and he passed with flying colors, just as he had done before. He was the healthiest eighty-year-old I knew—sharp as a tack mentally with a "physiological" age twenty years younger than his chronological age—the kind of elderly patient I liked to ask, only half joking, *What's your secret?* Whenever I asked Fred this question, he would just chuckle and say, That's a good question, a very good question. But he didn't say much about the phone calls. In fact, he didn't remember them very well. This concerned me even more. I talked to Martha privately about this. She couldn't put her finger on anything specific. But, she said, I've been married to this man for fifty-five years and there's something fishy going on—that's the word Martha used, "fishy"—because most of the time he's just his same old Fred and then, especially at night but not every night, he's . . . different . . . I know, I know, but that's the best I can do, Brendan, he's just *different*, I can't say how exactly.

Finally, Martha and I convinced Fred to see Katherine Armour, a professor of psychiatry at Dartmouth who, in her seventies herself, specialized in geriatric psychiatry. Fred wasn't crazy about this idea—in fact, that's exactly the way Fred put it, chuckling—but he went along when I reminded him that Martha was concerned about him. What's the harm? I said, and he reluctantly agreed. Just last week I'd heard that Dr. Armour hadn't found much either when she examined Fred. But now she'd begun to receive his phone calls at night, too. Uncertain what was going on, she was debating whether to hospitalize Fred on the inpatient Psychiatry service to observe him around the clock for a few days.

As my old Volvo huffed and shimmied up the next hill, I wondered whether Martha's frantic call this morning meant Martha wanted me to arrange the inpatient Psych observation, now. It seemed like a good idea, for Martha's sake as well as Fred's. As much as I was perplexed about Fred, I was concerned about Martha, too. She was the one with the bad heart.

I would need a plan. I checked the clock on my car's dashboard. It read 6:05. This was okay. Dr. Armour and her husband were avid bird-watchers, even in winter. They'd be up and about, even at this hour. And I could do my part. Fred and Martha would go along with what I recommended. They trusted me.

This didn't mean we were friends. I hadn't let that happen. When friends wanted to become my patients, I talked them out of it. And when patients wanted to become my friends, I put them off. This was awkward, sometimes—and often I wished I didn't have to refuse the dinner invitations or golf outings or theater tickets—but I didn't see any other way. Professional objectivity was impossible when caring for a friend or a relative. Love and loyalty, or guilt and regret, just get in the way. But maintaining a distance was a personal defense, too. After all, the "doctor-patient relationship" *is* a relationship. And, like all relationships, it can get complicated.

Across the road, heat rose from the chimney above Inge's house.

Pale wood smoke danced in the trees, beckoning. Was her husband away? In my mind's eye, I could see the sleek stone fireplace inside, the lush Scandinavian carpet on the hearth. Was she sitting there now, by the fire?

For a long time, I had seen Inge only at the office. In the beginning, it was usually for stomachaches or insomnia or other vague aches and pains. Soon enough, though, it became clear that she was depressed and lonely and needed someone to talk to. Her husband was a research scientist who studied cold climates in remote places like Greenland and the Antarctic, places too forbidding for a young wife and child. She was alone a lot. For a woman who looked like Inge, making friends in a small town wasn't easy. The men couldn't take their eyes off her. The women resented her for it. Antidepressant drugs made her worse. She didn't trust psychologists or psychiatrists. (They're all voyeurs, she said, they just get off on other people's troubles.) So she talked to me.

I hadn't seen her in several weeks when she called one day. It was winter. She asked me to come see her at home. She said she'd been so tired these past few weeks she hadn't been able even to leave her house. Her husband was away. Her son was at the babysitter's. I'm all alone, she said.

It took me a while to find her house. The sun had begun to set when I arrived. No one answered when I rang the doorbell. Soft evening light filled the downstairs rooms but Inge wasn't there. She was upstairs, lying on her bed. She wore a nightshirt, nothing else. She didn't get up. She just lay there. Her skin was translucent, white as the snow outside her window. Unnaturally white. When I touched her, her heart was racing. I put pillows under her long, bare legs to examine her. She moaned when I put my finger inside, but was otherwise unresponsive. The stool in her rectum was black as coal. I guessed she'd bled out almost her entire blood volume these past few weeks. I covered her with blankets and called for the ambulance. Had Inge been Martha's age, that stomach ulcer would have killed her, but within a few days she was well again. Her husband flew back urgently from Hudson Bay. In her white hospital bed she blushed pink and smiled wide when he promised he would be home more often now.

This morning, as the chimney smoke wafted into the gray pre-dawn, I hoped Inge's husband had kept his promise.

How complicated couples are! In my short career as a doctor, I had become impatient, even contemptuous, of people who gossiped and opined about other couples' relationships. No one can know what goes on between two people except the couple themselves. I couldn't even begin to imagine all the water that had passed under Fred and Martha's bridge. Fifty-five years! They'd been married almost twice as long as I'd been alive. How could I think I could help *them*?

But I was learning. On every corner in this town, down every street I passed this morning, there were stories like Inge's. The house calls, like the one this morning, took a lot more time than the phone calls ever did, and they took a bigger piece out of me, too. But I remembered them all and I learned something every time. The word doctor is derived from the Latin root *docere*—to teach—but, in my experience so far, the patients had taught the doctor at least as much as the doctor taught them.

At the crest of the hill, near the beginning of the Dartmouth campus, the old Westman house stood empty and dark. The path to the front door hadn't been shoveled all winter. Could it really be ten years since I had spent the better part of three days there, trying to help Ms. Westman die? Back then, I didn't know much about such things. I was new, fresh out of training, well equipped to deal with the heart attacks, cancers, and infections in the hospital. But helping old folks die at home wasn't part of the medical curriculum in my day.

Ms. Westman had just had her fourth stroke. Her son, who had run the local pharmacy since her husband died, knew that his eighty-nine-year-old mother didn't want to go back to the hospital. Ever. After I reviewed her medical records—she had been hospitalized thirty-eight times in the past ten years—I agreed with the son's request to try to care for Ms. Westman at home. When I arrived, my shiny black doctor bag in hand, the poor woman was lying on her bed, fully clothed, unconscious yet groaning, rolling her head this way and that as if trying to shake off a pain that not even coma could relieve.

I examined her as best I could. But, for the life of me, I couldn't figure out the source of her suffering. It was painful just to watch. Finally, remembering that I was here not to make a diagnosis but to make Ms. Westman comfortable, I gave her a shot of morphine. To my horror, this seemed only to make her worse. She was so agitated, so distressed!

I was about to give up—tell the son we had no choice but to call an ambulance—when the visiting nurse arrived. Peggy was an older Scotswoman, nearing retirement. She had visited Ms. Westman at home regularly for years. Peggy took one look at her, writhing on her bed, and said, Ah, now, what a shame. Such a fine lady she is.

Then Peggy saw that I was clueless, clearly over my head and at my wit's end.

Firmly but diplomatically—after all, I was the doctor and she the nurse—Peggy said, Ooh, doctor, yes, let's get her out of that girdle now, shall we?

I didn't know what she was talking about. A girdle? Such distress from a girdle? But I didn't have any better ideas. It took all that we both could do to get Ms. Westman, a large woman and dead weight, out of that brocaded dress and the heavy nylon stockings and the lacy garters with the metal clips and the rubber buttons and the tight elastic girdle and all the rest of it. When we were done, Ms. Westman was stark naked but she was still writhing and groaning.

Peggy looked at me expectantly, awaiting my order.

I didn't know what to do. I wasn't at the hospital. I couldn't just order some tests or X-rays or ask a consultant to see her. What to do?

Her tone deferential but firm, Peggy said simply, Dr. Reilly, she has to pee.

Before I could even register this idea, Peggy spread Ms. Westman's doughy white thighs and deftly slipped a catheter into her bladder. A torrential stream of urine shot out into a large metal basin, nearly filling it. Immediately, Ms. Westman (who remained peacefully asleep thereafter until her death three days later) let out such a prolonged and exuberant sigh of pleasure and release that she seemed in the throes of ecstasy. She even grinned, her face lopsided by her stroke but utterly satisfied, comatose or not.

Peggy watched her, then smiled and shook her head. She clucked her tongue pensively and said, It's quite something, is it not, Dr. Reilly?

What?

Well, now! How women of a certain age . . . and breeding, if I may say so . . . just can't . . . bring themselves . . . to . . . wet their pants! No matter what! Now, isn't it remarkable, that?

And so it was, at least to me.

This was how doctors learned. This was the people part of doctoring—the part the patients teach the doctors, not the other way around—and it was endless, the stuff of novels, not textbooks. I never did find an authoritative medical reference about how to handle my visit to Mr. Chadwick, an old angler with Parkinson's disease who asked me to remove a fishhook stuck painfully in his upper eyelid. He refused to go to the hospital. (That suggestion had made his head shake even more.) He apologized for bothering me about such a foolish thing and said that, in the old days, he would have just removed it himself, but his tremor was pretty bad now, both his head and his hands. So he talked me through the procedure, right there on his front porch, easy as pie.

The textbooks hadn't helped me much when I'd had to figure out what to do for Tim, either. Tim was a good man—orphaned as a five-year-old, he'd taught himself to become a fine auto mechanic—but he couldn't handle his beer and had been trying to stay on the wagon so he could win back his estranged wife and kids. Taciturn and hardworking, Tim asked me to sew his nose back onto his face at home at his kitchen table, so his wife wouldn't hear about how he'd passed out, face first on the floor, onto a jagged shard of beer bottle. His nose was hanging off his face, like a flag at half-mast. I'm no plastic surgeon and probably shouldn't have done what I did, but about a year later a permanently sober Tim, despite his odd-looking nose, was able to reconcile with his kids, if not his wife.

If only there were a book of life, somewhere I could just look up the answers. The intimidating breadth of clinical skill and experience that primary care requires is humbling, but these "people things" were the hardest part. Some involved classic issues in medical ethics;

these I could read about and consult with colleagues to help me. But so many others were judgment calls where there was no right or wrong answer, where I couldn't be sure what was the best thing for my patient or what were the appropriate limits of my responsibility as their doctor. These ambiguities were part of the job.

In the decade immediately preceding my early morning house call to visit Martha and Fred, luminaries in American medicine hotly debated the "boundaries" of our profession. Is medicine strictly a curing science, its purview limited to human biology and disease? Or is medicine a "helping profession" whose boundaries extend beyond biomedical science?

This debate continues today. Its arguments affect not only how our society spends its resources to improve its citizens' health but also what kind of help its citizens can reasonably expect to receive from the medical profession. Can a medical doctor like me help Laura Henderson, the grieving widow? (Medical doctors are trained to treat disease. Is grief a disease?) Do Fred's loopy phone calls mean he's ill? Or is he just getting more eccentric and forgetful in his old age? (If so, what can I do about that? And how can I help Martha, now sick with worry about Fred?) Did loneliness cause the bleeding ulcer that nearly killed Inge? If so, could better doctoring have prevented it?

For the past thirty years, the biomedical side in this debate has clearly held the upper hand. Its argument was articulated most famously by Donald Seldin, a distinguished physician-scientist, in his widely publicized address titled "The Boundaries of Medicine":

> Medicine is a very narrow discipline. Its goals may be defined as the relief of pain, the prevention of disability, and the postponement of death by the application . . . of medical science to individual patients. . . . A heritage which invests medicine with the priestly function of the counselor and comforter of the sick . . . has resulted [in] a tendency to construe all sorts of human problems as medical problems. This medicalization of human experience leads to enormous . . . frustration and disillusionment when medical intervention fails to eventuate in tranquility . . . and happiness.

Human problems . . . are medical problems and medical illnesses
only when they can be approached by the theories and techniques of
biomedical science.

Seldin argued that a clear boundary can (and must) be drawn between medical care and health care: Medical care is a part of, not a
synonym for, health care. Health is affected by many nonbiological
factors—social, economic, psychological, and cultural factors—but
these issues (including substance abuse, poverty, various forms of
mental illness, and the aging process) "lie outside the arena of medicine." Furthermore, *within* the arena of medicine, Seldin argued that
another boundary must be drawn that separates patients' problems
into those that biomedical science can and cannot solve. In his view,
it cannot solve problems like grief, worry, alcoholism, and risky behavior. (Such problems are the "turf" of paramedical professionals,
such as psychologists, social workers, and ethicists.) Medicine's task
is not to make people happy. Medicine's task, *in its entirety*, is to
understand, prevent, diagnose, and treat scientifically definable biological dysfunctions.

This is an enormous task but, as Seldin argued, also a "very narrow" one. Even if Inge's bleeding ulcer was caused by the stress of
loneliness, it's not her doctor's job to have prevented it. Like Laura
Henderson's grief, stress and loneliness are not *diseases*. These afflic-
tions cause patients real suffering—and may eventually lead to "real"
diseases such as bleeding ulcers—but they are not, in the biomedical
view, *medical* problems.

The contrary argument holds that this biomedical model works
well for researchers (a good fit for their reductionist methodology)
and for some practicing physicians (their job made easier by its narrower scope) but not for patients. This view was articulated best by
George Engel, a legendary professor of medicine (and a contempo-
rary of Donald Seldin), in the prestigious journal *Science*:

> Despite the enormous gains which have accrued from biomedical re-
> search, there is a growing consensus among the public . . . that physi-
> cians are lacking in interest and understanding, are preoccupied with

procedures, and are insensitive to the personal problems of patients and their families.

Medical institutions are seen as cold and impersonal; the more prestigious they are as centers for biomedical research, the more common such complaints.

In Engel's view, the biomedical model was winning battles but losing the war. The root cause of this failure was widespread misunderstanding about the difference between illness and disease. Long before medicine was remotely scientific—indeed, before the modern scientific concept of disease even existed—people who felt ill sought help from healers, because they believed that the healer might know why they felt ill and how to make them feel better. For the patient (the literal meaning of the word is "one who suffers"), the *illness* is everything. No less today than in prescientific times, what matters to patients is how they feel, the impact of their "ill-ness" on how they function, its portent for their future, how they live their life.

But the connection between illness and disease, even today when the explanatory power of biomedicine is so powerful, is tenuous at best. Some patients who feel ill have no definable disease. Other patients, who have definable diseases, don't feel ill at all. And, when one disease afflicts two different patients, their illnesses—how the disease makes them feel—may be completely different. Such discordance between illness and disease led Engel (and many others) to conclude that a purely biomedical model is inadequate to the goals of medicine. All too often, when doctors tell patients with ambiguous illnesses, "There's nothing wrong with you," the doctor really means that "There's nothing wrong with you that fits within my own, narrow biomedical model of disease."

But all human illnesses and diseases express themselves through their victim, a *person* who feels, communicates, and attributes meaning to those experiences in unique ways. The clinical "expression" of disease—the illness—*always* will vary with the individual characteristics, psychological makeup, and cultural background of the disease victim. Thus, Engel argued, doctors will never be able to diagnose and treat their patients effectively without understanding, and gaining expertise in, these nonbiological domains. To be effective, the physician must accept the responsibility "to evaluate whatever problems the patient presents and recommend a course of action, including referral to other helping professions."

During a few brief periods in the 1970s, and again in the 1990s, Engel's "biopsychosocial model" gained some traction in the United States. Young physicians like me embraced primary care medicine because we were inspired to help "the whole patient," notwithstanding the ambiguity (and hubristic zeal) this implied. Today, however, primary care physicians in the United States are in shorter supply than ever. The biomedical model of medicine is clearly dominant, propelled by its truly remarkable scientific achievements. In fact, the science has shown that some health domains once deemed not "biomedical"—such as substance abuse, mental illness, aging—do, in fact, have important biological underpinnings. Nevertheless, Engel's fundamental concern remains unanswered today: What happens to patients whose illnesses don't "fit" the biomedical model? Who helps them?

I stopped for a red light at the corner of Wheelock and Park streets, where the Dartmouth campus began. Hard ice covered the fine red clay tennis courts in front of the new athletic center. Across the street, construction on the new student housing complex had been halted temporarily, a rare concession to the brutal cold and heavy snows of January. These new dormitories would mark the beginning of the Big Change, Dartmouth's first bricks-and-mortar acknowledgment of societal changes it could no longer ignore. For more than two hundred years, Dartmouth had been a wealthy, world-class institution whose all-male Big Green alumni—"men of granite" who "bled green"—had given generously and fought hard to preserve its traditions. But recently the college trustees had recognized the female sex as a constituency they couldn't live without, one deserving more respect than it typically received at Dartmouth's infamous frat parties. Despite fierce opposition from rabid alumni, they had voted to admit women students to Dartmouth.

Women? At Dartmouth?

The first few pioneering females had been housed in temporary quarters, which most of them liked precisely because they weren't far removed from the men's dorms. But this advantage soon lost its luster, at least for some, who wound up coming to me. Dartmouth ran an excellent student health service, including an inpatient infirmary, but like the rest of the college it wasn't ready yet for female problems—or, at least, not the kind of female problems that found their way to me.

The Dartmouth women I saw seemed female analogs of Dartmouth men: clean-cut, athletic, attractive kids from Connecticut and California, kids from good families with bright futures who had had all the advantages and probably always would have. But, behind their practiced smiles and polished social skills, some of these young women were hurting badly, in ways they couldn't explain. One had intractable headaches. Another couldn't sleep. A third had constant pelvic pain that defied physical explanation.

The first one, Jennifer, was a tall, raven-haired all-American soccer star whose fine cheekbones, athleticism, and ribald sense of humor would have made her a big man on campus—if she'd been a man. Eventually we got down to why her headaches were happening, how the guys would show her (four or five at a time) what they really thought of her. She couldn't confide in anyone, including her own family. (That's why she was here: Her father and older brother and all her uncles had gone to Dartmouth.) She said there was just no way she could talk to them about it. After I'd figured out what was going on with Jennifer, it didn't take long to get to the bottom of Kylie's pelvic pains or Samantha's insomnia.

The traffic light turned green. I drove past the dormant Caterpillars at the construction site—excavators, front-loaders, and cranes glistening with ice. Directly across the street was the modest frame house where Hugh MacNamee and his family lived. A psychiatrist who specialized in adolescent mental health, a kind man with teenagers of his own, Hugh had seen Jennifer and Samantha and some of the other girls at my request. He had helped them. He never said anything to me about it—whatever they discussed was confidential—but I knew he had helped. And I suspected that the location of the new women's dormitory was no coincidence.

Hugh's elderly mother, Patty—a wizened, wise, delightful widow in her eighties who had a bad heart—lived in an oxygen-equipped apartment in the attic of Hugh's house. Sometimes, in the evening on my way home from the hospital, I would stop in to check on her. (Patty never asked for me—she always said she didn't like being a "nuisance"—but Hugh's wife would let me know when the swelling in Patty's legs or shortness of breath seemed worse.) In recent months, whenever I visited her, Patty had developed a conspicuous habit of looking out her attic window at the construction site across the street. With a twinkle in her eye, she would say to me: Isn't it fine that the Dartmouth girls will finally have a place of their own? Isn't it fine?

Once, just once, Patty had slipped. (I think. It was hard to tell with Patty; she was an ace poker player.) On that one occasion, Patty had said: *your* Dartmouth girls. Isn't it fine, Brendan, that *your* Dartmouth girls will have a place of their own? I never asked her what she knew, but, like Patty, I was glad for the girls.

My car approached the center of town. There, the Dartmouth green lay empty and white in the lifting darkness. In summertime, the green was a wide expanse of lush lawn bordered by giant leafy elms and grand stone buildings, each named for a wealthy alumnus. The professorial life at Dartmouth, a first-rate institution in a beautiful place, seemed pretty sweet. Its focal point was Baker Library, the stately brick edifice whose iconic bell tower was the north star of academic life here. But this star had begun to dim for some of the Dartmouth faculty, many of whom were my patients. More than a few had become restless and dissatisfied. After they had survived the gauntlet to tenure, they seemed to spend most of their time learning more and more about less and less. As their academic focus shrank, their personal horizons constricted, too. Bored, they poured their energy into hobbies or had affairs or drank too much or paid too much attention to their children (or, in some sad cases, not nearly enough).

Initially, I attributed faculty ennui to the small size and homogeneity of the college population, an insular culture that glorified bits of arcane knowledge that only a handful of people in the world cared about. But, in time, it seemed to me that the cause of their angst—which, in some cases, led to panic or depression and thence to me—wasn't that their life's work seemed useless. (They all knew from the start that unearthing new evidence about Shakespeare's mistress or Lincoln's sexuality wasn't *useful*, not in any practical way.) Instead, the problem seemed to be that the merits of their research, which required great effort and skill, could be judged only subjectively, decided by the prevailing opinion of expert peers like themselves. This was less true in the sciences (and in the business and engineering schools) than the arts, but even the chemists and geologists and economists never seemed sure that they weren't wasting their time. (These were the days when quantum mechanics and Thomas Kuhn were all the rage: Nothing was certain.) To compensate, many professors found solace in the beauty, if not the truth, of what they taught. Others found meaning in the process, if not the outcome, of their discoveries. But more than a few found neither. Of these, the ones I saw just seemed to feel smaller as they got older.

Medicine, it seemed to me, was different from these other pursuits in both its science and its practice. The science's power to prolong and improve people's lives seemed limitless. It was tangible, visible, its value objectively indisputable. A mere five years after HIV, a new disease, had killed thousands of people like Saul Henderson, medical scientists had isolated the murderous piece of RNA that caused it, a stupendous achievement. There was talk about eradicating HIV from the planet entirely, along with smallpox, polio, and other viral scourges. The pace and practical utility of such discoveries were breathtaking.

Although very different from medical research, the practice of medicine was vital, too. If you made the effort, you could find out what *really* happened. Did my diagnosis prove correct? Did my treatment work? When my patient died, did the autopsy show what I had missed, how I could have done better? Every day as a practicing doctor, I encountered an objective reality—*out there*, independent of my own wishfulness or bias or ego—actual things that happened to real people in real time, some of them the result of what I did or didn't do. And, like trees falling in a remote forest where no one can hear them, these things happened whether I knew about them or not. Finding out—actively, even desperately, tracking down *what had happened*—became an essential part of what I did. Whether the final factual reality proved me a success or a failure, finding out made me better and wiser. But only if I took the trouble—and had the guts—to find out. To look reality in the eye.

Personally, this was a godsend. I had grown up on denial. My own family was beset by many of the same problems (and blessings) that have long bedeviled (and saved) large Irish families: alcoholism (and romanticism); depression (and stoicism); religiosity (and puckishness); inbreeding (and wanderlust). Drink ruined my father's medical career and nearly killed him when I was eight, the second of five kids then aged one to nine. My mother never spoke about it. None of us kids visited Dad even once during the entire nine months he spent in the VA hospital just three blocks from our home. Afterward, my father had lived the life of a "dry drunk," working a menial medical job for the Pennsylvania Railroad, punctual and professional at the office but brooding and resentful at home. Mom denied her own alcoholism for years, and Dad, who figured he had no rights in the matter, did nothing about it until others intervened.

So I had seen up close the effects of creating one's own reality. Then, when I went to medical school, I saw that real shit happens to real people whether you want to admit it or not. And I learned that when you're trying to help those people, denial just doesn't cut it.

Fortunately, I married a woman who understood this. Ironically, Janice thought I was in denial, too—about my own habit, an addiction to medicine—and that, as a result, I was in danger of living the life of a "dry drunk" like my father. And, when you got right down to it, there I was, sitting in my car that February morning, waiting for a traffic light before sunup, stealing my precious vacation time from the people I loved most because I *needed* to find out about Martha and Fred.

The light turned green. As the road began its steep decline down the hill from Hanover toward Norwich, I looked west over the Connecticut River to the high meadows of Vermont. Even in winter, when the maple, beech, and birch are bare and the pastures pale with ice, it is some of the prettiest country in New England. Up there, on the south face of the slope, was an old weathered barn, too far away to see. That's where John would be now, out of bed hours ago, feeding and milking, tending the machines and the stalls, maybe even birthing a calf.

Compared to John Melby, my family and I knew nothing about denial. Dairy farming was backbreaking work, seven days a week, but John Melby loved it. So did his wife, Shane, until the trouble got out of hand. Ostensibly, the trouble was John's unshakeable conviction that he had colon cancer—even though two colonoscopies, a sigmoidoscopy, and two barium enema X-rays had proved he had no such thing. To look at him, John was the last person you would expect to be ruminating endlessly, anxiously, about a disease he definitely didn't have. Six feet three, 220 pounds of pure muscle, with a confident smile, cleft chin, and penetrating brown eyes, he looked, even at age forty, like a recruiting ad for the U.S. Marines, which, as it happened, he once had been. Fresh out of high school, where he'd been the football captain and married the homecoming queen, John had served two tours of duty in Southeast Asia in the early sixties, before Vietnam was called a conflict, much less a war.

Like most doctors, I hadn't learned how to help hypochondriacs like John, but he kept coming back to see me anyway. I didn't find out about the real trouble until Shane started coming to see me, too. After she got to know me, she told me about how John spent his nights.

Sometimes it's the moon, John said, when he tried to explain it.

The moon?

Yeah, somethin' about the moon, doc. Like . . . when it's about half full and . . . a little cloudy, you know?

Uh-huh . . .

Wet wood, too. Or wet leaves. When you burn them, you know? It's the smell.

Okay.

And the chopper. You know, when the helicopters come down over the river sometimes, transporting somebody into the hospital? The sound, you know? It's the sound of the darn thing.

Yeah.

Those were his triggers. Whenever he saw or smelled or heard those things, John would drop in his tracks. He might be in the barn or the kitchen or out in the field. He might even wake up with it and slip stealthily out of bed, careful not to wake Shane or the kids. Then he would crawl, on all fours, all night sometimes, out in the pastures, around the farm's outbuildings, on patrol, with a loaded M-60 in his hands and murder in his heart. Usually, Shane wouldn't even know until she found him in the morning—outside, asleep under the porch, covered in mud and manure, his rifle held tight to his chest.

His were the delayed kind, they had told him at the VA, the kind of flashbacks that don't start until years later. But he was getting worse and the kids were getting older and they didn't understand why their dad was the only dad who couldn't go on overnight field trips or to bonfires the night before a big game. John never said an unkind word about anyone, including the VA doctors (whom he didn't like) or the Vietnamese. (They were just fighting to keep their farms, you know, doc?) And he didn't blame the guys. (No, sir, I'm proud of what we did, I'm proud to be a Marine.) And he didn't blame Johnson. (But Kennedy would have stopped it, don't you think so, doc?) It was just one of those things, he said, what are you gonna do?

But, uh, doc, about those colonoscopies? I've been reading that they can miss the cancer sometimes, you know? So, do you think we should take another look up there, or what?

I drove across Ledyard Bridge into Vermont. Ice floes cracked on the riverbank below. I thought about Maggie, John's daughter, who had come to see me just last week. She was a lovely, healthy girl who was getting married in the spring. She worried that her father wouldn't be able to walk down the aisle with her. He couldn't handle a crowd, not even when it was just family and friends. It would break Maggie's heart if her dad couldn't give her away. I promised her I would try again to get John to take some medicine. I didn't tell her I was pessimistic. The wedding was only a few months away.

As I drove into Norwich, Hanover's quaint quiet sister town on the Vermont side of the river, it occurred to me that Fred and Martha were John's temperamental opposites. Martha was uncomplaining to a fault. And when I first met Fred, he'd had a fainting spell at home—passed out cold at his kitchen table—but he didn't seem concerned in the least. In fact, he was more intrigued by the experience than worried about his health. He'd never fainted before and found it "very interesting."

Fred was an engineer, a rather famous one. Before coming to Dartmouth to teach at its prestigious graduate school of engineering, Fred had worked for big corporations like Ford and General Motors, inventing (and patenting) all kinds of useful things. Like all engineers, he was fascinated by "how things work." But Fred admitted that he didn't know much about how the human body works, so he'd had a grand time in my office with the Dartmouth medical student who examined him before I came in, each of them bouncing ideas off the other about the various "mechanisms" that might cause a person to faint. In the course of their discussion, the medical student had consulted a textbook I had written about the diagnosis and treatment of common medical problems (including fainting), which became grist in their mechanistic musings. In the end, it wasn't clear why Fred had fainted—he wasn't injured, his examination was normal, and his many tests turned up nothing—but Fred liked me anyway and, because his own physician had just retired, he asked me to take him on.

I wasn't accepting new patients—I had too many already—but Fred won me over with his charm. He had returned to see me to review his test results and brought with him a copy of my textbook. (This alone would have won me over; then he said he'd actually read it.) He said he thought we were kindred spirits. He considered himself a "generalist" engineer, and he had the track record to prove it: He had invented everything from disc brakes for cars to navigation systems for airplanes. He'd even designed one of the first heart-lung machines for cardiac surgery. Fred liked the fact that I was an internal medicine doctor whose specialty was *not* specializing—not limiting my expertise to one bodily organ (like a cardiologist) or one disease (like a cancer specialist)—and whose goal was to take care of the "whole" patient. He had highlighted in yellow magic marker a phrase in my textbook's Introduction: "We generalists must know our own limitations . . . but we will remain vital in our efforts and proud of our work if we heed our patients' plea: *Be my doctor.*" That day in my office, Fred had simply pointed at those yellowed lines and asked, Can you do this for me?

It had been easy—Fred had never once needed my help—until a few weeks ago.

Hello?

Brendan, I've been thinking about what you said the other day . . .

Fred?

. . . and I've been working on this new idea . . . seems promising . . .

Uh-huh?

Well, when we did the new navigation system for the Electra . . .

Electra . . . ?

. . . it was heavier than the old direction finders. People thought it would eat up too much fuel if the plane had to carry the new, heavier device on long trips . . .

Okay . . . ?

Click-click.

Fred? For Pete's sake, Fred! Leave the man alone! Hang up the phone!

I turned left on Elm Street and began the climb up to Fred and Martha's place. Norwich had long been a quintessential Vermont town but change was coming. The town's public areas still included nothing more than a post office, a grammar school, a swimming hole, and Dan and Whit's general store. The store's motto, crayoned on a wood beam above an old-fashioned Coca-Cola-red freezer, read, "If we don't have it you don't need it," and this had been pretty much true for a very long time. But as I downshifted into the hill, I passed the pond and the paddock behind Joanie's McMansion. Norwich never used to look like that.

I'd been inside the McMansion only once, a few months ago, a weekend house call. Joanie was a divorcée with two little kids who'd moved to Norwich from New Jersey a year ago. She had a mild chest cold. Her father, who was visiting from New York, wanted me to hospitalize her. *You can't be too careful about these things, don't you agree, doctor?* He wore Gucci loafers with gold buckles, a Rolex the size of Staten Island, and a toupee that may have cost more than my house. After I'd examined Joanie and reassured her, he pulled me aside privately to push harder for his hospitalization idea, and waved a wad of fifty-dollar bills at me. He didn't know what to think when I declined, told him the house call was on the house, and left him spluttering at the front door. This wasn't New York.

I was paid a salary. No bonus. No incentives. No "skin in the game." I didn't make more money the more patients I saw, or the more tests I did, or the more referrals I brought into the hospital. The Dartmouth group was one of the largest multispecialty practices in the United States; we did everything for the people of northern New England from cutting-edge cardiac surgery to neonatal intensive care—and we did it cost-effectively and well. Our heart surgeons and neurosurgeons and orthopedists were paid higher salaries than mine—but not much higher (less than double), a remarkable thing given the fact that I, compared with internists in private practice, was grossly underpaid myself. It was a special group of doctors who had developed this model of medical care and sustained it for decades—one that put patients first, not the doctors or the hospital or the bottom line—and I felt proud to be one of them.

We were a team. My job was to do what I was doing now: be the front man, be available to people who needed help when they needed it, figure out what was wrong with them, and get them to specialists when (but only if) the patients really needed them. Above all, as with Fred and Martha, my job was to *be their doctor*—the one they could count on, no matter what, over the long haul. From patients' perspective, what I did was every bit as valuable to them as the great things our specialists did. The insurers didn't think so, of course; they reimbursed the specialists and surgeons at much higher rates than my services. But this was the genius of the Dartmouth model: The caregivers, as a group, cared more about serving patients well than kowtowing to what insurers valued. None of us was getting rich—I couldn't even afford to send my kids to private school—but we believed in what we did and we tried to do right by our patients.

This wasn't socialized medicine. It was medicine that made sense within a particular social context. Rural New England was a place where people were raised to value three things above all else: their independence (New Hampshire's state motto is Live Free or Die); their environment (Vermont is the Green Mountain State); and their neighbors. You helped other folks and they helped you; it was as simple as that. Ripping them off in the process, or putting a dollar value on everything you did, was a repulsive, foreign idea. To a city boy like me, doctoring and getting to know these folks—farmers and stonemasons, potters and carpenters, lumberjacks and weavers—had been a revelation.

But the change was coming and, as I chugged past Joanie's place and up the hill to Fred and Martha, I knew the old way wouldn't survive. New York and New Jersey had discovered New Hampshire and Vermont. Before long, money would gum up the works here, too. But it never occurred to me that one could actually *measure* the differences in quality and cost between the Gucci-loafers-fistful-of-dollars style of medical practice on Park Avenue and the very different style here.

But that's what Jack Wennberg was doing at Dartmouth, even way back then. I had last seen Jack a few months before, on a mountain-top. Together with friends from New York, Janice and I had climbed Cardigan Mountain to get an eagle's-eye view of the spectacular fall foliage down below. At the summit, we met Jack and his wife, who had climbed there many times before. After some small talk, they suggested we descend the mountain by a different route from the way we'd come up. The view is even better, if you can believe it, Jack said. This alternate route down would have left us several miles from where we had left our car at the bottom. But Jack said they were going down the way we had come up and they'd be glad to drive our car around to the other side of the mountain and leave the keys in the car. Delighted, we agreed. Our New York friends were astounded. Leaving your car unlocked with the keys on the front seat wasn't something people did in Manhattan.

Jack had grown up in Vermont, trained at Hopkins and Harvard, but then returned home to the place he loved most. His area of research at Dartmouth was called "small area analysis," a term he had invented and that no one else in medicine cared much about. Using data he had collected in Vermont and Maine, he discovered that more women who lived in particular towns in these two states had had a hysterectomy than women who lived in other towns. This did not make the evening news. But Jack cobbled together enough grant funding to investigate these "small area variations" further. He discovered that more men who lived in particular towns had had a prostatectomy—and more children had had a tonsillectomy—than those living in other towns. He also found that hospitalization rates for various medical conditions (like Joanie's respiratory infection) varied widely for people who lived in different areas. None of these variations seemed to make any sense. They couldn't be explained by differences in the towns themselves or the people who lived in them. Trained in sociology as well as medicine, Jack became intrigued by the idea that these variations somehow reflected differences in the "culture" of medical practice in these different locales. To understand this phenomenon better, Jack recently had broadened his sights and begun studying differences in physicians' use of hospital services in Boston versus New Haven.

At the time, I thought small area variations in medical care belonged in the same category of trivial academic esoterica as exciting new discoveries about art history or geology. Others, much wiser than I, knew better.

In 1975, Howard Hiatt, a physician and dean of the Harvard School of Public Health, published a provocative and prescient article titled "Protecting the Medical Commons: Who Is Responsible?" that cited Jack's work prominently. Using the analogy of a large grazing pasture shared by many dairy farmers, Hiatt argued that, if a single farmer increases his number of cows and consumes more of the pasture, this will have little effect on the overall welfare. However, if *all* of the dairy farmers do the same, that is, increase consumption of the pasture to maximize their own self-interest, this will destroy the welfare of all. Hiatt contended that U.S. society faced a similar dilemma about medical care.

Hiatt strongly endorsed the traditional principle that a doctor's primary responsibility was to "do everything possible for the individual patient." But this principle, applied in an era when costly new medical technologies and treatments were introduced almost daily, raised the specter of our society "reaching a point where marginal gains to individuals threaten the welfare of the whole." Societal medical resources—the medical commons, like the grazing pasture—are finite. Unconstrained use of those resources by individuals, which inevitably will limit the resources available to the rest of us, "is a luxury we can no longer afford." What to do? Obviously, priorities must be set. But Hiatt asked: *Who is responsible* for setting these priorities? Who will make these decisions?

> It is surely not fair to ask the physician or other medical provider to set [these priorities] in the context of his or her own medical practice....
>
> To protect the commons from useless, prematurely introduced, or otherwise inappropriate practices, the physician must join statisticians, epidemiologists, and economists to ensure that no practice is widely adopted without prior evaluation.

Hiatt identified several categories of medical practices whose incursion on the medical commons seemed problematic. He cited Jack's research because it dealt with the most important of these: practices whose value was unknown, negligible, or even negative (more harmful than beneficial). For example, pediatricians had long believed that as many as 90 percent of the one million tonsillectomy operations performed annually in the United States (in 1975) were unnecessary, a waste of medical resources. But this contrarian view was difficult to prove until Jack's research showed that the rate of tonsillectomy varied *tenfold* in different New England towns. And, Jack argued, avoiding unnecessary tonsillectomy procedures not only would save precious resources ($360 million in 1975), it would also reduce deaths from (tonsillectomy-related) general anesthesia. Jack's work had shown that *elective, unnecessary* tonsillectomies cost hundreds of millions of dollars and scores of kids' lives every year. In Hiatt's view, this exemplified the kind of "health services" research (rarely done in 1975) badly needed to help protect the medical commons.

Hiatt didn't stop there. A fervent supporter of biomedical science and technological innovation, he applauded the discovery of new, potentially valuable practices. In 1975, these novelties included computed tomography (CT scans), intensive care units (ICUs), and "prehospital rescue units" (ambulances with emergency medical personnel on board). But, ever mindful of the endangered commons, he insisted that new technologies and practices not be adopted until they are proven more effective—*and more cost-effective*—than the status quo.

Regarding CT scanning, for example, Hiatt cautioned that "already there is evidence of its being used for purposes for which much simpler equipment is adequate. Will we be able to establish guidelines for the purchase and use of this machine [1975 cost: four hundred thousand dollars] before it too becomes a prominent and unregulated occupant of the medical commons?" Intensive care units and emergency ambulances no doubt save lives, Hiatt argued, but how many lives—and at what cost? Will "universal implementation" of these promising new practices be cost-effective? Hiatt and others had good ideas about *how* to answer those questions (using rigorous health services research methods). But who would empower and oversee this process? Again, Hiatt's essential question was: *Who* is responsible to protect the medical commons?

In 1975, when Hiatt wrote confidently that "few would question . . . that we are approaching . . . a limit" to the resources our society can devote to the medical commons, health care spending in the U.S. amounted to 6 to 7 percent of the nation's $1.6 trillion gross domestic product. Thirty-five years later, in 2010, U.S. population had grown 50 percent (from 200 to 300 million) and health care spending had grown more than 2,000 percent (to 17 percent of the nation's $14.6 trillion gross domestic product). Newfangled curiosities in 1975, intensive care units and CT scanners and emergency medical ambulances are now ubiquitous. Today, there are more intensive care units than hospitals in the United States but their cost-effectiveness is not known. Seventy million CT scans are performed annually in the United States—all of them expensive and many of them unnecessary. (Worse, it is estimated that ionizing radiation from these CT scans will *cause* fifteen thousand to thirty thousand cancers annually—1 to 2 percent of all new cancers diagnosed.) Fifteen thousand

American communities now employ 850,000 emergency medical personnel to staff what Hiatt called "prehospital rescue units." No doubt these ambulance crews do fine work, but who is tracking their effectiveness and cost?

Since Hiatt's time, the one person in the United States who has been "tracking" medicine most carefully—and, arguably, doing more than anyone else to protect the medical commons—is Jack Wennberg. Forty years after he started asking questions about the "culture" of medical practice in rural Vermont, Jack's lifelong research has illuminated medical culture throughout the United States and around the world. His *Dartmouth Atlas of Health Care* chronicles the irrational variation, inequity, inefficiency, and potential for improvement of the U.S. health care system. Not incidentally, and largely due to Jack's efforts, many fewer kids today undergo—or die from—unnecessary tonsillectomy.

But if you met Jack today on a mountaintop in Vermont, he would be the first to admit that Howard Hiatt's urgent question—*Who will take responsibility* for protecting the medical commons?—remains unanswered. Neither the medical profession nor the politicians have done so. Is the "delivery" of health care in the United States today accessible and efficient? Does it provide a sense of security and continuity of care to all Americans? The national shortage of primary care physicians—the one doctor you and all Americans need—has reached unprecedented, crisis proportions. Countless sick patients are discharged from U.S. hospitals today without a follow-up appointment to see a doctor. Measles and other communicable diseases are on the rise due to spotty delivery of preventive health services. Perhaps naïvely, Howard Hiatt had hoped in 1975 that one day all Americans, when they need "enlightened advice" from a health care professional about an urgent medical concern, could just pick up a telephone "any time, day or night." How many people today do you know who can do that?

Fred and Martha could.

Rivulets of melting snow crisscrossed the road as my car began the steep part of the climb. I knew every foot of this hill. In the summer and fall I cycled in the Vermont mountains. Sometimes, at day's end, I would take a spin after work across the river and up this hill to the top where the paved road faded into a dirt path, centuries-old stone walls tumbling across a broad high meadow shaded here and there by copses of birch trees, their medallion leaves twittering green and gold in the evening breeze and urging me on, farther west into the sunset, and then down the back side of the high ridge, flying, heading for home. It was a special place—folks didn't call this God's country for nothing—and there at the peak of the hill stood Fred and Martha's house. Sometimes Fred would be out walking when I passed—Martha didn't get out much, the uneven ground hard on her arthritic knees and spine—and I would stop to say hello, panting and sweaty, and Fred would shake his head in his kind, avuncular way and say something dry about the folly of youth or offer an engineering suggestion about how to make my bike more aerodynamic and I would ask after Martha and then he would wave me on and wish me well and I would crest the hill past their house and spin across that glorious meadow into the western sky.

For me, the house at the top of this hill wasn't just Fred and Martha's place, it was part of a place I loved. During the long winter months, when I dreamed about summer—riding, with the wind at my back and the sun in my face and the river running fast far below—I would dream about the meadow at the top of this hill and there was Fred and Martha's house, in my dreams.

It was a modern house, flat-roofed and glass-walled, very different from most of the houses in this old Vermont town. Its design was elegant but simple, a sprawling fifties-style split-level specially renovated with two things in mind: convenient, elder-friendly living—and the view. Oh, the view! In every direction: across the river far below, east to the sunrise and the Dartmouth bell tower; north to the White Mountains and the Presidential Range; west to the Green Mountains and the sunset; south across my dreamy high meadow and beyond to Mount Ascutney.

It was a house that said a lot about the people who lived there. Before I'd seen it, Martha had seemed to me like so many other local well-to-do women of a certain age. Impeccably dressed, punctual, and polite—even formal, notwithstanding her martini-dry wit and the mischievous sparkle in her eye—Martha had seemed the type who would greet her guests at the foot of an imposing center-hall staircase just off a chandeliered dining room filled with antiques in the traditional upper-crust Upper Valley way. But Martha's house was wide-open Mies van der Rohe space with high ceilings, walls of windows, gleaming wood floors, Bauhaus décor. This all made more sense after I met Fred and learned about his accomplishments. But, as it turned out, the house had been Martha's idea, and after my first house call there, I couldn't help wondering about Martha, so attractive and youthful even in her seventies. She was more than twice my age and I didn't remember ever having such thoughts about an elderly woman before. Fred and Martha were a captivating couple wherever they went, in any company, but, in their own house, they seemed one of a kind, enviable, youthful despite their years.

Near the top of the hill the ice had not yet begun to run. I parked my car just below, about fifty yards from the house, and climbed the rest of the way. The sky across the river was beginning to brighten, a penumbra of blue rising up out of the eastern hills. It was going to be a beautiful day—Colorado weather, warm and sunny but plenty of snow—a great day to go skiing with the kids. I looked at my watch. It was 6:30, still plenty of time to get us all out to the skiway for the first run of the day.

In the few minutes it took me to reach the house, the blue had risen still higher in the eastern sky. Or so it seemed; maybe it was just the extra elevation.

In the summertime, two Adirondack chairs sat together here in the front yard, facing southeast, sunflowers all around. I would have liked to eavesdrop on those summer conversations, just the two of them, their memories and their jokes. Now the yard was three feet deep in snow, the triangular tops of tall wooden plant protectors barely breaking through its surface. The stone walkway tunneled toward the front door, walls of white up to my waist on both sides. It had been shoveled but . . . not carefully, not well. A whole section near the front door hadn't been shoveled at all.

This was odd. Fred was diligent about these things. He and

Martha had lived in the north country for a long time now and knew the risks of winter, especially for old folks like themselves. As I approached, I wondered when they had last been out of the house.

The outdoor lamps along the walkway and above the front door were dark. This was odd, too. They knew I was coming. Looking closer now, I could see that the house was dark inside as well. The windows were enormous, the lengthening blue glow from the east reflected there. But I saw no lights inside.

What the hell . . . ?

I stepped over the snowbank at the front door and rang the bell. No one answered. No lights switched on. Nothing.

I rang again.

Nothing.

I tried the door. It was unlocked. I stepped across the threshold into the foyer, my shoes caked with snow. It took a moment for my eyes to adjust to the dark.

Now, about twenty feet away, at the top of the two stairs that separated the living room from the foyer, I saw a white shadow, hovering.

Martha . . . ?

She didn't move. She didn't speak.

Martha, what . . . ?

She wore a long white robe over her nightgown. She held her cane in her right hand. With her left hand she made a gesture as if to wave me away.

I came closer.

What is it? Are you all right?

I could see her face now. She looked me straight in the eye, as she always did, but I wasn't sure she knew who I was. I saw in her gaze no sign of recognition or greeting. She was staring at me. But I wasn't sure she was seeing me.

It's Brendan, Martha.

She didn't speak. She tilted her head to the left with a weary, fed-up, what-can-you-do look on her face.

Immediately, I felt relieved. I had seen this expression many times before—whenever Martha would comment sarcastically about some hapless politician or an annoying side effect of one of her many medications. Good, I thought. This is Martha, not some shell of herself, suddenly impaired.

What . . . ?

She touched her hand to her lips. But still she said nothing. Then she made that motion again, a dismissive shooing motion that said something like Look-at-that-nonsense-over-there or What-more-is-there-to-say?

I don't understand . . .

She shooed me again: there, over there . . .

I looked where she pointed. The large open living room was empty. A corridor farther left led to the north wing of the house.

I walked down the corridor. Its walls were lined with family portraits and parchment copies of some of Fred's patents. Photographs of vintage airplanes and Kitty Hawk. Pictures of Fred smiling chummily with Harry Truman, Charles Lindbergh, Robert McNamara.

The door to the library was open. Sitting at his typewriter, an old black Underwood, Fred was dressed in a handsome green shirt and pressed khakis. His moccasined feet perched confidently atop the surface of his desk. His head leaned back against the chair as he looked out the big window toward the dawn. How long and languid his legs were. How contented he seemed.

Looking out the window, he hadn't turned to me yet. But I could tell he knew I was there. And his confident posture alone spoke volumes: Fred was sure he was right, whatever he and Martha had been squabbling about this time. His show of confidence made me doubt my own. What if he won't listen to me? What will I do then?

I braced myself for a difficult conversation.

Fred . . .

He didn't turn to me right away. Like his posture, this seemed intentional, a silent statement of control.

Fred, look . . . What's this about? Let's talk about it.

His eyes were closed. He seemed to be deliberating carefully about how best to begin, how to answer my question, how to stake out his own position on the matter. I was prepared for some of the same things I'd heard him say before, something about simple questions often being the most difficult ones, or about long marriages, or the challenges of old age that most people don't like to talk about. But he didn't. He didn't say any of those things. He had a smug little smile on his face like he knew a secret no one else knew. I looked at the typewriter in front of him but there was just a single blank page staring back at me and I don't remember which thing I knew first, the fact that he was dead or the fact of how he had died, because at the same time I saw that smile on his face and braced myself for whatever he would say I also saw how awkwardly his right arm was dangling down toward the floor where the gun lay on the carpet just below his limp outstretched fingers. It was a peculiar-looking thing—it might have been a piece of sculpture or a paperweight, something other than what it was, an antique German Luger with a tapered barrel and an elegant curved handle.

I couldn't see a wound. His clothes were pristine, no bloodstain spreading across his chest or abdomen. His face was unmarked.

Suddenly afraid, I looked quickly around the room, half expecting to see someone else there, lurking.

I don't know why I noticed it so quickly, such a small inconspicuous spot, no bigger than a pencil eraser. The cream-colored wallpaper was otherwise perfect, maybe that was why I saw it, and after I inspected it I knew where Fred's wound would be. The wallpaper had lifted up around the bullet hole and the paper's torn white edges were red and gray. Up close, the red was flat, the bloodstain still wet. But there was substance to the gray—clusters of tiny gelatinous globules, glistening like undercooked risotto, with pink striations of cerebral capillaries running through them. A few other lobules of gray matter were spattered on the wall nearby—they were sticky, not dripping—and as I turned back to Fred I traced the line from the wall to his head where the wound had to be. His hair was fashionably long and thick on the sides and even though it was snow white, still I had to tease it away to see the exit wound above his left ear. There was very little blood, just a small patch of red congealing against his pink scalp. The entry wound was in the same spot on the other side, just above his right ear. He couldn't have done it more cleanly if he'd used a stereotactic device, the kind neurosurgeons use to make sure they drill into the cranium in just the right place.

It was perfect: mission accomplished; minimal mess. And, judging from that little smile on his face, Fred knew it.

I don't remember much about the rest of that day. Martha's knees and back were hurting badly but still she couldn't sit down. She just stood there in the living room until the sheriff arrived. Norwich was a small town but the sheriff had been around for a while and he looked like he knew what he was doing. He asked Martha terse questions and let her talk, never interrupting but watching her closely as he listened. Occasionally he asked for clarification about this or that, as if he had his own version of what had happened—or maybe more than one version—and he was testing it against Martha's. She told him today was the day Fred was scheduled to be admitted to the mental health center for a few days of inpatient observation because he'd been acting so strangely lately. But these last few days he's been fine, she said, better than fine, really, he's been reminiscing about the kids and the old days and things we haven't talked about in a long time. He's been very affectionate, even frisky—that's the word Martha used, "frisky"—and she didn't bat an eye when she told the sheriff that she and Fred had made love the night before, something they hadn't done since she didn't know when. Fred got up early like he always did but this time he kissed her before he left the bedroom, and that was unusual, too, she said. She didn't make anything of it until she heard the single sharp sound from down the corridor a few minutes later.

The sheriff asked me if I'd touched anything—the gun, the typewriter, Fred—and I told him what I remembered. He looked at me funny when I told him I didn't know Fred was scheduled to be admitted to the inpatient Psych unit today. He wanted to know how that could be: You're his doctor, aren't you? I told him about the phone calls and the referral to Dr. Armour and how she must have arranged it but still he thought it strange that I didn't even know about it and he made a note of this on his writing pad. He called the coroner's office and arranged for the medical examiner to come pick up the body. Autopsies were required, he told us, in all cases like this. I wasn't sure what *like this* meant but when he said it to Martha he watched her reaction carefully and he seemed to do the same with me.

Martha didn't cry. Even after her daughter arrived and became hysterical in the library, Martha didn't cry. She just took her daughter in her arms and looked at me. I don't remember what I said to them. I stayed for a while longer, I don't remember how long. I called Katherine Armour, the psychiatrist. Then I just sat there in the living room thinking about what the sheriff had said. I didn't know what else to do.

When I left Martha and her daughter to drive home that day, all I could think of was a lecture given by Milton Helperin, the famous medical examiner in New York City, who had taught a class about autopsies in my second year of medical school. He told us a story about a Mafia assassin who had dropped dead on the stoop outside his mother's brownstone in Little Italy as he left the building after visiting her. He was a young guy with a lot of enemies, not the type who just keels over for no good reason on a sunny day. But after they had examined his heart and aorta and other internal organs, the pathologists doing his autopsy didn't have a clue what had killed him until they looked more carefully at the top of his skull. There, clean as a whistle, was the small hole where the bullet had entered his cranium and traveled straight down through his brainstem and spinal cord. Whoever had offed the guy from the rooftop of that brownstone—five floors directly above the stoop where the guy had been standing—knew what he was doing.

That's what I remember best about the rest of that day. I don't remember whether Janice had given up and taken the kids skiing without me, or whether I went with them. And I don't remember anything about the rest of my week vacation or how soon the weather turned frigid again. But I couldn't stop thinking about how clearly Fred had known what he was doing, how carefully he had planned it. Martha's daughter told the sheriff about the gun. Fred's father had brought it back from Germany as a souvenir after the armistice in 1919. Fred restored it himself, several years ago, in his machine shop. He wanted to make sure it worked, he had explained. He told Martha and his children that if he ever started to lose his marbles, the old Luger would solve that problem nicely. They all thought this was just talk, Fred's way of making philosophical banter. I hadn't known a damned thing about it.

So, for the next few weeks, this was why I blamed myself—for not knowing what Fred had said about his marbles and his gun—especially when his behavior and personality had changed so inexplicably. I should have asked. This was a no-brainer, Psychiatry 101: Have you thought about killing yourself? Have you made a plan? Do you know how you would actually do it?

Who knew what would have happened to Fred if it had gone the other way, if he'd made it into the hospital Psych unit that morning? Something bad was happening—major depression, incipient dementia, *something*. And whatever it was, Fred *was* losing his marbles, something he flat-out didn't want to live with. So I felt guilty about not doing my part better—and I vowed I would never let it happen again—but I didn't blame myself for Fred's death. He was the one who pulled the trigger.

So, I got on with my life.

That was the plan, anyway.

Chapter 6

THE POSTMAN RINGS TWICE

Appearances to the mind are of four kinds.
Things either are as they appear to be; or they neither are,
nor appear to be;
Or they are, and do not appear to be; or they are not, yet
appear to be.
Rightly to aim in all these cases is the wise man's task.

—Epictetus (second century C.E.)

March 1985

I didn't notice the letter until the end of the day. Maureen, my assistant, had slit open the envelope, as she did with all my mail. Then she'd left it there in the pile together with the laboratory reports, medical journals, letters from patients, correspondence from doctors around New Hampshire and Vermont about patients we shared. It may even have lain there for a few days before I saw it. Maureen always alerted me when something looked important. This didn't.

I received lots of autopsy reports. This one from the county medical examiner looked no more interesting than any other. Not that I was uninterested in autopsies. To the contrary, I always tried my best to get the family's permission for an autopsy whenever a patient died under my care. But I rarely needed the official typed report to know what the autopsy had shown. I already knew. Almost always, I went down to the morgue in the basement of the hospital while the pathologists were doing the autopsy. They answered my questions about what they found. I answered their questions about what we were looking for. Then I told the family what we had learned.

In Fred's case, I wasn't looking for anything. I knew the answer to the question his autopsy was intended to answer. The postmortem examination had been performed in the county coroner's office, so, unlike those performed at the hospital, I didn't attend it personally. But I didn't need his autopsy report to know what had killed Fred.

It was evening. I was in my hospital office. The internists and I who worked in the Section of General Internal Medicine (a division of Dartmouth's Department of Medicine) each had two offices, one here in the hospital and one across the street in Fowler House. The latter was a rambling two-story Colonial with large airy rooms, fine hearths, and a grand wraparound porch, the former residence of a local family donated decades ago to serve as the primary care practice site for people who lived in Hanover and Norwich. In the old days, Dartmouth's Fowler House doctors saw all of their patients there. In recent years, this had changed. As more patients from all over northern New England sought their medical care at Dartmouth, the size of the internal medicine faculty had grown and the proportion of its work devoted to the local population had shrunk. Still, several of us worked in both sites, serving the Hanover and Norwich people at Fowler House (and, not infrequently, in their homes), seeing the rest of our patients in our hospital offices.

Logistically, this was easy to manage; I could walk from Fowler House to my office in the hospital in less than two minutes and, from there, my hospitalized inpatients were just an elevator ride away. Recently, however, I had begun to think about closing Fowler House. The medical center's bean counters were asking smart questions and I, as the administrative chief of our section, had to admit that, financially, it was very costly to run duplicate practice sites—redundant clerical and nursing staff, phone systems, medical records. Some of my colleagues thought Fowler House was worth the cost; it preserved an old-fashioned, small-town ambience for the local townspeople. Others were more fatalistic, knowing we would concede sooner or later to the new economic realities of modern medicine. And some of us were uneasy about the inequity of offering "Cadillac" primary care (including house calls) to the relatively affluent, entitled residents of Hanover and Norwich but not to our patients who lived nearby in neighboring towns. A decision would have to be made about this—either we draw a line and defend it or we erase the line altogether—but, for now, my colleagues and I saw two different patient populations in two different offices. Local residents like Martha, Inge, and the Dartmouth girls came to Fowler House; folks like Saul, the man who died of AIDS, came to my hospital office.

That particular evening, I was running late—my mail unopened, my dinner uneaten—because it was my turn to staff the evening walk-in clinic at the hospital. Every weekday from 8:00 a.m. to 8:00 p.m., I or one of my colleagues, working together with physician assistants, saw patients who "walked in" to the medical center asking to see a doctor without an appointment. After a short wait, these unscheduled patients saw an experienced internist who could not only diagnose and treat their (usually minor) illnesses efficiently but also identify quickly the ones whose problems were more serious. This service kept many patients out of Dartmouth's emergency room—on busy days, the walk-in clinic might treat seventy-five to one hundred patients in twelve hours—saving them from the longer waits (and much higher bills) that emergency room care would entail. It was also appreciated by our specialists, who, as in all tertiary care referral centers, sometimes were asked to see patients who didn't really need their services. When I or my colleagues called them about a "can't wait" patient we were seeing in the walk-in clinic, the neurosurgeon or orthopedist or cardiologist on the other end of the line knew it was the real deal. Like many other aspects of the Dartmouth health care model, this team approach made sense to everyone—patients, doctors, even the insurance companies.

Like my colleagues, I saw outpatients in my office(s) for ten four-hour "sessions" per week—8:00 a.m. to noon and 1:00 p.m. to 5:00 p.m.—with nine of these sessions on weekdays and the tenth every Saturday morning. (All of the Dartmouth doctors worked Saturdays.) Before, after, and during these office sessions, we answered phone calls, responded to patients' test results from the lab or radiology, dictated charts, and handled sundry other unscheduled tasks. More often than most of my colleagues, I would also run up and down stairs to see my patients on the hospital wards. Typically, I had five or ten patients on the wards or in the ICU on any given day—the excellent Dartmouth house staff made my work with inpatients a lot easier, but I was the attending physician—and I saw most of these inpatients both before and after office hours (and more often if the patient was very sick).

I did more inpatient work than most of my colleagues because, during my year as chief resident at Dartmouth, I had helped care for many patients with life-threatening illnesses. When I decided, at the end of that year, to forgo my previous commitment to do further subspecialty training in Boston at MGH (Massachusetts General Hospital, also fondly known as "Man's Greatest Hospital") and instead join the faculty at Dartmouth as a "general internist," I continued caring for many of these very sick people from all over New England. In the ensuing ten years, many of these patients had died—hence my frequent receipt of autopsy reports—but other sick patients then took their place, referred to me by relatives or friends or local doctors.

This seemed to me the right job description for an internist. It combined primary care practice—managing chronic diseases (such as diabetes and emphysema), episodic minor illnesses (such as chest colds and back strains), and preventive medicine (such as Pap smears and blood pressure control)—together with acute-care, hospital medicine. Traditionally, internists had always done both—skill in hospital medicine made you better in the office, and vice versa—and I was following that tradition. I tried to convince my colleagues that they should do the same. This was a hard sell; they all knew I worked longer hours and more weekends than they did mainly because I had more sick patients in the hospital. I wondered whether I could re-engineer all of our job descriptions to sustain both our outpatient and our inpatient skills. Could our group function even better as a team? With this question in mind, I organized an experiment. Paul, a superb internist who was expert in primary care but also brilliant with sick people in the hospital, agreed to my request to spend one month doing *only* hospital practice, taking daily attending responsi-bility for all of our group's inpatients (who, on any given day, totaled twenty to twenty-five patients). If the pilot project proved successful, each of us could do this intensive inpatient job in monthly rotations. This would allow all of us to sustain our hard-won hospital skills—and our pride as "complete" internists—even as we focused more exclusively on our outpatient practices most of the year.

My "hospitalist" experiment, a proven success in Great Britain and other countries but rare (in 1985) in the United States, was a resounding failure. Paul, exhausted at the end of his month in hospi-tal, announced to our group that continuity of primary care was too important to interrupt for weeks at a time purely in the interest of "group efficiency." He reported that his own primary care patients had complained bitterly about his lack of availability to them (even though I and my colleagues cross-covered his office practice during the month to help him out). This disappointed me greatly. I thought Paul was lazy and regretted choosing him to take the lead on this. But every one of my colleagues strongly agreed with Paul. They didn't want to spend long, tiring days and nights in the hospital caring for sick inpatients, most of whom they'd never met before. They were primary care internists—top-notch, every one of them—and they thought that was good enough.

Certainly, it was good enough for our patients. We cared for adults of all ages—many were elderly but the youngest were six-teen—and we did pretty much everything they needed except deliver their babies and do surgical procedures. We spent a full hour with new patients. We examined every square inch of them. We didn't send them to an ophthalmologist to check their eyes; an audiologist to check their hearing; a cardiologist to listen to their heart murmur; a dermatologist to check them for skin cancer; an orthopedist to examine their swollen knees and sore shoulders; or a gynecologist to do their breast and pelvic examinations. We did it all—it was one-stop shopping—and, in the process, we got to know our patients as people, too. We were their doctors. Occasionally, we referred them to subspecialists, but only when we felt we were over our heads (which wasn't often) or when the patient needed a procedure only a specialist could do. And, when our patients came back to see us with a new problem or to follow up on an old one, we gave them thirty-minute appointments. Often, we didn't spend the whole half-hour with them, in part because every day we squeezed in other, unscheduled patients who called with urgent problems. But our patients knew they could have the whole half hour if *they* thought they needed it.

This was the tradition and culture of the Dartmouth model: provide *all* patients with longitudinal, comprehensive, personalized primary care enhanced by subspecialists' timely assistance *when medically necessary*. This model didn't pretend that primary care internists knew as much as their subspecialist colleagues. But excellent internists prided themselves on knowing "90 percent" of each medical subspecialty. If I diagnosed a thyroid problem or an intestinal disease or a heart rhythm disturbance in one of my patients, would a consulting endocrinologist or gastroenterologist or cardiologist add "value" to the patient's care? In some cases, certainly, but not all. In the Dartmouth health care model, more care was not necessarily better care.

This sounds simple enough, but it isn't. Sometimes, not even an autopsy can tell you whether you've provided the best care. But, that evening in my office, as I opened the envelope containing Fred's autopsy report, I didn't expect it to tell me anything I didn't already know. Not anything instructive, anyway. I knew that Fred's case would never make it to M&M.

"M&M"—Morbidity and Mortality (M&M) Conference—occurred weekly at Dartmouth, as in most teaching hospitals. Presented in a large amphitheater and attended religiously by senior and junior physicians, M&M analyzed the care of a patient who recently had died in hospital and whose autopsy results served as the final arbiter of whether his doctors had made the correct diagnosis and the best treatment decisions. The results of each M&M patient's autopsy were known beforehand by only a few people attending the conference: the pathologist who did the autopsy, the patient's attending physician, and one or two residents who had viewed the autopsy immediately after the patient died.

Just a few weeks before, I was in the know at M&M. I'd been

in the morgue myself with Donald Pease, my patient for ten years before he died, when the pathologist poked a dissecting probe into that hole in Don's perforated aorta. Then and there, I knew that his case would come to M&M.

As usual in M&M, Don's case was presented as an unknown. A senior resident described the facts of Don's final hospital admission as they unfolded over the course of those fateful thirty hours. The M&M moderators—the chief medical resident, with occasional comments by the chairman of medicine—interrupted the case presentation at crucial junctures and asked randomly selected senior physicians in the audience what they thought, what they would have done, how they would have responded as new developments and complications occurred. The mere fact that the patient was being presented at M&M meant that there was something unusual or "educational" about the case. Often, it meant that the autopsy had revealed unexpected findings. And sometimes it meant that the doctors in charge had blown it.

Everyone in the packed M&M amphitheater listened intently, trying to anticipate what the autopsy would show, what mistakes might have been made, and how they might have managed the case differently themselves. Intended to be instructive, this format sometimes degenerated into a preening contest among Monday-morning quarterbacks. In Don's case, I was expecting the worst.

The facts were straightforward. Don was a stoical sixty-five-year-old Vermonter with long-standing emphysema who came in to see me early one morning because he had developed abdominal and back pain during the night. Maureen, who knew Don never complained about anything, added him to my schedule without even asking me. When Don arrived, it wasn't clear what was wrong but it was obvious that he was acutely ill. He almost fainted as we lifted him from his wheelchair onto the examining table. His pulse was fast, his blood pressure low, and he was breathing even harder than usual. I drew some blood for testing, did an electrocardiogram, and wheeled him down to the emergency department, where it would be easier to monitor him and get a CT scan of his abdomen. His blood tests showed that he was losing blood from somewhere but his physical examination didn't reveal the source of bleeding, so I wasn't surprised when the CT scan showed a large retroperitoneal hematoma (a hemorrhage located in the rear compartment of his abdominal cavity). Among his many other medications, Don took blood-thinners for his heart and, even though our tests showed that his blood-thinner dose was properly adjusted, this kind of internal bleeding was a well-known complication of such drugs. The usual treatment is to transfuse plasma and other blood products to reverse the blood-thinning and replace the blood loss. We did this in the emergency department, after which Don felt better and was admitted to the hospital.

At this point in the resident's M&M presentation, the chief resident interrupted and pointed to the image of Don's CT scan projected on the big amphitheater screen. The large ugly hemorrhage, which compressed and displaced Don's internal organs, even looked painful. This was teaching point number one in today's conference: what such hemorrhages look like. Teaching point number two was what to do about them. To answer this question the chief called on a senior hematologist in the audience, a well-known expert on Don's blood-thinner drug, who eloquently expounded on the treatment of its bleeding complications. The chief thanked him and then called on Dr. King, a respected senior surgeon in the audience, and asked whether there was any role for surgical evacuation of this massive hematoma.

Tall and handsome with a full head of snow-white hair, Dr. King had a stentorian voice with a southern accent. His answer was quintessentially surgical, the kind of terse, cut-to-the-chase thinking that made surgeons indispensable and laughable at the same time.

Depends on what's bleedin', King said.

The audience laughed nervously.

The chief resident nodded, encouraging King to continue.

King pointed at the CT scan on the big screen.

Young man, I'm not seein' somethin' I need to see.

The chief nodded again. Like? he said.

Like? Like the damn aorta! King boomed.

At the podium, the chief resident nodded again and pushed a

button. Now a new image appeared on the amphitheater screen, a close-up CT scan image of the aorta, the main artery that carries blood from the heart to all other organs in the body. Just below the kidneys and above its bifurcation into the lower extremities, the aorta appeared slightly dilated, a small balloon beginning to bulge in the otherwise pipe-straight, cylindrical vessel. The aneurysm was small, only four centimeters in diameter. A thin, irregular line of white chalk outlined its interior—this was calcium deposited in the wall of the big artery, a sign that it was diseased and sclerotic—and there, right there at the tip of the chief resident's pointer, was a visible break in that thin white line. There was no way to tell for sure whether this was the cause of the bleeding, whether the aneurysm had leaked and then temporarily sealed itself. But it was awfully suspicious.

Dr. King? the chief resident asked.

Godlike, King stood up, gathered the crowd in his gaze, and addressed them.

If this patient's not in the operatin' room soon as you see this picture, he's a dead man.

Murmurs rippled through the audience. They knew what was coming now. After all, M&M was a "mortality" conference.

The resident continued his presentation of the case.

The patient's vital signs and abdominal pain improved after his admission to the inpatient ward, the resident said. He received more blood products and remained stable until 1:00 a.m. that night, when he developed worsening abdominal and back pain. Throughout the night his blood pressure continued to drop despite multiple blood transfusions. He was not transferred to the ICU or taken to the OR. He was treated with morphine. He appeared comfortable before he stopped breathing at noon the next day. CPR was not performed. Permission for autopsy was obtained.

The crowd's murmurs grew louder. The chief resident stepped down from the podium, giving way to the pathologist.

Dr. Faulkner began with the photograph he had taken in the morgue when I was there with him, his dissecting probe peeking through the hole in Don's ruptured aortic aneurysm. Certainly, he told the audience, this was the cause of death. He showed pictures of Don's lungs and heart and other diseased organs, and he listed all of the autopsy findings on a final summary slide. He then briefly summarized the results of several studies showing that about one-third of all patients with ruptured abdominal aneurysms die before they reach the hospital; another one-half make it to the hospital but die before they can have surgery. Of the remaining small minority who survive long enough to reach the hospital and undergo surgery, at least half die during or soon after the operation. Overall, then, and despite best efforts, only about one patient in ten survived this kind of catastrophe.

Don could have been one of those few lucky ones. We could have saved him. This was the take-home message for the M&M audience that day.

When the chief resident identified me as Don's attending physician and asked me to comment about the case, most of the eyes that turned my way were accusatory. Dr. King shook his leonine head silently. This kind of case was the raison d'être of large teaching hospitals like this one: to make a difference, to save a life, when others can't. Why did we fail? Why did I fail?

I asked Dr. Faulkner to return to the podium and tell the audience more about Don's lungs and heart. He repeated that the patient had bullous emphysema, severe pulmonary hypertension, and right ventricular overload. I asked him if he had ever seen worse. Faulkner, a very fine, experienced pathologist who had been doing autopsies for more than forty years, hesitated for a moment, then shook his head and said, No, I can't say I have.

A few in the audience turned to me and nodded, beginning to understand. But the rest were unimpressed, even after I told them that Don wore an oxygen mask twenty-four hours a day, lived in a wheelchair because he couldn't walk five steps without gasping for breath, and swore he would never do it again after spending four brutal weeks in the ICU on a mechanical ventilator last year to get him through a bad pneumonia. Don knew we weren't sure whether his bleeding was from the blood-thinner or his aorta (or both); that the only way to find out for sure—and maybe save his life—was to operate. But, whether it was the surgeons or I or the pulmonary specialists who talked to him that day, Don listened patiently, huffing and puffing in his bed, and asked all of us the same question: *So, if I get . . . through this operation . . . doc . . . I'll be on the . . . ventilator machine . . . right?* The surgeons tried to reassure him that the ventilator would be only temporary. The pulmonary specialists, more circumspect, told him he could "probably" be weaned off the machine again, as he had been last year. I told the audience what I knew about Don's life these past few years. How tired he was. How ready he was to let go. How even his grandchildren and beloved Red Sox didn't make it all worthwhile anymore.

Most in the audience were unmoved. As they filed out of the amphitheater, the consensus was that we had blown it. The autopsy proved that Don had a curable disease that, untreated, is *always* fatal. Certain death versus a chance to survive? Did the patient *really* understand this? Did I push hard enough to try to save his life?

I didn't tell them that when Don finally decided, late on that fateful day, not to have the surgery, he said, *I'll take my chances, doc. Maybe it's just the blood-thinner caused the bleeding. But if this doesn't go my way, I'd like you to see for yourself what was what. Maybe it will help somebody else someday.*

So, the day before he died, Don requested permission forms for a postmortem examination. The autopsy was his own idea.

Don's request followed some famous footsteps. Sir William Osler, the most renowned and revered physician since Hippocrates, had requested his own autopsy, too. Osler told family and friends that, given his lifelong interest in the case, he wished he could attend his own autopsy to see it for himself. Typically Oslerian, this choice of words was as precise as it was good-natured: The word "autopsy" literally means "to see for one's self." Osler died at his home in England after a protracted battle with bacterial pneumonia in 1919, nine years before the discovery of penicillin. (In his renowned preantibiotic-era textbook, *The Principles and Practice of Medicine*, Osler had dubbed pneumonia "the captain of the men of death.") Osler wanted his own physician, Dr. A. G. Gibson, to know why he had died, in the hope that this knowledge might help other patients in the future. So, as

Osler famously had done more than a thousand times for his own patients, Osler's doctor performed Osler's autopsy. In the kitchen of the Osler family home.

In Osler's time, autopsies were bellwethers and benchmarks. A high autopsy rate strengthened a hospital's reputation; it indicated that the medical staff wanted to learn as much as possible about their sickest patients—the ones who died—in an effort to improve doctors' diagnostic capabilities, perhaps gain scientific insights, and avoid error in the future. Since 1761, many hospitals had operated busy "autopsy theaters" where plaques on the wall read: *Hic est locus ubi mors gaudet succorso vitae* ("This is the place where death rejoices to come to the aid of life"). Through the first half of the twentieth century, about 50 percent of all patients who died in U.S. hospitals had autopsies; most major teaching hospitals exceeded that rate. In fact, in many teaching hospitals as recently as the 1970s, interns and residents openly competed to achieve the highest autopsy rate among their patients who had died. At M&M Conferences around the world, premortem diagnoses and treatments were compared with the indisputable gold standard, the patient's postmortem examination findings. In the days before CT scans and MRI machines, this was how doctors, young and old, looked inside their patients and "saw for themselves" why their patients had died. And, in some cases, how they might have been saved.

Osler's own autopsy revealed no surprises. It showed that his doctors had done all they could have done, given the (primitive) state of medical science at the time. In this regard, Osler was luckier than most. In his era, autopsies frequently revealed misdiagnoses and missed opportunities to save the patient.

Remarkably, despite spectacular advances in medical care, such misdiagnoses remain commonplace today. In 1983, researchers at Brigham and Women's Hospital in Boston—by all accounts, then and now one of the best hospitals in the world—asked whether autopsies were still worth doing. Conventional wisdom thought not. Medicine's diagnostic armamentarium had grown dramatically since Osler's time. Powerful new imaging technologies—ultrasound, nuclear scanning, computed tomography (CT), angiography—had transformed the practice of medicine, allowing doctors to peer inside living patients more clearly than ever before. Because autopsies are labor intensive, cost money (today, about two thousand dollars), and sometimes make patients' loved ones uncomfortable, regulatory agencies eliminated minimum mandatory autopsy rates as a criterion for accreditation of U.S. hospitals. The Brigham hospital researchers weren't sure this change was a good idea and designed a study to examine whether modern diagnostic technologies had made misdiagnosis a thing of the past. They reviewed postmortem examinations performed at the Brigham in 1960, 1970, and 1980 to compare the "yield" of autopsies in those decades.

These researchers found that autopsies in 1960 had revealed a major missed diagnosis in 22 percent, almost one in every four patients. Of these, about one-third (8 percent) showed that a correct diagnosis premortem could have led to the patient's cure or improved survival. The remaining two-thirds (14 percent) found diagnostic errors that contributed to the patient's death but probably could not have been treated successfully (in 1960). In other words, one of every twelve patients dying in 1960 at one of the world's best hospitals could have been saved had their doctors made the correct diagnosis. *In addition, another one in seven patients* who died had diseases that, unrecognized by their doctors, contributed to their death. Little wonder that doctors at the Brigham in 1960, like those in Osler's time, tried hard to obtain permission for autopsy whenever a patient died. This was how they learned. Doctors learned from their mistakes.

But what shocked many in the medical community was the finding that the rate of missed diagnoses documented by autopsy at the Brigham hospital hadn't decreased at all twenty years later! In 1970 and in 1980, the rate of major missed diagnoses was 23 percent and 21 percent, respectively, no different from rates in 1960. This lack of improvement did *not* mean that the Brigham doctors were failing to learn from their autopsies. Clearly they *were* learning, because most of the fatal diagnoses missed in 1960—blood clots in the lungs, bacterial infections such as pneumonia or meningitis, various cancers—were missed much less frequently in 1980. But, during those twenty years, medical progress had created new diagnostic challenges. For example, previously rare infections had become increasingly prevalent as complications of new treatments (immunosuppressive drugs) and new diseases (AIDS). As a result, autopsies in 1980 revealed significant changes in the specific type, but not the overall rate, of major missed diagnoses. The Brigham researchers concluded that, despite medical progress—indeed *because of* medical progress—the "autopsy remains a vital component in the assurance of good medical care."

And yet today, three decades later, the autopsy rate in U.S. hospitals is less than 5 percent. Many hospitals perform none at all. In 2004, a new generation of researchers found that fatal diagnostic errors have declined somewhat in the past forty years but estimated that, if autopsies were performed on 100 percent of patients who die in U.S. hospitals today, the rate of major missed diagnoses would range from a low of 8.4 percent (one in twelve deaths) to a high of 24.4 percent (one in four deaths). Even if one accepts the lower estimate in this range (8.4 percent), it means that more than 70,000 people die in U.S. hospitals every year with major missed diagnoses; about 30,000 of these patients would leave the hospital alive if their diagnosis were not missed. More chilling, these potentially preventable deaths are *not included* in the Institute of Medicine's sobering estimate that up to 98,000 patients die annually in U.S. hospitals due to medical error.

The implications are grave, and not just because autopsies are an indispensable quality improvement tool in hospitals. Autopsies establish the cause of deaths, thus ensuring the accuracy of national vital statistics. Today, in the absence of autopsies, it is estimated that at least one-third of all death certificates are incorrect. Autopsies also keep medical educators honest, showing medical students and physicians-in-training the final truth about their patients who die. Autopsies reassure family members of the deceased; protect against false medico-legal liability claims; evaluate the effectiveness of new treatments; improve our understanding of the natural history of disease; and identify new or emerging diseases. Research about Alzheimer's and other brain diseases, for example, depends on autopsies. (How else can one study cells deep in the brain, inaccessible during life?) Societal responses to public health threats, whether new diseases (such as HIV and SARS) or bioterrorism attacks (such as anthrax outbreaks), depend critically on autopsy findings, too.

Experts at the Mayo Clinic have concluded that "a wide range of medical, legal, social, and economic causes" are responsible for the decline of nonforensic autopsies and proposed no fewer than forty-six interventions to reverse this trend. But much of this problem, like other ills afflicting U.S. health care today, boils down to three things: money; public misinformation; and doctors' conflicts of interest.

First, follow the money. Payment for autopsies was built into Medicare's reimbursement to hospitals decades ago, because Medicare beneficiaries account for 75 percent of all deaths in the United States. Perversely, then, hospitals can increase their profits by *not* spending those resources on autopsies. Pathologists also can make more money by *not* doing autopsies, devoting their time instead to more lucrative services for the living.

Second, the public doesn't care, because the public doesn't understand the importance of autopsies. Many people refuse to consent to autopsies, believing that the postmortem examination disfigures the body (it does not) or delays funeral arrangements (it need not). When doctors take the time to explain these things, autopsy rates tend to rise.

Finally, many doctors are conflicted themselves about the risks and benefits of autopsies. The risks to the doctor may seem obvious: If an autopsy shows that the doctor missed an important diagnosis, this would seem to increase the likelihood of medical malpractice complaints. In fact, lawsuits are *less likely* when deceased patients undergo autopsies. And, despite all evidence to the contrary, many doctors continue to believe that the accuracy of modern diagnostic testing is so great that it renders postmortem diagnosis largely superfluous. In the majority of cases, they're right, since about 80 percent of autopsies confirm the accuracy of doctors' premortem diagnoses. But is this as good as we can do? Certainly not. We can and must do better.

Niels Bohr, the legendary Nobel laureate in physics, defined an expert as "one who has made every imaginable mistake in a very narrow field." Ultimately, this is the most important benefit of autopsies: to improve doctors' diagnostic expertise by letting them "see for themselves" their diagnostic mistakes. The quickening disappearance of the medical autopsy today poses a critical, unanswerable question: How will doctors achieve greater diagnostic expertise—how will we learn, and improve—if we don't know what we're missing?

Osler is turning over in his grave.

Fred, too, maybe.

Fred would have understood immediately the implications of his own autopsy results; they showed that his medical problem was more about engineering than biology. Had we found it when he was alive, surely he would have wanted to see it for himself, to watch it bounce and oscillate in his heart like . . . well, not like anything, really. Fred's problem is unique in nature, a truly rare anomaly—a right atrial myxoma, a benign tumor of the heart. Only about one in ten million humans will have one like it. Fred would have gotten a kick out of his had we found the tumor in time and cut it out of his heart. He might have kept it in a bottle of formalin on his desk. It looked like a little finger, but swollen at its tip, like a mushroom on a stalk. Surely Fred would have shown it to his friends, especially the engineers. To illustrate, Fred might have put his right index finger inside his left hand and wiggled it there, the finger fluttering gently in his palm as he opened and closed his fist around it, pumping his fist rhythmically like the human heart. *What a machine!* he would exclaim to his friends as he opened and closed his fist. *Can you believe the heart is only as big as my fist? That's some piece of engineering!* Then, suddenly, he would jam his fluttering index finger hard into the top of his fist, which now, seized up in a fierce clench, shuddered and shook, unable to relax and open and free the finger trapped inside. *It's like a jet engine that sucks in a flock of flying geese,* he might say to his engineer friends. And then, just as suddenly, he would pull his trapped finger back into his palm; his fist, now unseized, would resume its rhythmic pumping, opening and closing, his index finger fluttering gently again in his hand. *If you get lucky,* Fred would say, *the jet engine ejects that flock of birds and resumes operating just like before. If you're lucky.*

I got lucky, Fred would have said, grinning.

The county coroner's office didn't do all the fancy tests and microscopic examinations typical of a twenty-page university hospital autopsy report. Fred's autopsy report was only three pages long. Most of it described the appearance of the entry and exit wounds and the bloody mayhem left behind in his brain. There were the usual incidental findings, unsurprising in an eighty-year-old man: cholesterol plaques in his aorta, a spot of asbestos in his lung, a few cancer cells in one lobe of his prostate, a noncancerous nodule in his thyroid gland. I scanned quickly over these and other "incidental findings" because I was more interested in what they had found in his brain. But the report said nothing about the areas undamaged by the bullet, whether there were signs of Alzheimer's or any other brain disease that would explain why Fred was losing his marbles. It was only on my second reading that I noticed incidental finding number 4: "Right atrial myxoma, pedunculated, 1.7 X 2.1 centimeters." Like most doctors, I'd read about these tumors. But I'd never seen one. And this myxoma was in the right atrium, the rarest kind of all. How interesting! I thought, sounding just like Fred.

And then it hit me.

This was why Fred had come to see me in the first place. This was why Fred had fainted.

I could see him sitting in my office in Fowler House, the young Dartmouth med student at his side. Fred had his finger in my textbook, marking the page where a long, complicated diagram summarized how to diagnose the cause of syncope (fainting). He had been glad to read the part that said fainting usually isn't serious and, in many patients, doesn't require much diagnostic investigation at all. But Fred (and his med student) was intrigued by Fred's fainting spell because, according to my textbook, it had some "worrisome" features. Benign fainting usually happens when people are standing up; Fred's had happened while he was sitting down, eating dinner with friends. Most people begin to feel woozy and sweaty before they pass out; Fred lost consciousness all of a sudden, with no warning symptoms at all. More worrisome, Martha and their friends noticed that Fred looked blue in the face while he lay there with his head slumped over in the mashed potatoes. Most people who faint lose all color, look pale and clammy; Fred's blue color, called cyanosis, suggested that something suddenly had gone wrong with his heart or lungs. Last but not least, Fred was old. When old people faint for no obvious reason, and especially if they weren't habitual "fainters" when young, the cause is more likely to be something serious. On closer questioning, Fred admitted he might have fainted once before, a few months previously. On that occasion, he'd been alone, sitting in his front yard. Back then, he figured he'd just nodded off. Now he wasn't so sure. *Could be*, he said. *Very interesting!*

And so, the engineer in him wanted to know more about the system's circuitry and cybernetics. The med student had told him that fainting generally results from a temporary decrease in blood flow to the brain. Fred wanted to know all the components of this system, where in the system such a problem could arise, what kinds of feedback mechanisms usually compensated when the system broke down here or there. In the end, Fred agreed to all our tests because his fainting spell didn't make sense to him either. *Something* strange had happened—we had eyewitnesses to prove it—and it sounded like it might be a problem with his heart or lungs. But Fred had felt fine. He had no symptoms of ill health, before the fainting spell or now. Even at age eighty, he could climb the steep hill to his house and never stop to catch his breath. His physical examination was completely normal, no sign of any problem with his heart or lungs or circulation.

Interesting, Fred said.

We should have made a list. If we'd done that, maybe we wouldn't have missed it. It was all there, right where Fred's finger was stuck inside the textbook on that day in my office, all the different causes of fainting—the common and rare ones, the neurological causes and the cardiopulmonary causes, even a separate table listing the "Less Common Causes of Cardiac Syncope." And there it was, in black and white, just below pericardial tamponade and just above pulmonary embolism: atrial myxoma. Table 10-6B in my textbook noted that the history in patients with a myxoma doesn't help much and the physical examination and electrocardiogram are usually normal. Just like Fred. If we'd done it by the book, listing *all* of the diagnostic possibilities and then eliminating them one by one with our tests until only one or a few possibilities remained, we might have tripped over it. Had we done so, we might have said, Okay, finding an atrial myxoma is as rare as winning the lottery but what else could it be? It's the only diagnosis left on our list, the only one we haven't excluded.

But when his blood tests and chest X-ray and electrocardiogram came back normal, I didn't check things off a list. And when the twenty-four-hour continuous recording of his heart rhythm, and his nuclear lung scan, and the M-mode and 2-D ultrasound examinations of his heart were all normal, I didn't go back to Table 10-6B in the book to see what was left, what other diagnoses I should look for. I already knew what was written in Table 10-6B. I was the one who wrote it.

If I'd been smarter, even looking back now, would I have tried to convince one of our cardiologists to perform cardiac angiography to look for an atrial myxoma? Maybe. But, if I had, would the cardiologist have agreed to perform *two* of these procedures: first, an angiogram of Fred's arteries to see the left side of his heart (where 90 percent of myxomas are found); and second, an angiogram of his veins to visualize the right side of the heart (where Fred's myxoma happened to be)? I doubt it, because, unlike cardiac ultrasound, these invasive heart tests carry risks of their own. Cardiac angiography will *cause* a stroke in one of every one thousand patients who undergo the procedure. Does it make sense to take this one-in-a-thousand risk when the chance of finding an atrial myxoma is only one in a million? Logically, this would mean that diagnosing *one patient's* myxoma justifies causing *one thousand patients* to have a stroke. Try selling that approach to a patient—or a cardiologist.

That night, as I read Fred's autopsy report in my office, its main lesson was nothing new to me: Playing the risk-benefit odds was the right thing to do. Especially in Fred's case. Even exhaustive diagnostic testing does not reveal the cause in at least one-third of all patients who faint. By the odds—overwhelming odds—Fred should have been one of those.

But Fred's autopsy contained other lessons, too. For one, I had learned what the story of a patient with a right atrial myxoma sounds like—something I hadn't known, hadn't experienced personally, before. I would remember this story if I ever heard one like it again. As Don Pease had said about his own autopsy, it couldn't help him but it might help somebody else someday. At the same time, I kicked myself for not asking more about that *other* time Fred thought he might have fainted. *I was alone,* he had said, *sitting out in the yard. I figured I just nodded off.* As Fred had read in my own textbook, elderly patients with recurrent syncope—repeated episodes of fainting—will almost always have a demonstrable cause. After all of Fred's tests came back normal, I told him that if he ever passed out again, we would need to investigate further. Now, in hindsight, I suspected Fred had already had a recurrence of fainting when I first met him. I would remember that, too.

But the most important message I took away from Fred's autopsy was one more painful reminder of the fallibility of diagnostic testing. It wasn't just the machines that were responsible for these errors. True, the cardiac ultrasound machine had flat-out missed Fred's myxoma. I went back and reviewed the pictures with an expert ultrasonographer after I received Fred's autopsy results. Nothing there. How could the echo machine possibly have missed something that big? (Fred's myxoma was about the size and shape of a Tootsie Roll lollipop.) This was a well-known limitation of cardiac ultrasound technology in those days; its visualization of the right side of the heart was not nearly as accurate or reliable as its visualization of the left side. The important message, then, wasn't about the limitations of the machine. The important message was about the limitations of the doctors who relied on the machine. Like all technology, medical technology is only as smart as the people who use it. And, in Fred's case, I hadn't been smart enough.

Fred's cardiac ultrasound test result is called a "false negative." The test was negative—it found nothing wrong—but its result was false. That Tootsie Roll Pop was in there, bouncing around with every beat of Fred's heart, but the ultrasound machine missed it. Doctors know that *all* tests in medicine have a "false-negative rate"; every test will fail, in some proportion of cases, to find the abnormality it was designed to detect. *Every test.* Knowing this, doctors, upon receiving a negative (normal) test result, must ask themselves: *Is this a true-negative result?* If so, I can move on, confident that the patient's problem lies elsewhere. *Or, is it a false-negative result?* If so, I'm not finished here, I must pursue this possibility further. Many patients don't know this about diagnostic tests. Understandably, they assume that diagnostic technology is accurate and reliable. (Why would doctors use it if it weren't?) Patients don't realize that the accuracy and reliability of diagnostic tests are imperfect. Knowing this, expert doctors acquire a healthy skepticism about all test results.

Sometimes this skepticism helps. Sometimes it doesn't. On my way home that night, Fred's autopsy report ringing in my brain, the recent memory of another patient, Jeannette, and her angry, accusatory voice butted in. She had called from North Carolina for the second time that week. The first time, she had insisted that Maureen interrupt me—I was busy in the walk-in clinic—because it was an emergency.

I barely remembered her, having seen her only once for a routine physical examination a few months before. She was in her forties, an accomplished Dartmouth professor with tenure, a statuesque blonde well aware of her physical charms. Her history and physical examination were completely normal, as were her routine screening tests—Pap smear, mammogram, cholesterol—and she was glad to be told that all was well. Now, on sabbatical in North Carolina, she had begun to have headaches and pains in her neck and back. I couldn't tell much about this over the phone, but there was no obvious explanation for her complaints and she sounded very concerned, so I arranged for her to see an internist I knew at the university hospital in Chapel Hill. A week later, Jeannette called me back, irate and tearful.

I have metastatic breast cancer, she said. It's in my spine and my skull. They tell me it's so advanced that I must have had it for many months, maybe years. I saw you just a few months ago. How the hell did this happen? Why the fuck didn't *you* find it? What kind of operation are you people running up there?

She didn't want to hear about false-negative mammograms. I reviewed hers with three radiologists, each of them unaware of Jeannette's subsequent diagnosis, and they all read it as normal. She was premenopausal, her breasts large and still youthfully firm, the classic profile of a woman whose breast cancer is most likely not to show on a mammogram X-ray. Jeannette didn't know this—just as many women, even today, don't know it—but the false-negative rate of a screening mammogram is about 25 percent overall (and even higher than that in premenopausal women like Jeannette). In other words, when a mammogram is done for routine "screening" purposes— when there is no family history of breast cancer and no lump can be felt in the breast—one of every four breast cancers will be invisible on the mammogram. One in four.

Even in hindsight, we hadn't done anything wrong. Like many other women her age, Jeannette had been falsely reassured by a false-negative mammogram. Almost certainly, she had breast cancer when I examined her, a cancer that neither she nor I could feel and that the mammogram couldn't see. After the fact, Jeannette was furious. I didn't blame her. Not only had she been struck by a terrible disease, but both I and modern medical technology had failed her. So, she blamed me. Back home at Dartmouth, she went out of her way to tell anyone who would listen to steer away from me (and the rest of Dartmouth's medical center). In Jeannette's shoes, I might have reacted the same way.

There is no way to protect yourself from false-negative "screening" tests like mammograms, which are done to detect unapparent abnormalities. If no abnormalities are found, no further search is done (as when you pass the security "screen" at an airport). But *diagnostic* tests, which are done to evaluate a known abnormality, are entirely different. For example, had I felt a suspicious lump in Jeannette's breast, I would have dismissed her normal mammogram as probably a false negative. Why? Because I would have *known* an abnormality was present: I could feel it with my fingers. Despite a negative mammogram, further diagnostic tests (a biopsy of the palpable lump) would have been done. This was the opportunity I had missed with Fred. His cardiac ultrasound examination was a diagnostic test, not a screening test. It was done to look for specific heart diseases that can cause fainting spells (including, rarely, atrial myxoma). To correctly *disbelieve* a diagnostic test result—to dismiss it, decide it is "false," overrule it—is a big part of what separates truly expert diagnosticians from the rest of the pack.

I had learned this lesson years before from Mr. Kerr. He wasn't my patient. I saw him on rounds one day with the residents as their team's teacher that month. Each day, for an hour or two, they would present to me patients on their team—none of them patients I knew—who were interesting or challenging in various ways. Mr. Kerr, a seventy-five-year-old man from southern New Hampshire, had had fevers every day for the past few weeks. He'd had lots of unrevealing diagnostic tests before he was referred to Dartmouth and now, after a few days in the hospital here, the cause of his fever was still a mystery. This is a well-known syndrome in medicine, appropriately called "fever of unknown origin" (FUO), whose list of possible causes is very long. These causes include common diseases such as tuberculosis and cancer (which, in some cases, are difficult to find) as well as rare diseases that most doctors never see. The first steps in evaluating FUO always are a tediously detailed history—looking for subtle symptoms, forgotten medications, exposure to unusual infections from animals or foreign travel—and a meticulous physical examination. In Mr. Kerr's case, this hadn't helped; his only symptom or sign was fever. Unlike Fred—whose fainting history, at least in retrospect, suggested a problem with his heart or lungs—Mr. Kerr's history and examination hadn't helped his doctors narrow down their diagnostic search at all. And Mr. Kerr's doctors knew that, as with some cases of fainting, the cause of FUO is never found in a significant minority of patients. His doctors had begun to think that Mr. Kerr might be one of those; they were running out of ideas.

So was I. As I interviewed and examined Mr. Kerr in his hospital room, accompanied by his residents and medical students, I kept coming up empty. From skin rashes to shortness of breath, from dental problems to diarrhea, from joint aches to headaches, he denied them all. He looked a little thin—he had lost about ten pounds—but he didn't look sick. Still, we examined every inch of him, including the retinas of his eyes with an ophthalmoscope. Finally, we brought the big textbook of medicine into his room, propped it open to the page-long, tiny-font table of one hundred or more known causes of FUO, and walked through them all, one by one. None of them made sense in Mr. Kerr's case. It looked to me as if the team should send him home, as I had done with Fred, tell him we would investigate his problem further only if it didn't go away.

We closed our textbook, put away our instruments, and prepared to leave. As we did, an orderly knocked on the door, entered Mr. Kerr's room, and placed his lunch tray on the bedside table. It was noon. Hungry myself, I began to praise the hospital's food service (which was uncommonly good), if only to offer Mr. Kerr an encouraging word about something. But what I saw, when I lifted the plastic lid from his dinner plate, struck me as odd. It was a "soft" diet: mashed potatoes, pureed squash, applesauce. No meat or poultry or fish, no bread or salad, no solid food of any kind. It was the kind of diet ordered for patients recovering from abdominal surgery or old people who don't have teeth. Mr. Kerr was neither. I asked the residents why Mr. Kerr was on a soft diet.

He isn't, the intern answered. He's on a regular diet.

I pointed at the food on his tray.

The intern shrugged. We all looked at Mr. Kerr.

I prefer soft food, he said.

Why?

He pointed to a place under his right ear.

My jaw bothers me when I chew. So . . . I don't chew.

After a few more questions and a reexamination of Mr. Kerr's mouth and jaw, it became clear that he had jaw claudication, a very unusual symptom, which meant that the blood supply to the muscles of his jaw was compromised. (When asked why he hadn't mentioned this before, he said he figured he was just getting old.) In an elderly patient with fever, the symptom of jaw claudication could mean only one thing: Mr. Kerr had temporal arteritis (sometimes called giant-cell arteritis), an inflammatory disease of arteries that can cause permanent blindness when it involves the arteries of the eye. This disease can be cured with steroid drugs, but, because steroids also cause serious complications, it is always wise to *prove* that the diagnosis is correct before committing to the treatment. This requires a biopsy of the temporal artery, the blood vessel whose pulse you can feel in your temple just lateral to your eyebrow.

Jim Morgan, a Dartmouth rheumatologist who treated many patients with temporal arteritis, saw Mr. Kerr a few hours later and agreed immediately with our diagnosis. *Has to be*, Jim said. He recommended starting high-dose steroid treatment immediately, pending the results of the biopsy.

The next day, Mr. Kerr felt like a new man. For the first time in almost a month he had no fever. He wolfed down a thick cheeseburger for lunch, happy to chew again. Temporal arteritis was not a rare diagnosis at our medical center but it was the first time Mr. Kerr's residents and students had seen it. They told many of their colleagues about their "great case."

But, later that day, the results of the biopsy returned from the lab. Our pathologists, who knew a lot about this disease, had examined more than one hundred different sections of Mr. Kerr's surgically excised right temporal artery. Cold normal, every one. The residents and students were crestfallen.

Now what do we do? they asked Dr. Morgan.

Jim didn't miss a beat.

False negative, he said.

So?

Biopsy the other one, Jim said.

So they did, but only after convincing Mr. Kerr to go along. He couldn't understand why we needed "another piece" of him, especially now that we seemed so confident about what was wrong with him. The next day, one of the med students showed him a picture of his second biopsy, proudly pointing to the giant cells swelling inside his inflamed left temporal artery.

Great, Mr. Kerr said, as he pulled on his pants and got ready to go home. But you already knew that, right?

Mr. Kerr had a point, one that many patients don't understand about diagnostic tests in medicine. Tests can't make diagnoses; only doctors can. When using a test to help make a diagnosis, doctors must combine the test result with other things they know about the patient.

In fact, when interpreting *any* test result—a blood test, ultrasound, CT scan, tissue biopsy—expert diagnosticians don't interpret the patient based on the test, they interpret the test based on the patient.

In Mr. Kerr's case, for example, we didn't exclude the diagnosis of temporal arteritis after his temporal artery biopsy showed normal (negative) results. We assumed that Mr. Kerr had temporal arteritis (based on his compelling symptoms), *notwithstanding* the negative biopsy result. (False-negative biopsies occur in 10 to 15 percent of patients with subsequently proven temporal arteritis.) Medical diagnosis is all about interpreting test results in light of *everything else* the doctor knows about the patient. Most of the time, these two sources of information agree: The diagnostic test result is concordant with the doctor's clinical suspicion. It's when the test result is *discordant* with the doctor's clinical suspicion, as in Mr. Kerr's case, that expert diagnosticians show their stripes. To posit that a diagnostic test result is wrong, that is, falsely negative or falsely positive, requires the clinical confidence to disregard the result as if the test had never been done at all. When experts do this, they're right more often than wrong.

Mr. Kerr not only accepted this idea, he also questioned why his second biopsy should be done at all if its result wouldn't change how his doctors thought about and managed his care. Remarkably, this is *exactly* the question expert diagnosticians ask before recommending *any* diagnostic test: How will the result of this test affect my decisions about this patient? In essence, Mr. Kerr was asking: Why do another biopsy when you've already decided what's wrong and how to treat it?

Mr. Kerr's smart question had two answers. First, the results of the second biopsy, whether positive or negative, would *not* have affected our treatment decision. We would have treated Mr. Kerr with steroid drugs either way, because even two biopsies—one of the right temporal artery and one of the left temporal artery—will miss the diagnosis in a small number of patients (fewer than 5 percent) with temporal arteritis. In addition, the large potential benefit of steroid drugs (they prevent blindness, if Mr. Kerr has temporal arteritis) outweighs their potential harm (if it turns out he does not have temporal arteritis). Treatment with steroid drugs would be the wise decision in Mr. Kerr's case whether the second biopsy proved the diagnosis conclusively or not. Second, however, the biopsy results *would* change how Mr. Kerr's doctors managed his illness in other ways. A positive biopsy would clinch the diagnosis, bringing closure to the diagnostic search. In contrast, a second negative biopsy would be unsettling—not enough to stop steroid therapy but enough to cause us to remain vigilant for alternative diagnoses we might have missed. When Mr. Kerr understood this rationale for the second temporal artery biopsy, he readily agreed.

Most diagnoses are probable, not certain, something most laypersons don't know and some doctors don't appreciate. Furthermore, as in Mr. Kerr's case, how probable the diagnosis needs to be before the doctor accepts it as "true" (and treats it) depends on the relative harms and benefits of the treatment in question. On one end of this spectrum, antibiotics frequently are prescribed for patients whose need for them is highly uncertain, because the potential benefit of antibiotic treatment is great (if the patient has a treatable infection) while its potential harm is small (if the patient doesn't have a treatable infection). At the opposite end of this spectrum, cancer chemotherapy is almost never initiated unless the diagnosis of cancer is 100 percent certain. Why? Because the potential harm of chemotherapy is great while its potential benefit is relatively small (for many types of cancer). As a general principle, then, the greater the potential harm of a treatment in relation to its potential benefit, the more certain a diagnosis must be before that treatment is begun.

In this regard, Fred's case was the flip side of Mr. Kerr's. If the ultrasound tests had detected a myxoma in Fred's right atrium, our cardiac surgeons would *not* have accepted this diagnosis as "true" and recommended surgery. Why not? Because cardiac surgeons don't crack open the chest of an eighty-year-old man and cut into his heart unless they're damned sure they'll find what they're looking for. The potential benefit of surgical treatment for Fred's myxoma would be great, but so would its potential harm if it had turned out that Fred didn't have a myxoma at all. Because ultrasound tests can be "falsely positive" (that is, the ultrasound detects a myxoma that, in fact, isn't there) as well as falsely negative, the surgeons would have insisted that further diagnostic testing be done preoperatively to make sure the myxoma was "real." Just as we had disbelieved a normal temporal artery biopsy in Mr. Kerr's case, we would have disbelieved a cardiac ultrasound diagnosis of myxoma in Fred's case.

Such skepticism about diagnostic test results isn't easy to muster. Humans are inclined to trust technology, often blindly. Doctors tend to believe that diagnostic tests—whether they are abnormal ("positive") or normal ("negative")—mean what they say. The wise use of diagnostic tests requires more than smart technology. It also requires doctors' awareness of the technology's imperfections, a tricky business given doctors' imperfections, too.

Early in World War II, during the Nazi bombing of London, British defense ministers experimented with a new technology called radar. By stationing radar operators along the southeast coast of England, they were able to detect incoming Luftwaffe bombers in time to alert the air wardens in London to sound the alarms. Countless lives were saved as a result. But these radar defenses were imperfect. Sometimes they missed low-flying Messerschmitts that destroyed wide swaths of London neighborhoods, killing many people who lived there. At other times, radar detected Nazi bombers entering British airspace that, in reality, were nothing more than large flocks of birds wheeling innocently in the skies above Dover Beach. (Then, the alarms would sound and Londoners would scurry to underground shelters, awaiting an attack that never came.) When the British radar operators were right, their "true positive" diagnoses saved lives and their "true negative" diagnoses prevented further anxiety in a city under siege. But when the radar operators were wrong, their "false-negative" diagnoses cost lives and their "false positives" (false alarms) caused additional, unnecessary anxiety.

Churchill's ministers dealt with these imperfections in Britain's air defense by learning from their mistakes. They improved the performance of their technology by studying its "hits" and "misses"; then they recalibrated their radar receivers to discriminate better between German warplanes and flocks of birds. They improved the performance of radar operators by giving them daily feedback about the success and failure of each positive or negative "call" they had made. By continually comparing their radar defense performance with an indisputable "reference standard"—what actually happened on the streets of London—they learned and improved.

The result of these efforts was the development of "receiver operating characteristics" for radar defenses, an explicit measurement system that allowed the British radar operators to know the likelihood that a positive (worrisome) radar signal was true positive (the real thing) versus false positive (a false alarm), and the likelihood that a negative radar signal was true negative (safe) versus false negative (trouble). Perfect accuracy was unachievable. But continuous improvement became the explicit, shared goal of British air defense—and it made all the difference.

Today, the accuracy of medical diagnostic tests is measured by the same method. All medical tests have "receiver operating characteristics" that, when depicted on a graph (called an ROC curve), show the likelihood that an abnormal test result is a "hit" (true positive) or a "false alarm" (false positive), and the likelihood that a normal test result is an "all clear" (true negative) or a "miss" (false negative). Armed with these "likelihood ratios" of diagnostic tests, doctors can decide more confidently whether, given all *other* aspects of the case, a diagnosis is sufficiently likely or unlikely (after the test result is known) to move on to the next step. This decision is *never* certain, never black or white; it is *always* a judgment call, based on how much diagnostic uncertainty is tolerable in a particular situation. And, as with radar defense systems, the best decisions in medicine are made by experienced "operators" who understand the accuracy (and limitations) of the diagnostic technology they use.

Fred understood these things far better than I. An aviation expert in the years preceding World War II, Fred knew a lot about radar and the limitations of technology. One of his most important patented inventions was the "automatic direction finder" that used radio signals to provide accurate directions for airplane pilots. His invention improved the sensitivity and specificity of radio signal detection on board the plane—it reduced the false-negative and false-positive rates of previous direction finders—thus allowing pilots who were flying in a storm or over the ocean always to know where they were going. No doubt Fred's invention saved lives, before and after the war.

So, Fred knew all about "false negatives." Had our roles been reversed—had he been the doctor, not I—might he have questioned whether his own diagnostic tests had missed something important? I have often wondered.

More than his autopsy report, it was the second letter about Fred that changed everything. The return address on the envelope got my attention first. It read "M. Coover" from a town somewhere in Ohio. Had Martha left town? Fred was born and raised in Dayton. I wondered if Martha had gone to stay with family or friends.

I hadn't told Martha or her children about the autopsy report or Fred's myxoma, because it seemed to me esoteric medical stuff, trivial compared to the tragedy they were dealing with, irrelevant in the larger scheme of things. I filed it away as just one more learning experience, one more example of the pitfalls of technology and my own fallibility. During the few weeks that followed, work and winter went on as before.

I had stayed in touch with Martha after Fred died to make sure she was able to sleep and eat and manage at home. Her daughter was staying with her temporarily and, by all accounts, Martha was getting along, as she put it. We didn't talk about Fred. Martha didn't bring him up and neither did I. I hadn't gone to Fred's funeral. I never went to my patients' funerals unless my presence was personally requested by the family, which rarely happened. Some doctors appear at their deceased patients' services uninvited—a sign of respect, they think, a gesture of closure—but I always felt uneasy about this. It seemed to me intrusive and self-serving, an opportunity for the doctor to receive polite but perfunctory thanks from grieving family and friends "for all you did to help Charlie." I mean, what else would people say?

But now, after opening the letter from M. Coover, I knew what Mark Coover, Fred and Martha's son, would have said to me at Fred's funeral. It wouldn't have been perfunctory. And I wasn't sure if it would have been polite.

I'd heard about Mark, a successful engineer and inventor like

Fred, but I'd never met him. (I knew his brother and sister well; both lived in New England and, like Fred, became patients of mine after Martha got to know me.) Mark had sent his letter to me in a big brown envelope, the kind you use if you don't want to fold the paper inside. It was several pages long, typed expertly on thick bond paper. It could have been a research paper submitted to a scholarly journal. A carefully worded argument supported by references with foot- notes, its tone was professional and detached. But clearly, beneath the surface of that fine white paper, its author was deeply troubled.

He thanked me for taking care of his mother and father, who spoke highly of me. He wrote this without a trace of irony. But then he respectfully raised questions about Fred's death and proposed his own, carefully reasoned explanation for it. In short, it was my fault. Mark's letter didn't say this explicitly but that's how I read it: Fred's death was my fault.

As the administrative chief of Dartmouth's group of general in- ternists, I received occasional angry letters complaining about care given by one of us. In some of these letters, it was immediately clear that the writer was unhinged, upset about a loved one's medical trag- edy but obviously irrational and mistaken about its cause. In others, it was hard to tell: The distraught writer would describe unfortunate clinical events and troubling professional behavior that I, knowing the people involved, thought might be true. But, after investigating the allegations in these cases, I would almost always conclude that there was no way to know the truth; it was "he said, she said" stuff that could never be resolved objectively. Typically, this resulted in carefully worded written replies to the complainants, empathizing with their loss and thanking them for taking the time to bring these issues to our attention. But in ten years of writing these letters, I had felt compelled not even once to admit fault or culpability. This was no cover-up. I worked with a very capable, dedicated group of doctors and my investigations of these matters, while often thought- provoking, only made me appreciate my colleagues—and the difficulty of the work we did—even more.

After reading Mark's letter, I immediately concluded that Mark was rationalizing his father's death, looking for something or someone to blame, anyone but Fred himself. In theory, Mark's argument was plausible. But, in reality, I was certain it wasn't true.

Mark, it seemed, had confused his father's medical care with his mother's. His letter claimed that Fred had died, delirious and suicidal, as a side effect of a drug Martha took for her heart condition. Mark didn't explain why Fred would be taking Martha's pills. And even if Fred had taken Martha's medicine—which I had no reason to believe—this would have been an irrational act itself. Thus, it might have been an *effect* of Fred's losing his marbles but certainly not its *cause*. Both factually and logically, Mark's letter made no sense to me.

Still, it troubled me. Unlike most such letters I'd read, this one was about me. You can't help but be shaken when you suddenly discover that someone out there thinks, however incorrectly, that you've failed to live up to the sacred oath every physician has sworn since Hippocrates: *First, do no harm.* All doctors know that medicines can harm, confuse, even kill people. But Fred didn't take any medicines. I knew this for a fact. Certainly, if Fred *had been* taking any medicines, it would have been my responsibility to question whether this might be the cause of his altered mental state. Mark's letter cut to the heart of what I did, who I was: I was Fred's doctor.

Mark's letter also rattled me because it was expertly written and tautly argued, complete with authoritative references from the medical literature. This was 1985, pre-Internet. Mark must have spent hours, maybe days, researching his facts in a medical school library. I knew that grieving relatives sometimes grab at straws when devastated by tragic events. But I was troubled that such a capable, intelligent person (as Mark clearly was) would pursue and then articulate his theory so confidently without first vetting the one fact critical to its credibility. Why would Mark go to such lengths to posit that his father had died from "digitalis delirium" without confirming that Fred ever took digitalis? Fred *didn't* take digitalis (or any other medicine). I knew this. *Martha* took digitalis (for her rheumatic heart condition). Sadly, I thought, I could have saved Mark a lot of heartache if only he'd asked me about it before he jumped in and started assigning blame.

I was even more rattled by the fact that I had never heard of "digitalis delirium." I knew a lot about digitalis. The drug had been widely used for centuries to treat patients with congestive heart failure and common cardiac arrhythmias such as atrial fibrillation. Medical schools and residency programs taught extensively about digitalis drugs, not only because doctors prescribed them so often but also because their side effects could be very serious, even fatal. Scores of my own patients took these drugs. I took great care to monitor the levels of digitalis in their blood, even if they didn't complain of side effects. I made sure that the level of potassium in their blood was always optimal—if too low, it could contribute to "dig toxicity"—and I was careful not to prescribe other drugs that could interact with digitalis in harmful ways. In other words, like most internists, I was expert in the use of digitalis drugs. But I didn't know digitalis could cause confusion, agitation, or other neuropsychiatric side effects.

Mark did. His letter quoted extensively from the writings of John King, a physician in Baltimore who, in 1950, had reported six convincing cases of digitalis-induced delirium—ranging from mild disorientation and confusion to frank psychosis requiring physical restraints—all completely reversed by stopping the drug. I could see why Mark was so taken with his theory. Some of Dr. King's patients—and a few other reports Mark had found, dating back to 1921—sounded a lot like Fred.

I couldn't help but wonder: If Mark, a nonphysician, knew things about digitalis that I didn't know, was it possible he also knew things about his father's medical care that I didn't know? Could I be wrong?

I put down Mark's letter and looked up digitalis in the current editions of the authoritative textbooks of medicine and pharmacology. I found not a word there about delirium or neuropsychiatric side effects. This reassured me: I'd never seen it; I'd never heard of it; and the major textbooks didn't mention it at all. The literature Mark had dug up was ancient, anecdotal stuff—stories, not science—which, on closer examination, began to look pretty flimsy. None of it would pass muster with any self-respecting medical journal. Mark himself questioned the "scientific value" of these reports but confessed that they had "made a powerful impression on me." They made an impression on me, too. So, to reassure myself further, I looked again through the long lists of known digitalis side effects in the textbooks.

And then I saw it.

I hadn't missed what I was looking for. I found nothing in the books about delirium. But all of the lists included "visual disturbances" as common side effects of digitalis, including scotoma (blind spots) and yellowish penumbras around objects in the patient's visual field. I was familiar with these side effects. I had cared for many digitalis-intoxicated patients with such symptoms. But they had nothing to do with . . .

Angels?

I could still hear Fred's voice on the phone that night, before Martha got on the extension and shushed him.

Yeah, you know, cherubim and seraphim . . .

Oh, shit.

I've been thinking about haloes . . .

That's what he had said, I was sure of it. *Haloes.*

Could it be? Could Fred's crazy phone call about angels have been related to digitalis? Was he seeing, and then ruminating deliriously about, digitalis-induced haloes? Could it be?

I didn't want to bother Martha about this. She would feel even worse if she found out that Fred had been taking her pills—and that this might have had something to do with his death. I hoped Mark would keep it between us, at least until I responded to his letter.

I called Westman's, the local pharmacy. If Fred had been using Martha's digitalis pills, Martha might not have noticed but she would have had to refill her own prescription more frequently. George Westman, the pharmacist, knew me well—I spoke with him almost daily about patients and I'd been his mother's doctor before she died—and he was glad to help, no questions asked. He scanned his records quickly and reported that Martha's digitalis prescription had been refilled about every two months, appropriate for a bottle of sixty pills, one taken each day.

Relief washed over me. Fred hadn't been using Martha's pills.

Then George said, Hmmph. Funny you should ask, doc. Looks like Fred refilled *his* prescription early.

My heart began to race.

Fred?

Yeah, Martha's husband. Passed away recently. Too bad. Nice guy. I guess he wasn't yours, huh? Scrip was written by a Dr. Beringer. Don't know him. A resident at the hospital, maybe.

Now my heart was hammering.

Fred? What's the prescription for?

Digoxin 0.25 milligrams, once a day, fifty pills, George said. Started it in late December. Shouldn't have needed more until mid-March. But he refilled it early, in late January.

I didn't tell George why it mattered, or that I was Fred's doctor, or that Fred wasn't supposed to be taking any medications. My anxiety had morphed into anger. Why the hell would Doug Beringer, a senior resident at the hospital, write a prescription for Fred? And why didn't I know about it? And how could Fred's son in Ohio know about it when I didn't?

I called Doug Beringer. He was an excellent third-year resident, soon to begin fellowship training at Johns Hopkins. He didn't remember Fred. He seemed embarrassed by this after I told him he had written Fred's prescription in December, just a few months ago. The hospital was very busy over the Christmas holidays, Doug told me, and you know we write a lot of prescriptions for digitalis. He said he'd go down to Medical Records in the hospital basement and investigate.

I did the same. I walked over to Fowler House, dug out Fred's medical record. It was all there: Fred's initial visit after his fainting spell, his follow-up visit to review his normal test results, the last recent visit when I'd brought him in to check him out after he started making the crazy phone calls. But there was nothing about prescriptions. Nothing about Doug Beringer.

It didn't make any sense.

But now Mark's letter made perfect sense. The crazy phone calls had started in early January, soon after the date of Fred's first digoxin prescription. Why hadn't I asked Fred about drugs when I checked him out soon thereafter? Drug side effects were the *first thing* you wonder about when an elderly patient shows a change in mental function or behavior. I didn't ask because I already knew. Fred was my patient. Fred didn't take *any* drugs.

And now I remembered my conversation with Katherine Armour, the geriatric psychiatrist, when I asked her to evaluate Fred in mid-January.

Any new meds? Katherine had asked me over the phone. It was the obvious question.

No, no, he doesn't take any medications at all.

So Katherine hadn't asked Fred about it either.

Later in the day, Doug Beringer appeared outside my hospital office while I was seeing patients. He handed me a thin sheaf of paper with Fred's name all over it.

I found it down in Medical Records, Doug said. Mr. Coover was admitted to the hospital over the Christmas holidays. He stayed for only two days and I was off the day he was admitted. He came in after a syncopal episode. All I did was discharge him and write out his prescription. I guess that explains why I don't remember him. His hospital discharge summary hasn't been signed off yet, so it was downstairs in medical records in the "pending" pile. Took us a while to find it. You don't look so good, Dr. Reilly. Is anything wrong?

I bet I looked a lot worse when I finally went in to see my next patient. I kept her waiting while I read through Fred's hospital chart not once, but twice, thunderstruck.

Fred had done exactly what I'd asked.

If it happens again, Fred, we'll need to investigate further.

It was the day after Christmas. This time, Fred had passed out at the breakfast table, blue in the face, out cold for a full minute or two. At the hospital, he looked and felt fine but was noted to be in rapid atrial fibrillation, a fast irregular heart rhythm common in the elderly. The onset of this kind of cardiac arrhythmia can sometimes cause a fainting spell, and in the absence of any other demonstrable cause, the team concluded that this was the most likely explanation. After a few doses of digitalis, Fred's atrial fibrillation had not only slowed down nicely but also converted back into normal sinus rhythm, the best result possible. Appropriately, they had kept him on a daily digitalis pill as a precautionary measure. If the arrhythmia recurred, as atrial fibrillation often does, the digitalis pill would keep Fred's heart rate slow enough to protect him from passing out again. In the hospital, they had repeated all the tests. The cardiac ultrasound, Fred's second, was completely normal. As previously, the ultrasound lab had noted, among two full pages of other (normal) comments about Fred's heart, that "the right-sided cardiac chambers are sub-optimally visualized, but with no apparent abnormality seen." This was the standard disclaimer about the technical limitations of the test. But there was no hint of that lethal lollipop, Fred's myxoma—the real cause of his fainting spells and, almost certainly, the cause of his atrial fibrillation, too. We had missed the diagnosis not once but twice.

During this time, I was away with my family, visiting my parents over the Christmas holiday. Paul, doing my "hospitalist" pilot project for our group that month, had been Fred's attending physician during his brief hospital stay. As usual, Paul had analyzed Fred's problem insightfully and overseen the appropriate evaluation and treatment. The diagnosis of myxoma didn't occur to Paul, either, but this was no surprise. Paul was as pragmatic as he was brilliant. You don't look for a one-in-a-million diagnosis when you already have a diagnosis that's sensible and common. (There's an old saying about medical diagnosis: When you hear hoofbeats, think horses—not zebras.) At Paul's request, a cardiology consultant had seen Fred in the hospital and agreed.

And there, in Paul's chart note on the day of Fred's discharge from the hospital, was the explanation for why I had never heard anything about this: "Patient's primary care physician is Dr. Reilly. Patient will arrange outpatient follow-up with Dr. Reilly to monitor dig level and assess progress next week."

This was the plan for Fred's posthospitalization follow-up. He would call and make an appointment to come in and see me.

Who knows? Maybe that's why Fred started calling me at home. Maybe he had become confused, digitalis-delirious, and although he knew he was supposed to contact me, he couldn't remember why. That would explain why we talked on the phone about haloes and airplanes, not about his recent hospitalization and the new heart medicine he was taking. And when, finally, I had dragged him into Fowler House to evaluate his peculiar behavior, I had his outpatient chart—the only medical record I knew about—but the rest of it, the inpatient chart, was sitting in a big pile of more than a hundred charts in the hospital basement awaiting Paul's signature. Paul had been our group's "hospitalist" for the whole month of December. Now, overwhelmed with his own patients who had missed him during his month in the hospital, Paul was slowly working his way through that pile of hospital charts, a few at a time. Fred's was on the bottom.

Paul groaned when I told him. Fred was his first experience with a right atrial myxoma, too. Paul knew a lot about suicide—he had a keen interest in "psychosocial" medicine—and he sympathized about Fred's death. He knew that almost any drug can cause confusion in an elderly person, but, like me, was unfamiliar with digitalis delirium.

I guess we'll never know for sure, Paul said. The digitalis may have had nothing to do with it. If only he'd made it into the hospital that morning! That's when he was scheduled to be admitted to the Psych unit, right? Then we would have known! The Psych guys would have stopped the digitalis. Or, if they didn't know about it, he wouldn't have received it. Either way, then we would have known. Don't go crazy about this, Brendan. Many elderly people who develop delirium have underlying cognitive dysfunction, Alzheimer's usually. It's a tragedy, for sure. Terrible for the family. But who knows? If Mr. Coover was beginning to develop Alzheimer's, he may have saved himself from an even worse fate. We'll never know now.

Paul apologized for forgetting to tell me about Fred's hospital admission. But then he shook his head.

It's a flawed model, he said with great conviction. Discontinuity of inpatient and outpatient care . . . this experiment we just tried with me covering all of our patients in the hospital? . . . It's a disaster waiting to happen. Who knows whether it contributed to Mr. Coover's death? But, if it didn't hurt him, it will hurt others. Convenient for doctors; bad for patients. Sorry, but I think it's a bad, bad idea.

I didn't know what to tell Mark. I could have told him that he was probably right. I could have told him that I and others had missed Fred's underlying diagnosis, a surgically curable benign tumor that caused not only his fainting spells but also his atrial fibrillation—and his treatment with digitalis. I could have told him that, if I had made the correct diagnosis in the first place, none of this would have happened. I could have told him that I also failed to diagnose Fred's delirium—a very common problem in elderly patients—as well as its most common cause, a drug side effect. I could have told him that I didn't even know about Fred's hospitalization—or his treatment with digitalis—because, despite Dartmouth's exemplary commitment to continuity of patient care, I had personally championed a "hospitalist" experiment that had undermined this continuity and claimed Fred as its first victim. And I could have told Mark that a tiny flaw in Dartmouth's otherwise excellent medical records system had denied me my best chance to learn the truth in time.

Or I could have made excuses. In hindsight, Fred's fate seemed star-crossed. A rare diagnosis. A rare miss, not once but twice, by a powerful diagnostic technology. A rare drug side effect in a man whose rare charm and wit, unwittingly, hid it well. A rare, coincidental experiment about hospitalists with unintended consequences. A rare glitch in a superb medical records system. A lethal weapon, restored and preserved for its exact eventual purpose, forgotten by all but its forgetful victim. So many blind spots—Fred's, mine, Katherine Armour's, Martha's, the "system's"—each overlapping with the others. None of us, nor all of us together, had seen it coming.

Had I said such things, it wouldn't have made Mark any less troubled or sad. But it might have helped him. It might have comforted him to know that his father didn't choose to die, didn't want to leave Martha and Mark and the rest of their family bereft and bewildered, without explanation. It would have meant that Fred didn't do it, that he didn't kill himself. It would have meant that I, and fate, and the "system" killed Fred. It might have helped if I'd told Mark that.

But I didn't tell him that.

I wrote Mark to tell him it was possible that his theory was correct but that we didn't know—we couldn't know—for sure. The autopsy couldn't prove it one way or the other. I had contacted the county coroner's office, asked if they could do further analyses, toxicology tests to look for digitalis in Fred's remains. Too late, they said, and it wouldn't matter anyway. If the tests were negative, they might be false negative. And, if they were positive, they would confirm only what we already knew, that Fred was taking digitalis, not whether the drug had caused his delirium or his death.

As Paul had said, we would never know.

So I offered Mark my condolences. I told him I wished I had done better. Maybe it would have made a difference, I didn't know.

Martha and I never talked about it. Not really. I remained her doctor (and her family's doctor). But we never had a heart-to-heart about Fred. For some time afterward, I assumed I was the impediment to our clearing the air, setting the record straight, assigning responsibility where it belonged. I assumed it was my own sense of shame—and my propensity for denial—that, combined with Martha's silent stoicism, prevented any confrontation or confession or closure between us.

But Martha was wise and, in time, I came to see that the reality of the situation was more complicated. Martha felt guilty, too. Superficially, whenever the subject arose with me or others, Martha's attitude was Yankee philosophical, a terse blend of Calvinist predestination and existential resignation. No point crying over spilt milk, she once said to me, especially when you don't really know how it got spilt.

But, deep down, if Martha blamed anyone for Fred's death, she blamed herself. She knew him better than anyone. Looking back, she saw how obvious it was that something was seriously wrong. She never forgave herself for those nights when she told Fred to hang up the phone and leave me alone. And she knew all about the gun. Fred had told her about the gun long ago.

In the months that followed Fred's death, Martha and I saw each other less often. Only when necessary, always in my office, never at her home. We maintained our connection, in some ways stronger than ever. We had become unindicted codefendants, tacitly codependent, uncertain of our guilt or how to think about each other. Years later, long after Martha died, her daughter told me that Martha had loved me. So, there was that, too. We were like an estranged couple who still shared children, treasure, memories. We needed each other, felt sorry for each other, and avoided each other, always regretting the reasons why.

During the months that followed, I don't know how Martha managed in that house, reminders of Fred all around, their Adirondack chairs empty now in the garden, the sun setting into that glorious meadow every day.

As for me, I kept my distance. I rode my bike elsewhere, not up that hill. I stayed away.

Until I couldn't.

Chapter 7

LOST MARBLES

Ring them bells Sweet Martha . . . for the chosen few
Who will judge the many when the game is through
Ring them bells, for the time that flies
For the child that cries
When innocence dies.

—Bob Dylan, *Ring Them Bells* (1989)

June 1985

It would have been easy to walk away, recuse myself, as the lawyers say, plead nolo contendere or take the Fifth, so many ways to bow out forthwith. No one would have blamed me, not even Martha—oh, she might have loved me less, but she would have understood—and her children would have accepted my withdrawal without complaint, including Mark, who drove east from Ohio. It would have been easy for me to ask Paul, already complicit in the irony if not the guilt of Fred's death, to take over for me and help get Martha through this thing, whatever it was.

When I first heard about Martha's illness, it seemed right up Paul's alley, a classic example of psychosomatic medicine, his specialty. She won't get out of her chair, Martha's daughter told me. She even sleeps in it. She says she can't walk or even stand up. I don't know what to do, Margaret said.

It was easy to leap to the kinds of hypotheses that Paul might entertain—paralyzed by grief, immobilized by loneliness, that sort of thing. Freud himself had marveled at Charcot's work on hysteria more than a century ago, most of his patients women with "hysterical paralysis" resulting from various subconscious conflicts. If this were Martha's problem, it would be a delayed reaction, but shell-shocked soldiers weren't the only victims of post-traumatic stress disorder. Martha was a setup.

Or was she? Martha's heart had been weak before it was broken, but she'd survived the winter without complaint. So, why now, in June? Here in the north country, June is lilacs and every shade of green and a soft golden light that lingers deep into evening time. Winter, not June, was when folks hunkered down, conserved their energy, insulated themselves against the cold and the past. That was when the widows nursed their memories and the dreamers their disappointments—in winter, when the dark came early, the long snowy nights silvered by moonshine, the planet oblivious to everything but its own gravity. Not now, not in June. Even subconsciously, why would Martha cry out now?

Back then, not knowing better, I tried to make sense of such things, look for the logic where none could be. I had a lot to learn about medicine's mysteries.

The ambulance people brought her in a wheelchair. Martha had never used a wheelchair before, but she had refused to be transported on a stretcher. *I can't lie down*, she had told them. When they wheeled her into my office she shot me an embarrassed smirk and said, *Look at the mess I've dragged you into this time*. Martha's demeanor was the opposite of what I would have expected if she were giving up and hunkering down. She wasn't withdrawn or passive, limp with resignation. She was the Martha I had always known: self-deprecating but feisty, sarcastic, her world-weary shrug more protest than surrender. So I decided right then and there, correctly or not, that if Martha says she can't walk or lie down there's probably a damned good reason for it. And it's my job to find it.

But my confidence ebbed after I examined her. I found nothing new, nothing to explain her complaints. Her vital signs were normal and, despite her grief, she hadn't lost weight. Her heart was enlarged but it always had been and she swore that her breathing had nothing to do with her inability to walk or lie down. With great conviction, she said the problem was in her legs. But her pulses felt no feebler than expected in an old lady with a bad heart, and the arthritis in her knees and lower back seemed no worse than before. Her strength had always been surprising and it was no different now: When I asked her to bend her knee up to her chest and resist me, I couldn't push her down, left or right, and I found no sign of a neurological cause of her symptoms. But when, finally, I asked her to stand and try to walk, she said, *I can't do it, Brendan.* I said, *I know, I'm sorry, Martha, but I need to see for myself,* and she said something about Doubting Thomas and sticking my hand into her wounds but she said it in the kind, knowing way a mother admonishes her child and then she raised herself up out of the wheelchair and stood there with her back bent over and her legs trembling and when I asked her to take a step she seemed stuck to the ground, grimacing, and when she straightened up to try to walk she moaned and fell back heavily into the wheelchair.

I'm sorry, I can't do it, please believe me, I just can't do it.

I asked her to tell me what she felt when she tried to walk, what she was feeling that made her sit back down. All she could say was *It's my legs, my legs,* and when I asked about her knees and hips where the arthritis was bad, she said, *No, it's not there, it's my legs,* and she ran her hands along her thighs from her knees up to her waist and said, *Here, it's here.* I checked the feel and strength of her thighs again and they were normal, cold normal, no different from yours or mine, just older. *No,* she protested, *they don't bother me when I'm sitting, it's only when I try to stand and walk,* and at first this didn't make any sense to me. She must have seen this in my face—more than puzzlement, she saw doubt, disbelief—because she said, *All I can tell you is what I feel, Brendan, I'm not making it up, you know,* but then she saw that that's exactly what I was wondering, against my better judgment: Maybe this really was one of those "conversion reactions" I had read about in Freud but never seen myself. Martha looked at her daughter and then she looked at me and she said, *You must believe me, you two especially, you must believe me.* I said something lame like *Of course, we believe you* but now I wasn't sure if she believed me.

So there we were, the three of us in my examining room, and I'd swear that each of us, if asked, would have acknowledged that we weren't three, but four. Right there, over there, the ghost in the corner. His name was Fred.

I sent Martha downstairs to get a series of X-rays on her hips and knees and lower back, knowing they wouldn't show me the answer, but it bought me some time to see my other patients and think about what to do. When she returned from Radiology, I saw no option but to put her in the hospital. Her X-rays showed the same severe osteoarthritis she'd had in her knees and hips and spine for years but nothing that explained what was happening to her now. I was reluctant, in fact almost ashamed, to admit a patient to the hospital when I didn't have a clue what was wrong, especially if it turned out to be all in her head. Martha didn't like the idea either. She almost refused, despite her daughter's pleas. This worried me even more. Clearly, she wasn't seeking attention. She preferred to go home and sit in her chair and see what tomorrow would bring. So, finally, I played my ace of spades. I told Martha that if we'd gotten Fred into the hospital in time, things might have turned out differently for him. *Let's not miss our chance again, okay? I don't think I could handle that, Martha.*

It was the first time since Fred had died that I had mentioned the ghost in the room. Martha just lowered her head, quietly nodded, and said, *Okay.* I think she did it more for me than for herself. But I think it made her begin to doubt me, too.

God knows she had good reason. Whatever had happened to Fred, I hadn't helped. And she could see now that I wasn't sure if I could help her either. I was confident enough about my ability to diagnose physical disorders, notwithstanding my recent failure to diagnose Fred's. But it was the other side of the "biopsychosocial" sphere that intimidated me, the dark side, that murky realm of desire and wish that makes every person a mystery. Martha could see that I was straddling the fence between a physical, biomedical explanation for her illness and a "psychophysiological" explanation, the paralyzed-with-grief hypothesis. And, though she didn't say so, Martha was offended by the very idea. She wasn't the "type" to have a conversion disorder. *Pshaw!* she would have said if asked—she actually used old Yankee words like that—*I know what's in my own head! Whatever this foolish thing is, it's in my legs, not my head!*

I sent Martha and her daughter down to the hospital admitting office and I paged the admitting resident on call. I wasn't looking forward to our conversation. He or she would be very busy, running around admitting new patients, and even though residents aspired to autonomy and said they wanted to figure things out for themselves, they also wanted to get their work done. So, when presented with a new admission from the clinic, most of them listened politely to the senior physician but then blurted out what they really wanted to know: So, what's wrong with this lady? Why are we admitting her? I wasn't looking forward to the answer I would have to give about Martha: She's an old lady with a bad heart who says she can't walk but I haven't found any obvious physical explanation for this yet and I'm beginning to wonder if it's because she's carrying a ghost on her back.

Luckily, it was Jim Henshaw who answered my page. Jim had come to Dartmouth from Duke, planning to return to Duke for a cardiology fellowship after doing his medicine residency here. Recently he had begun to wonder instead about a career in primary care, in part because of his experience with a patient we had shared several months before. Mrs. Jardin was an elderly French widow who lived near the Canadian border in northern New Hampshire. She traveled down to Hanover every year to have her checkups done at Dartmouth. She was remarkably healthy and wanted to do everything she could to stay that way. She was always pleased when I announced every year, after examining her carefully and doing various tests, that she would probably live to be a hundred. *Don't be so pessimistic*, she would say with a twinkle in her eye, reminding me that her mother had lived to 107.

Jim got to know her when, last winter, Mrs. Jardin had come to see me complaining that something was wrong with her legs and I had admitted her to the hospital on Jim's team to find out what was wrong with her. Mrs. Jardin never complained about anything. But for the past week she had noticed that climbing the stairs and even rising from a chair seemed difficult somehow and she knew for sure that something was wrong. I agreed with her. When I tested the strength in her upper legs as she lay on my examining table, I was able to overcome her resistance; I could easily push her knees, first her left and then her right, down from where I had asked her to flex them hard up against her chest. She was a seventy-eight-year-old 105-pound woman; I was a thirty-five-year-old 170-pound man. But I knew that this weakness was abnormal for her. I had done this same strength test every year on Mrs. Jardin, most recently just several months ago, and every time before now she had passed with flying colors. Her weakness was subtle but it was real, and the pattern of her weakness suggested that she had a muscle disease. More worrisome, her complaints were only a week old, so I couldn't tell how fast her muscle weakness might be progressing. I had seen a patient with polymyositis, the disease that I worried she might have, worsen so rapidly that he couldn't swallow or breathe within just a few weeks after his initial symptoms began. I admitted Mrs. Jardin to the hospital for careful observation and arranged her muscle biopsy for the next day.

Jim, a junior resident at the time, was a bright, confident guy not many years younger than I. Given our trivial age difference—and knowing I didn't mind—he took some liberties with me that he dared not try with older faculty physicians. After examining Mrs. Jardin himself in the hospital, he had called me on the phone and joshed me about her good-naturedly. *She's the healthiest old lady I've ever seen*, he said. *She wouldn't make it into the hospital at Duke, I'll tell you that. I'll bet you a pizza we find nothing.* He wasn't impressed when we repeated her examination together and demonstrated the subtle weakness in her legs. Jim said, *Come on, we're big guys, we're a lot stronger than she is, of course we can overcome her muscle resistance!* But he changed his tune three days later when Mrs. Jardin was so much weaker she couldn't get out of bed and her muscle biopsy showed changes typical of polymyositis. When Jim brought the pizza down to my office that day he looked as if he'd just witnessed a miracle of some kind. Starry-eyed, he wanted to know how I'd done it.

It ain't rocket science, I told him. *It's as simple as this: I know her. I'm her doctor. Having examined her so many times before, I knew this was abnormal. For her. That's all there is to it.*

This was not something a new physician-in-training, even one as talented as Jim, could know. It was a new idea for him: A doctor could be so prescient, so sensitive to subtle but important changes, *entirely* because the doctor knew the patient well? They didn't teach this stuff in medical school. Jim began to rethink his career plans. He began to think he'd like to be able to do the same thing.

So Jim didn't miss a beat when I told him now about Martha. *We're on it*, he said. I told him I wouldn't bet a pizza on this one. I had an idea what might be going on but I honestly wasn't sure. *See what you think after you examine her yourself*, I told Jim. I didn't tell him about Fred. I was pretty sure Jim would find out after talking to Martha (and, if he didn't, I'd give him a hard time about it). Jim couldn't learn from this case—and we couldn't get to the bottom of it—if we didn't talk about the ghost in the room, along with everything else. Later that day, when Jim called in all the consultants we thought we might need—Vascular Surgery, Orthopedics, Neurology, Cardiology, Anesthesia, Rehab Medicine—he called Psychiatry, too. I wasn't looking forward to explaining that last one to Martha. But I needed all the help I could get. I didn't pretend to know 90 percent of what psychiatrists know. I wasn't sure I wanted to, either.

Just down the hall from Martha's hospital room lay the most recent example of my inexperienced ineptitude in the twisted mysteries of the mind. Alice Quinn had refused to talk to the shrinks at all. She told them I didn't know what I was talking about. She told them I was incompetent, completely wrong about what was wrong with her, and that she wanted a different doctor. Until that happened, she would speak to no one, especially not psychiatrists. I'm not the crazy one, she said. Reilly's the one who's crazy.

There had been more than a few moments this past week when I had thought she might be right. Alice was way out of my league. When it came to patients with factitious illness—people who purposely made themselves sick—I was a babe in the woods. I'd read about such patients. I'd seen patients in psychiatric hospitals who had cut or burned themselves. But this was different. This was the big time and Alice was right about one thing: I *was* over my head.

She was young, in her twenties, plain-looking and grim, not one to have lots of boyfriends. Her doctor had sent her to me from Frankfurt, one of the last remaining factory towns in northern New Hampshire, famously repugnant for the sulfurous rotten-egg odor belched continuously from its smokestacks into the surrounding countryside. It was a hardscrabble, hard-living town that had seen better days, a place where a girl like Alice could get lost or worse. Her fevers had started two weeks ago. Her blood cultures had grown *Staphylococcus aureus*, a bad bug, but her doctors couldn't find where the infection was coming from. Alice herself knew a lot about such things; she worked as a technician in the Frankfurt hospital's microbiology laboratory. When, after a week, her doctors admitted they were stumped, it was Alice who asked to be transferred to Dartmouth. For the first few days, we were stumped, too. She didn't have a fever, her examination was normal, and all of her tests, including her repeat blood cultures, were negative. We concluded she didn't need to stay in the hospital, thinking she might have had a harmless "transient bacteremia" from a tiny skin sore that was now no longer apparent. I was glad for her. It could have been much worse, a dangerous infection in her heart or bones. I thought it odd that she wasn't enthused by my good news—she remained quiet, passive, rarely making eye contact—but she agreed to call her parents so they could come take her home in the morning.

That night her temperature spiked to 105. The next day her blood cultures, drawn during the night, were growing *Staph* bacteria. Clearly we were missing something. We certainly couldn't send her home. Again, she took this news in stride, not a hint of emotion. She was a strange duck, I thought, but so were a lot of people and again I made nothing of it. Then, for the next three days, she was fine—no fever, no abnormalities on her new tests, negative blood cultures. I called her doctor in Frankfurt. He said, Yeah, the same thing happened here, too. Puzzled, I discussed this with Alice.

That's why I'm here, she said.

And that night her temperature spiked again.

The next day I felt like a petty thief as I closed the door behind me and rummaged through the clothes and luggage in her hospital room. I wasn't exactly sure what I was looking for but I'd sent Alice downstairs to have another set of X-rays so I could snoop around on my own. After picking through her private possessions—frilly underwear and pink hair curlers, a romance novel and toiletries—I'd found nothing and felt like a peeping Tom. As I prepared to leave and rethink the case all over again, I lifted up the mattress and found her pocketbook hidden there. The syringe was in a zippered compartment, thick yellow pus filling its 10 cc barrel more than halfway, its attached needle carefully capped. I took it down to the lab, asked the techs to stain and culture the pus, and then compare it to the *Staph* bacteria we'd grown intermittently from Alice's blood. For sure it would be identical. This was the stuff she'd been injecting into her own bloodstream to make herself sick. It was a dangerous game she'd been playing, Russian roulette for real, and it meant that her (potentially fatal) infection was the least of her problems. She was crazy. Crazy enough to risk killing herself just to get attention. There was no way I—or any psychiatrist—could cure that.

But I could make it worse. And, not knowing any better, that's exactly what I did.

We were alone, in her room, the door shut to the corridor. I hadn't done what you're supposed to do when you have an important conversation with a patient. I hadn't sat down next to her bed, met her at eye level, tried to make more personal contact. I stood over her, towering above, looking down. I hid the syringe in my closed fist. Then, slowly, I opened my hand in front of her face and showed it to her.

At first I said nothing. Neither did she, not even after I told her that the pus in the syringe showed sheets of *Staph* bacteria just like those in her blood. She didn't feign innocence. She didn't ask where I got the syringe. She didn't accuse me indignantly of rifling through her private possessions. No, she didn't say anything.

I pushed her. I demanded an explanation. I wanted to hear her confess, apologize. Instead, in a smug unemotional voice, she explained that she had developed a boil on her skin during one of her fevers and she had aspirated the pus herself into a sterile syringe to help the doctors identify the cause of her fever.

I thought I gave it to the doctors, she said with a shrug. *I guess not, huh?* and then she looked me straight in the eye.

I knew this wasn't true. Under the microscope, we had found no white blood cells—human cells—in the syringe, proof that the pus hadn't come from a person. It was a pure culture of *Staph* bacteria, grown in a petri dish, presumably in the hospital laboratory where she worked. Or, who knows? Maybe she grew the stuff at home, in an incubator in her bedroom. Anything was possible. She was nuts.

But she was good. She didn't miss a beat. She simply shrugged again and said she'd aspirated the boil more than a week ago, so the white blood cells in the syringe would have lysed by now. *That's why you can't see them under the microscope. The white cells are dead.* Then she pointed to a place on her left arm, badly bruised from the multiple needle sticks she'd had for her many blood tests, here and in Frankfurt. *It was here, the boil was here,* she said, *but you can't see it anymore.*

I wasn't about to argue with her. I asked her to think more about this. I told her we wanted to try to help her. I recommended that our psychiatrists come talk to her. She said nothing. I told her that if she refused our help we would send her home in the morning. And, yes, I would have to tell her doctor in Frankfurt. She said nothing. I asked if she understood me. She simply turned away.

Late that night, I received a phone call at home from the intern taking care of Alice. Her temperature was 104 degrees. Her blood pressure was unobtainable. She was in shock, near death. We moved her to the intensive care unit, gave her large doses of IV antibiotics and powerful drugs to support her blood pressure. She made it through the night. In the morning the intern showed me what he had found in her bed after I told him about the syringe. It was another syringe, this one plunged empty, spittles of pus still visible at the bottom of its barrel. When they moved her into the ICU, they found the needle marks in her groin.

She'd had another one. When I found the first syringe, I hadn't been smart enough to look for others. Out of spite, or whatever it was that motivated her, she'd shot the whole barrel of pus into her femoral vein after I'd confronted her. This huge bolus of virulent bacteria, injected directly into her circulation, had induced a catastrophic inflammatory response. Now she was alive, but barely. She would have critical care doctors taking care of her now, not psychiatrists.

I showed her. So then she showed me.

Alice lived in a world like no other. She knew what she was doing but she didn't know why. She wasn't a malingerer, someone who purposefully fakes illness or causes disability to achieve material gain. She didn't even have a motive, not consciously anyway. All I had accomplished by confronting her, like an avenging prosecutor, was to make myself feel better at her expense. Once discovered, her back to the wall, she had no choice but to fight back the only way she knew how. She'd show me, even if it killed her.

No one knows how this happens. But almost certainly, Alice's Munchausen psychopathology was about nurture, not nature. It's not about biology. It's about people feeling hurt, deep down. Abusive parents? Malicious peers? A talented, timid dreamer wasting away in a dying town? Who knows?

This was what worried me about Martha. I had just proved that I was way over my head with Alice, a patient who was consciously hurting herself for subconscious reasons. Was Martha hurting for subconscious reasons, too? If so, she might be even more of a challenge than Alice, one I certainly wasn't qualified to meet.

And yet, if Martha's pain was all about Fred, who better able to help than I? Was Martha hurting because she feared that Fred had known *exactly* what he was doing? If so, he would have known that, in killing himself, he was breaking Martha's heart. Could Fred have done that? Mark's theory about digitalis, impossible to prove, said emphatically, No, Fred didn't do that. Could I cure Martha, then, simply by siding with Mark and telling her so? If it would help Martha, why not tell her I had screwed up with Fred?

But there it was again, the doctor's golden rule: *First, do no harm.* At this point, it was equally plausible that Martha's pain was caused by an undiagnosed physical disorder, nothing to do with all these psychological babblings. I even had an idea what that disorder might be. If I was right, it would be hard to prove—and even harder to fix. But if Martha's problem was physical, the last thing she needed from me right now was some soulful confession about Fred's death. That would only make her feel worse. Still learning, I had begun to see the wisdom of the old saying, inverted: Don't just do something, stand there.

So that's what I did. During Martha's first two days in the hospital, I didn't do anything. This was awkward but painless—both for Martha and for me. She seemed comfortable enough propped up in her hospital bed or sitting in her bedside chair. She didn't ask for pain medicine, although she tired easily from the frequent parades of medical students, residents, and specialists who came in to interview and examine her. I stayed in the background, Martha's attending physician-in-charge, content, even relieved, to share the burden of responsibility with my colleagues. For now, I was off the hook, my role mainly to clarify consultants' opinions for Martha and her children.

John and Margaret, both patients of mine, hung on my every word. They were very worried, especially because Martha's illness had followed so soon after Fred's death. John, a psychologist, said something about how it never rains, it pours. Margaret kept a stiff upper lip in Martha's presence but, outside her hospital room, broke down a few times. Mark was worried about Martha, too, but he seemed at least as worried about me. Mark didn't mention Fred or our correspondence about him. But he questioned everything I said. He pushed me to reconcile each consultant's findings with the others. As it turned out, this wasn't easy to do.

The Vascular guys thought that poor circulation in Martha's legs could explain her pain but she couldn't walk even a few steps and they thought this peculiar. The cardiologists didn't think Martha's heart was the problem but they worried about it for other reasons. Along with her digitalis and other heart drugs, Martha took blood-thinners to prevent clots from forming in her enlarged heart. If Martha needed any invasive tests (such as the angiogram of her leg arteries that the Vascular guys had recommended), her blood-thinners would need to be stopped, thus exposing her to the risk of a stroke. The cardiologists also weren't sure if Martha's heart could handle major surgery, if it turned out that's what she needed. The Anesthesiology guys agreed, rating Martha's surgical risk from general anesthesia as high, an off-putting "4" on their risk scale of 1 to 5. The orthopedists agreed that the arthritis in Martha's spine and hips and knees was bad but they doubted it was causing her inability to walk. They changed their tune when the Neurology guys raised the possibility of spinal stenosis, a narrowing of the spinal canal (usually caused by spinal arthritis) that pinches the nerves in the legs when the patient stands or walks. Could be, the orthopods said, but the only way to know was to perform a myelogram, an invasive procedure that requires a spinal tap and injection of dye into the spinal canal. Worse, in Martha's case, the spinal tap and injection would have to be done in her *neck*, not her lower back, because her lower spine was so badly deformed by her arthritis. A cervical myelogram was a tough procedure even for young patients, requiring them to lie still on a hard table for a long time as the table tilted severely up then down, again and again, turning the patient on her head and then upright, to allow the dye to travel the entire length of the spinal canal and image it on X-rays. Many patients refused this procedure, especially when warned that one of the (rare) complications of cervical myelography was bleeding into the spinal cord. If this happened, it could cause the patient to become quadriplegic (even if she wasn't taking blood-thinners, as Martha was).

Last but not least, on Martha's second day in hospital came the Psychiatry consultants. Their conclusion: "Possible reactive depression. No evidence of major affective disorder. Cannot exclude the possibility that the patient's current pain syndrome is related to somatization."

Predictably, at the end of that second day, Martha was mad at me. She was worn out from all the consultations and tests. But the psychiatrists were the icing on the cake, as Martha put it. We were alone in her hospital room. Her children had gone home for the evening, resting up for the family conference we had arranged for the next morning to discuss what to do, given the conflicting opinions and risks raised by the various consultants.

Martha just shook her head.

Do you know what they asked me, Brendan?

The Psych guys? I can guess.

They asked me about Fred.

Mmm.

They asked me how I felt about Fred's death.

Yeah.

You know what I told them?

What?

I told them I loved Fred from the first time I met him. Fifty-seven years ago. I told them he was the best person I ever knew. I told them we were happy together for a long, long time. And now he's gone.

Yeah.

So I asked them: How do you think I feel?

Apparently, this had ended Martha's conversation with the psychiatrists. They wouldn't answer her question, so she didn't answer any more of theirs. They told her they'd be back to see her again tomorrow. Martha said, *I don't know what's making me hurt, Brendan, but it's not Fred. Let the poor guy rest in peace, for Pete's sake. I'll do whatever you say but let's skip the psychiatrists, okay?*

We agreed to talk more about it in the morning.

But Martha couldn't sleep that night. She told her nurse that she was hurting, even just lying in bed. She couldn't get comfortable. Around midnight, the nurse called the intern, who checked Martha, found nothing new, and ordered some pain medicine and a mild sleeping pill. According to the nurses' notes, Martha then slept fitfully through the night.

It was early when I came to see her. The night nurses were huddled with the day nurses, doing their change-of-shift report. Martha was alone. The smell in her room was suffocating. Fistfuls of wet feces dripped off the walls around her bed. Her arms and hands and nightgown were covered with it. Her bed was wet with urine, soiled with excrement. She was tossing shit all around the room. She cackled when she saw me.

See that one, Fred? I got him! Oh! Watch out! Fred! Get your head down!

Martha . . . ?

You go, Fred. You go find Electra. I'll stay here. Oh! Oh! Look there! So many . . . so many Japs!

Martha, I'm not . . .

Fred, you promised me! You said you would take care of the babies! When I'm gone, the babies . . .

Now she was crying, her shoulders shaking.

Martha, let me . . .

I told you! Fred, I told you! It's not your fault! It's her own damn fault! Who does she think she is, flying around in men's pants? It's her own damn fault!

I don't . . .

She's gone, Fred! She's gone! Don't you see? It doesn't matter anymore. It's not your fault!

Sobbing, Martha buried her head in her hands, smearing her face with feces. She gasped.

I ran out to the nurses' station, got some help. We had to lift Martha out of her bed to clean her up, change her sheets. She fought us, screaming at Barbara, one of the nurses.

See what you've done? You did this! Fred didn't do it! You're a selfish bitch! All you care about is yourself!

Barbara, a pretty young woman, was stunned.

Mrs. Coover, I don't . . .

Fred! You saw it! She did it!

Martha, I'm not Fred . . .

Now Martha was sobbing again, her head thrown back in despair. *I don't care! I don't care! You want to go with her, you go ahead! She's crazy, Fred! Amelia Earhart? So what? She'll kill you, too! The babies, Fred! You promised me you'll take care of the babies!*

A couple of hours later, I didn't tell Martha's children about the mess or the real reason we'd moved her to a different room. What they saw for themselves was bad enough. Martha was drowsy now but still delirious from the pain medicine and the sleeping pill she'd received the night before. She didn't recognize her children at all.

John frowned. Margaret began to cry. Mark didn't know what to think.

Now Martha was just like Fred.

Delirium can happen to anyone. And it does, frequently.

Today, at least 20 percent of the 12.5 million people aged sixty-five years or older who are hospitalized annually in the United States develop delirium. In some hospitals, the incidence of delirium exceeds 50 percent. This problem adds billions of dollars to annual Medicare costs and causes untold suffering for patients and their families. It also kills people. In fact, the in-hospital *mortality* rate for patients with delirium ranges from 22 percent to 76 percent, higher than the death rate for patients with a massive heart attack or overwhelming sepsis. There are many reasons for this stunning statistic, including the fact that some deathly ill patients become delirious because they are deathly ill. But, in many cases, delirium is preventable; for this reason, national hospital accreditation agencies have recently mandated that prevention and treatment of delirium become an essential quality improvement priority in all U.S. hospitals.

Better late than never. This has been going on for a long time.

Nearly fifty years ago, Z. J. Lipowski called delirium the "Cinderella" of American medicine: "taken for granted, ignored and seldom studied." He noted that delirium often seems harmless enough, as when "a delirious patient walked into a hospital emergency room and was found fumbling in a refrigerator where drugs were kept; it turned out he believed himself to be at his house and was looking for a bottle of beer." But other cases that Lipowski described were not so amusing:

> A middle-aged lawyer, hospitalized for acute pancreatitis, wrote a note to his wife urging her to bring him his gun to the hospital. . . . It turned out that the patient had hallucinated [intruders] entering his room through a hatch in the ceiling. They [his doctors] marched around his bed making threatening gestures. He wanted a gun to defend himself.
>
> A young woman hospitalized for a viral infection . . . complained . . . about anxiety and nightmares. These complaints were ignored and . . . the patient wandered away from her bed, slipped into a laundry hatch on the ward and fell several floors, sustaining multiple fractures of the spine and legs. . . .
>
> A barbiturate addict . . . mistook her [hospital] room for a prison cell from which she expected to be taken to be executed. She was caught opening a window [high above street level] in an attempt to escape.

Yet, for every one of these frightful cases, Lipowski noted that there are many more "'good,' i.e., quiet and compliant, delirious patients

[who] do not *bother* anybody." Like Fred, these patients "hide their delirium under a façade of pleasantness, cooperativeness, or by parrying with humor." How common is this?

Today, the prevalence of delirium among very elderly people in the United States (eighty-five years and above) who are *not* in the hospital is 14 percent. *One in seven* of the 6 to 7 million very elderly people living in the community suffers from delirium. Most of them "hide" it, one way or another, eluding discovery like Fred.

Delirium occurs when patients with particular *predisposing conditions* are afflicted by specific *precipitating events*. The most common predisposing conditions are elderly age, prior cognitive dysfunction (especially dementia), daily use of psychoactive drugs, immobilization, and visual or hearing impairment. Because these conditions are increasing in U.S. society today, so is the incidence of delirium. But even a young healthy person may become delirious if the precipitating event is severe enough. For example, classic medical experiments about the effects of fever showed that artificially raising body temperature to 104 to 107 degrees Fahrenheit caused delirium in more than half of normal young human subjects. But it is the *interaction* of susceptibility (predisposing conditions) with precipitating events that results in most cases of delirium. (The most common precipitating factors are drugs, infections, chemical imbalances, sleep deprivation, and surgery.)

Anticipating these interactions can prevent delirium before it happens. Instead of sleeping pills, patients in the Yale Delirium Prevention Trial were given warm milk or herbal tea, relaxation tapes, and bedside massages; nighttime noise in their hospital corridors was reduced. These and other "low-tech" commonsensical interventions reduced the incidence of delirium in the Yale patients by one-third. Similar preventive studies have reduced delirium in elderly patients hospitalized for hip fracture, *one-half* of whom developed delirium (lasting an average of *three days*) if they didn't receive such interventions.

Although targeted interventions can prevent many cases of delirium, they require hard work and cost real money. The average additional cost of labor and equipment to prevent *one* case of delirium in hospital during the Yale study was $6,341 (in 1999 dollars). Even if we make this investment, the prevalence of delirium likely will continue to rise, given the increasing life expectancy and prevalence of dementia in elderly U.S. adults. Although one-third of delirium cases in hospital may be preventable, the remaining two-thirds are not. Whether precipitated by the patient's acute illness (for example, an infection) or its treatment (drugs or surgery), delirium is an unavoidable outcome for many patients in hospital. For this reason, although prevention is desirable (and, in some cases, feasible), early recognition and treatment are equally important.

The Achilles' heel of such efforts is that the early recognition of delirium— by definition, an *acute change* in the patient's mental status—requires familiarity with the patient's usual mental status. In acute care hospitals, where so many patients are cared for by doctors and nurses who have never met them before, hospital staff will be far less likely to recognize the telltale *changes* in affect or behavior that herald the onset of delirium. Worse, when elderly hospitalized patients develop florid delirium—agitated, wandering, disruptive behavior—hospital staff often assume that the patient has *dementia* (that is, long-standing, irreversible cognitive impairment). A vicious cycle then ensues: Psychoactive drugs (tranquilizers, antipsychotics, sleeping pills) are given to calm the "demented" patient's agitation, which drugs often only make the patient's delirium worse.

It happens all the time.

When my father was eighty-five years old, I flew him to Chicago (where I worked) to undergo risky lung surgery. I knew that Dad's risk of developing delirium in hospital was high; he had become floridly delirious the last time he was in the (same) hospital when he had major surgery to remove a cancerous kidney. We took precautions to prevent it, but, immediately after his (successful) lung operation, I received an urgent call from the head nurse to come see Dad in the surgical ICU. When I arrived, both of his hands had been restrained (painlessly) with soft straps to prevent him from pulling out his IV or bladder catheter or chest tube, all of which Dad still needed immediately after surgery (but none of which he wanted). In protest, Dad had told the head nurse and everyone else in the ICU that "your commanding officer does not have the prerogative, under the terms of the Geneva Convention, to issue orders pertaining to me or my troops."

Dad recognized me when I arrived in the ICU but he said, spluttering with exasperation, "What the hell kind of army are you running here, Bren?" Dad was convinced that he was the commanding general of the South Vietnamese Armed Forces; he was not at all pleased that "the Americans are throwing their weight around again." Because I was wearing the same "uniform" (a long white coat) as most of the other "troops" in the ICU, Dad thought that I was an American army officer. For the next two days, Dad's delirium was managed successfully by minimizing the drugs that had precipitated it—and by suggesting that the hospital staff salute whenever they approached him.

Dad's delirium was diagnosed quickly and treated with dispatch because I knew him. Like many other members of our Greatest Generation (he served in World War II, not Vietnam), Dad was normally reserved and polite, a good listener, never one to call attention to himself. His behavior when delirious was dramatically different from the "real" Dad. Interestingly, the *content* of Dad's delirium had an internal logic of its own (like some dreams): The medical staff in the ICU *was* indeed an allied foreign "army" pledged to help Dad through a life-or-death battle. And Dad's officious behavior when delirious reflected his proclivity, when "himself," to state his opinions authoritatively (even when there was plenty of room to disagree). Only someone who knew Dad could see these tangential connections between his normal and delirious behavior.

But even when the patient has one doctor who knows him well, delirium can easily elude detection. When Dad developed delirium for a third time, I was smarter than before—but not by much. In the aftermath of his lung surgery, we reduced Dad's daily medications to virtually none. From time to time, however, he would call me in Chicago and ask me to phone in to his local pharmacy on Shelter Island a prescription for an antibiotic. Dad's bladder cancer and catheter caused symptoms intermittently (bleeding and urinary discomfort) that resembled symptoms sometimes caused by a bladder infection.

A retired physician, Dad wanted to "stay ahead" of any possible infection by treating it early. This seemed to me harmless enough. In fact, I suspected that the antibiotic had a placebo effect on Dad; he invariably reported that it quickly made him feel much better. But, after several requests for these prescriptions, I discovered just how much of a placebo the antibiotic really was: It made Dad high. (Mild euphoria is one of the "quiet" forms of delirium.) My initial reaction was permissive—given Dad's depressing medical condition, I figured he could use a few "highs"—but soon it became clear that the drug also slurred his speech, unsteadied his gait, and accentuated his irascibility. I stopped the antibiotic and tried to find other ways to lighten his load, give him some laughs. (Because Dad was legally blind, audio books and comedy shows on the radio helped the most.) But none of them matched the high he got from that antibiotic. When I took it away, he missed it.

I had missed it, too. So had the local pharmacist. Neither of us knew that this particular antibiotic could cause delirium. In fact, any drug can do it. *Any drug.* Little wonder, in our "pharmaceutical" society, that so many old people today fall and break their hips.

Or lose their marbles.

For those next few days, Martha's delirium persisted. If we were going to pursue a physical cause of her symptoms, she needed a myelogram. But, given the risk and discomfort of that procedure, we needed her permission to do it, and she was in no condition to consent to anything. Most of the time she was sleepy or quietly confused, especially during the day, but at night she drove the nurses crazy with her agitation and hallucinations. That first night her children took turns staying with her in her hospital room, hoping it would help. But all it did was scare them even more. The next night, they stayed away. It can take a few days, I told them, for the effects of the drugs to clear.

So we waited. While we did, the orthopedic and neurological consultants coalesced around the spinal stenosis hypothesis as the best explanation for Martha's symptoms. Nerve pain is the worst pain of all. If the nerves to Martha's legs were being pinched every time she stood to walk, it made perfect sense that she was refusing to get out of her chair; it would hurt like hell. If this was her problem, strong pain medicine clearly wasn't the answer; the resulting delirium would be even more debilitating than not being able to stand or walk. We couldn't just treat Martha's symptoms. We had to find the cause. All agreed that the myelogram was the logical next step.

But if we found the cause—if the myelogram proved the diagnosis of spinal stenosis—what would we do? In those days, surgery for this condition required a team of orthopedic surgeons (experts about the bones and ligaments of the spine) and neurosurgeons (experts about the nerves and spinal cord). It was a big deal: complex, lengthy surgery, risky for any patient. But an eighty-year-old woman with a bad heart who needed blood-thinner drugs? Who, delirious and bedridden, now looked like hell? The cardiologists and Anesthesia guys didn't say much; they just rolled their eyes, reiterated the risks, and waited for the rest of us to decide.

It was the radiologists who brought us all together. They said we're not doing the myelogram unless we know it will make a difference. Why put the patient through the risks of a cervical myelogram, Peter Spiegel asked me, if you're not going to fix what you find? Spiegel, Dartmouth's chief of Radiology, was right about this. And even if I had thought he was wrong, I knew I couldn't convince him otherwise. Spiegel was an old-fashioned radiologist, one who saw himself as an integral part of a team trying to do the right thing for every patient. He was proud of radiology's remarkable, and growing, contributions to scientific medical care. In Spiegel's view, radiologists weren't simply highly paid technicians who interpreted body images to help the "real doctors" make diagnoses and plan treatments. For him, radiologists were real doctors, too; they also needed to see the big picture, understand the complexities of the patient's problem, to decide how best they could help. Spiegel refused to let the internists or the surgeons take him (or any of his radiologists) for granted.

I had learned this lesson several years before when caring for a patient with life-threatening pulmonary embolism (blood clots in the lungs) who wasn't responding well to treatment. I was worried, not only because the patient was a medical malpractice attorney from Washington, D.C., but also because I wasn't absolutely sure I had made the correct diagnosis. In the middle of the night, I asked Spiegel (the on-call radiologist) to come back into the hospital to perform a pulmonary arteriogram, a difficult invasive procedure not often done (but the only way to be certain about the diagnosis). After listening to my dilemma on the phone, Spiegel agreed to get out of bed and spend most of the night in the hospital on one condition: if I agreed to be there with him. He didn't need me (and I couldn't help him) to do the arteriogram test itself. Spiegel insisted that I have a sleepless night, too, because he wanted to find out how badly I thought the patient needed the procedure—right now, at midnight. As it turned out, the arteriogram made all the difference for the patient, and not a minute too soon. Spiegel and I both learned some things that night.

So now I couldn't just stay on the sidelines, waiting for the specialists to do their thing with Martha. I had to step in, orchestrate their various opinions and risk assessments and leanings. While we all waited anxiously for Martha's head to clear, I met repeatedly with the orthopods and the neurosurgeons and the cardiologists to get consensus about what to do. We needed a plan. We needed a commitment, shared by the whole team: Go or no go?

Every day, Mark asked me about Martha's digitalis. He knew she needed it, an essential medication for her heart condition. I reassured him that we had stopped all "psychoactive" medications, including the pain medicine and sleeping pill that seemed to have precipitated Martha's delirium. But, each day, Mark questioned whether we were doing enough. I sympathized—how could I not?—but I didn't stop Martha's digitalis. She had used it for years and she needed it now more than ever. But this didn't make my wait any less fretful.

After three days of delirium, Martha seemed herself again. She still looked like hell—seventy-two hours of hallucinations, agitation, and sleep deprivation take a lot out of you at age eighty—but she knew where she was, she knew me and her children. It took a while to explain to her how she had lost three whole days but finally she took our word for it. The surgeons and cardiologists didn't like what they saw, but, in the end, they agreed to give the myelogram a go because they took Martha's word for it. In fact, as it turned out, it wasn't just that they believed Martha. They believed *in* Martha.

Dick Saunders, the chief of Neurosurgery, and Pete Hall, the orthopedic surgeon on the case, agreed that spinal stenosis *could* explain Martha's pain, but the only way to know for sure was to see whether Martha improved after surgery. Even if the myelogram test could be performed safely—and even if it clearly showed stenosis of the spinal canal—this wouldn't prove that spinal stenosis was the *cause* of Martha's pain. In the past several years, improved CT scan machines had shown that many patients—especially elderly patients like Martha with severe arthritis—have stenosis of the spinal canal that causes *no symptoms at all*. Merely seeing a narrowed spinal canal on a myelogram doesn't mean it needs fixing.

In the end, what sealed the deal was common sense. Saunders and Hall, the surgeons, wanted to know one thing: Why now? Martha had had arthritis in her spine for decades, but she began experiencing her current symptoms just a few weeks ago. Why now?

The surgeons couldn't ask Martha, so they asked her daughter, In the time leading up to your mother's current illness, did anything unusual happen that might explain a worsening of her arthritic spine? It seems so obvious, so easy, after the fact. But asking the right question at the right time needs knowing *why* it's the right question—and sometimes that's not easy at all. After Margaret remembered that Martha had taken a fall eight weeks ago in her bathroom, we asked the radiologists to reconstruct the computerized images of Martha's spinal CT scan and saw a fracture through one of her spinal joints. These images couldn't show for sure whether she had spinal stenosis—only the myelogram could tell us that—but they showed *why* Martha might have developed the symptoms of spinal stenosis so recently. (Afterward, Margaret said it never occurred to her to connect the two: Martha's back pain from her fall had improved before her legs ever started hurting.)

This was good enough for the surgeons. Now it all made sense. So, if the myelogram showed something fixable, they agreed to try to fix it. As they delivered this opinion to Margaret, both surgeons looked admiringly at Martha, dozing fitfully again. If your mom gutted it out at home for eight weeks with a fractured spine, Saunders told Margaret, and she never even asked for help, the least we can do now is give her the benefit of the doubt. Let's do this.

The next day Martha was higher than a kite again, stoned on pain medicine. Spiegel and his radiology team had had to give her lots of drugs just so she could tolerate the contortions they put her through during the myelogram procedure. But she had done well, no bleeding or other complications.

Mark wanted to see the pictures himself. Saunders and Spiegel showed him what a normal myelogram looks like. Then they showed him Martha's. Mark didn't need any convincing. An engineer could see as well as a neurosurgeon where the nerves to Martha's legs were being pinched inside the spinal canal, the column of X-ray dye twisted and constricted by a perfect storm of old degenerated discs, protuberant arthritic bones, and the latest insult: scarring, swelling, and slippage around that recently fractured spinal joint.

What Mark wanted to know was whether Saunders and Hall could fix it. And whether Martha would survive the operation.

The answer to your first question is Yes, I think so, Saunders said.

And will she make it through the surgery? Mark asked.

I can't answer that, Saunders said, and neither can anyone else. Clearly, there are major risks. But if your mom decides to give it a go, we'll do our best.

We were lucky to have surgeons like Saunders and Hall, skilled technicians who were willing to operate on high-risk patients if, on balance, this made sense to the patient. The surgeons at Dartmouth were not unique in this regard. The post–World War II surgical culture had produced many surgeons willing to "do our best" even when they knew that their best might not be good enough. But this culture had begun to change recently. Many surgeons wouldn't have touched Martha with a ten-foot pole. She was old, she was complicated, and the odds were high that she wouldn't do well. Even if the surgical procedure itself went well, Martha could easily end up crippled, stroked out, or dead. Many surgeons didn't want their fingerprints on cases like those. (Insurers had begun talking about publishing "report cards" of surgeons' success rates to help patients decide who the "best" surgeons were. An unintended consequence was that many surgeons then began shying away from the high-risk cases.) But for Saunders and Hall and many other Dartmouth surgeons it wasn't about ego or statistics showing their operative "success rates." It was all about the patient.

I wasn't a surgeon but I knew how hard this could be. You don't spend the best years of your life working tirelessly to become a surgeon so you can use your hard-won skills on hopeless cases. You do it because you want to fix people; you want to help them. So, when you ask a surgeon to join a battle that might lose the war, it can be a hard sell. Had Martha's case been hopeless, even Saunders and Hall would have refused to operate. Surgery, like all medical treatment, is about probabilities; it takes guts—and a special kind of selflessness—to offer a patient hope when surgical success is improbable but the nonsurgical alternatives are even worse.

Just a few weeks before, I had asked the heart surgeons to do this for Joe Blackburn. Joe's chances had been even worse than Martha's, but the principle—and the admiration I felt for my surgical colleagues—was the same.

Joe was a retired oil executive who had moved to Vermont five years ago. He was a tall, slow-talkin' Texan who'd had his aortic valve replaced ten years before by Dr. DeBakey's famous surgical team in Houston. He was otherwise a healthy, happy-go-lucky guy who loved to fly-fish and hunt in the Green Mountains. Until this past summer when he began to feel tired, he'd never needed more from me than an occasional checkup. Just a few weeks later, Jim was in Dartmouth's coronary care unit, dying.

At first, it hadn't seemed serious at all. Over the summer, Joe had looked okay, his heart sounded fine, and he had no fever or abnormal blood tests. We tried stopping several medications he took that can cause fatigue as a side effect, one at a time, to see which one was making him tired. But when he came back a few weeks later, he looked terrible—gaunt, fearful, ten years older. I put him in the hospital. His prosthetic heart valve was infected—probably it had been infected for weeks—and now, despite the appropriate antibiotics and maximal medical therapy, he was failing. His infection, called subacute bacterial endocarditis, wouldn't clear. Fluid was backing up into his lungs. His kidneys had begun to fail. His only hope was to surgically replace his infected heart valve with a new one, an operation that rarely succeeded because the new valve, when sewn into ratty infected heart tissue, often became infected, too. In Joe's case, the chance of successful surgery was maybe 10 percent. But it was his only chance, because without surgery his probability of survival was zero.

As usual, this all came to a head late at night. Joe had gone into pulmonary edema—he was drowning in his own body fluids—and we'd had to put him on a breathing machine. He was awake but couldn't talk with the breathing tube down his throat, so he wrote notes to me and his wife to answer our questions about what he wanted to do. We could snow him with morphine and he would die painlessly or the surgeons could take him to the operating room tonight, where the ultimate outcome would likely be the same. I could offer Joe this choice only because Bob Sargent, the cardiac surgeon on call, had just told me over the phone, *We'll give it a shot if he gives the okay. Just make sure he and his wife understand the odds. Call me back.*

Joe made it out of the operating room but died twenty-four hours later. His wife was expecting the worst—Sargent had prepared her—but she was grateful beyond words. She told Bob that DeBakey couldn't have done better and Sargent was grateful for that. Joe became a negative statistic in Sargent's surgical success rate for aortic valve replacements. But Sargent had known this was likely to happen when he agreed to operate. It was Joe's only chance, so Sargent put Joe's interests ahead of his own.

Saunders and Hall could have said no to Martha, too. Too risky, they could have said. But they didn't say that.

Instead, they asked me: *What does Martha want to do?*

Martha had given the go-ahead for the myelogram. But now she was delirious again from all the drugs she'd needed to get her through the procedure. So we waited again.

Her days of delirium—and the uncertainty about her future—had been torturous for her children. Lying in her hospital bed, disheveled and confused, Martha looked even older than her eighty years and much frailer. Her grip on life itself seemed no less tenuous than her grip on reality. She had a catheter in her bladder now, her urine draining into a bag by the side of her bed. The nurses rolled her over frequently and checked her, cleaning her up when she soiled herself. She had intravenous lines in both arms, one to hydrate her with fluid and nutrients, the other to give a continuous infusion of blood-thinner for her heart. Her arms were black and blue from all the blood tests. An oxygen cannula in her nose dangled awkwardly from her ears. To Margaret and Mark and John, Martha not only didn't act like their mother, she didn't look like her either.

Margaret was terrified that her mother would die, either from the surgical procedure itself or from postoperative complications. As Margaret watched Martha now, so diminished in her delirious state, she could feel her mother slipping away. Would it be so bad, Margaret asked me, if Mom didn't have the operation, if she had to live a bed-to-wheelchair existence? Her arthritis is pretty awful anyway, Margaret reasoned, and she couldn't walk much even before her spine got this bad. Why take the risk of surgery? She might have some good years left without the operation.

Mark saw it differently.

Look at her, he said to Margaret. This is Mom's future? If she can't walk, how will she get to the bathroom? She'll wind up with a permanent catheter, infections, more drugs, maybe this horrible confusion all over again. She'll go stir-crazy, confined to that house, like she does every winter even now. Mom has always valued her independence more than anything else. She'd be miserable knowing she's a burden. She'd rather be dead . . .

Margaret's eyes grew wide.

Mark!

. . . like Dad, Mark said.

Mark! How can you say that!

John, the psychologist, stepped between them. Fighting about it won't help, he said. You're both right. You're both right.

John looked at me.

So what do we do, Brendan?

We don't do anything, John. It doesn't matter what we think. What matters is what your mom thinks.

So, a few days later, when Martha was Martha again, we went through it all with her. The diagnosis: likely correct, but uncertain until she walked again. The surgical option: dangerous, a difficult and prolonged recovery, an unclear prognosis. Her many medical risks: infection, heart failure, stroke, bleeding, delirium, the unknown. The nonsurgical options: physical therapy, a wheelchair, live-in help, some of Mark's gloomy scenarios. And, finally, the generic salve about there being "no right or wrong answer here."

Martha, her wry witty self again, listened carefully to all this, occasionally clucking "Lucky me!" or "Won't that be fun!" She asked a few pointed questions. She asked her children what they thought. They told her. Then she turned to me, a twinkle in her eye.

Well, here we are again, Brendan. Another fine mess I've gotten you into. I think I know what your answer will be but I'm going to ask anyway . . .

Martha . . . I began.

What would you do, Brendan? If you were me?

I wanted to tell her. I'd never thought the doctor should merely lay out the options and then let the patient decide. That's what doctors are for: *to help patients decide.* I knew Martha wouldn't make her decision purely on the basis of my recommendation, as some patients tend to do. She just wanted to know how I saw it. She would weigh my opinion together with the many other factors she considered. But she was struggling. She'd been through an awful lot. Her own children were divided, their emotions fraught. Martha knew this might turn out badly whatever she decided and she didn't want guilt or regret or recrimination to be the legacy she left her family, not after what had happened to Fred. In asking my opinion, Martha was looking for a crutch, a helping hand. A friend.

I couldn't do it. Not there, not then, Margaret and John looking on, holding their breath, Mark staring me down.

You'll want to sleep on this, Martha. It's your call.

But late that evening I returned. Her children had gone home, awaiting Martha's decision. I had come back to make sure she wasn't flying again. Delirium can be intermittent, punctuated by lucid intervals when the patient appears completely normal. I needed to make sure that Martha had fully recovered—and that her decision, whatever it would be, was clearheaded. Although I tried to conceal my examination of her mental status as simple chitchat, Martha knew I was checking her out to see if she had all her marbles.

She was clear as a bell. This established, Martha smiled her wry little smile and looked around her private room.

So, finally, we are alone, she said.

Mmm.

She looked me straight in the eye.

It would help me to know, Brendan. If you were in my shoes, *what would you do?*

I wanted to help. I thought I owed her that much. So I told her what I would do.

The next morning, Martha signed the surgical consent forms. Margaret was in tears. She and John gave Martha a hug. Mark looked as if he hadn't slept much. He seemed a lot less sure of himself than he had before.

I suspect that Martha had been leaning toward surgery before I leaned that way, too. But I didn't ask her about this. And she didn't tell. She kept it to herself, right to the end.

One year before Fred died, David Hilfiker, a family physician working in rural Minnesota, electrified the medical profession by confessing serious, sometimes fatal errors he had made in caring for his patients. Published in the *New England Journal of Medicine*, "Facing Our Mistakes" describes in heartrending detail Hilfiker's discovery that he has mistakenly aborted a live thirteen-week-old fetus (whose parents badly wanted the child) and his struggle to deal emotionally and spiritually with his guilt about it. Clearly a competent, dedicated, and caring doctor, Hilfiker finds that he cannot forgive himself for his error, despite "reassurances from the pathologist that it is statistically 'impossible' for four consecutive pregnancy tests to be negative during a viable pregnancy," the facts in this tragic case. Devastated, he concludes that no post facto reconstruction of the events "can obscure the hard reality: I have killed their baby."

Worse, after confessing his culpability in this and other cases, Hilfiker admitted:

> The medical profession simply seems to have no place for its mistakes. There is no permission given to talk about errors, no way of venting emotional responses. Indeed . . . I lapse into neurotic behavior to deal with my anxiety and guilt. Little wonder that physicians are . . . defensive about our judgments . . . blame the patient or the previous physician when things go wrong . . . yell at nurses for our mistakes . . . have such high rates of alcoholism, drug addiction, and suicide.
>
> At some point we . . . need to find healthy ways to deal with our emotional responses to those errors.

A year later, Hilfiker had left medical practice. He took time off, wrote a book. Its conclusion:

> Ultimately, I believe there is no solution to the problem. All of us who attempt to heal the wounds of others will ourselves be wounded; it is, after all, inherent in the relationship. . . .
>
> We can either fight against the pain, and in so fighting, bring ourselves to a numb cynicism or a fragile despair, or we can accept it, become one with it, and allow it to minister to others.

For centuries, medicine had been considered more than a "helping profession"; it was a vocation, akin in many respects to religious ministry. But, in our increasingly secularized society, even the (non-religious) "Samaritan" role of doctors—empathizing with and helping others, selflessly—has been devalued, sometimes even ridiculed in the ascendant business culture of medicine. This new culture has even changed our vocabulary. Doctors and nurses have become "providers" of medical care, itself now a "commodity." Patients have become "customers," the "consumers" of medical care.

Yet health providers still feel guilty when things go wrong with their patients. Guilt is about self-disappointment, the anguish I feel when I fail to live up to my own standard of what I ought to be. This feeling is a moral phenomenon: Guilt is all about "ought"—one's sense of good and bad, right and wrong. But doctors' mistakes are not *moral* failings (except in very rare cases in which a doctor's misdeed is intentional or callous). Surely these mistakes deserve discovery, remediation, and, if feasible, prevention. But do they require *forgiveness*? "We forgive the *wicked*," a wise man said, "but we *excuse* the ignorant." Making a mistake, even a "stupid" mistake, doesn't make a doctor wicked.

Nevertheless, many doctors, like Hilfiker, have become the "second victim" of medical error. Some of us, guilt-ridden and gun-shy, may be too far gone to help.

Fewer than 10 percent of all U.S. medical school graduates today become primary care physicians for adults, a precipitous (and accelerating) decline from a few decades ago. Hardest hit have been the ranks of family medicine doctors (a group that has contributed disproportionately to the care of patients in underserved areas). Many of these doctors, especially those who serve in rural communities where specialists' help is far away, suffer the same wounds and bear the same burdens that David Hilfiker bore decades ago. These folks, in my view, are the unsung heroes of American medicine. The *breadth* of their responsibilities—they deliver babies, staff emergency rooms and ICUs, perform minor surgery, help dying patients pass peacefully—makes theirs the most demanding job any doctor can do. It can also be the most rewarding job—emotionally, not financially.

And yet we're losing the doctors who do this work—and we're losing them fast. Simply throwing more money at them won't fix this. As a society, we must also encourage them, appreciate them, thank them for their service. And, yes, sometimes, we must forgive them, too.

I left Dartmouth not long after the events described here. I didn't uproot my family and my work because I couldn't live with the mistakes I'd made. What happened to Fred and Martha became a part of me, a part I didn't want to forget or deny. Certainly, I wished I had done better for them. But, for me, the question became *how* I could do better, having learned that even dedicated, gifted doctors inevitably harm some people in the process of helping others.

Perhaps later than some in my profession, I had seen how utterly audacious are the ambitions of modern medicine. To unravel the mysteries of biology and human disease—the product of eons of evolution—and then to dare to *intervene?* Mess with Mother Nature? Have the balls to battle the dragon of death? This was hubris beyond hubris, the stuff of Sophocles and Icarus. For me, now a scarred veteran in a brave new post-Hippocratic world, medicine's venerable first principle had become an empty shibboleth, an inside joke. *First, do no harm?* Oh, please. *Of course, we do harm.* If we didn't do harm, we couldn't do good.

I gave up primary care, largely because I had too much respect for it to think I could do it well part-time. I took a job as the chief of medicine at one of the University of Rochester's teaching hospitals, where my other responsibilities precluded full-time clinical practice. Naïvely, I thought I could still be a "real doctor" while devoting a lot of my time to teaching, administration, and research. For the first two years, I managed a small panel of my own primary care patients. These folks were easy to find and happy to have me; our hospital served Rochester's impoverished inner city, where many people had no doctor at all. But I found out soon enough that I was kidding myself. Unavailable to my patients too often, including times when they needed me most, I found I couldn't do the job of a "real doctor" part-time.

Fred and Martha helped me through this transition. They had taught me that it was the medical care "system" that had failed them, not just one doctor. And so, I, together with many colleagues, tried to build a better system for inner-city Rochester. We created a neighborhood network of about twenty primary care practices with a shared clinical information system. We funded patients' preventive health care with millions of dollars in government research grants. We hired and trained inner-city folks to help their neighbors "navigate" our health care system more effectively. As a result, more African-American women got mammograms. More black and Latino babies got immunized. More elderly and ill folks talked to their doctors about end-of-life care. And my own former panel of primary care patients got doctors who were always there for them. I maintained my own clinical skills by carving out stretches of time to work on the hospital's busy inpatient service. I became a "hospitalist"—the name itself wouldn't be invented until several years later—the same role I had hoped Paul would pioneer at Dartmouth. Inner-city Rochester was a long way from the Ivy League and Fowler House, but my years as a real doctor had prepared me well for my new role in my new place.

I lost touch with Margaret and her family until several years later, when she wrote me a letter after I had moved to Chicago to become chief of medicine at Cook County Hospital, the famous (and sometimes infamous) "mother" of American public hospitals. In its heyday the largest and busiest hospital in the United States, County was a huge, sprawling enterprise that struggled to care for the vast underserved patient population of Chicagoland's poor and ethnic minorities. Even Margaret, still living in bucolic Vermont, knew that County must be, as she wrote, "quite an adventure." She enclosed photos from a recent family wedding. There was the flower garden in front of Fred and Martha's house. Those twin Adirondack chairs. Mountains in the distance, the river valley far below, the high meadow of my dreams. One of the photos is a group portrait of twenty-eight people that includes all of Fred and Martha's children, grandchildren, and great-grandchildren. (Margaret provided a "key" to the photo that identified them all, from grandson Fred to great-granddaughter Molly.) Martha herself is in the back row, lovely as ever in a violet dress and a string of pearls, standing next to Mark. No wheelchair for Martha even now, almost ten years after her spine surgery. Nearing ninety, she didn't look it. She was smiling ear to ear, cracking a joke just as the photographer said cheese.

The only one missing was Fred.

I wrote back, told Martha and Margaret a little of what I was doing in Chicago, how my experience with Fred had opened my eyes to new challenges and opportunities. As I had done in Rochester, I was trying to improve the system in Chicago, too, working with a team of smart, dedicated colleagues. A big part of this involved learning how to deliver care more cost-efficiently—we were dealing with limited resources, staggering demand, and political gridlock in the County government—all the while trying to preserve the personal, trusting doctor-patient relationships that had made County Hospital a special place for generations of Chicagoans. Working together, we were learning to embrace what we didn't know, admit our ignorance and mistakes, share these lessons with each other, all in an effort to do more with less. We won some and we lost some. I told Margaret and Martha that I thought Fred was looking over my shoulder.

Time passed. As my own mother began to lose her memory, when it became clear that Mom had Alzheimer's disease, I often thought of Fred. Mom's strange behavior over the previous several years—the occasional gift that seemed odd, inappropriate; those letters or cards that weren't quite right, not like Mom at all—finally made sense to me, in hindsight. So I wondered, looking back, when did it *begin*? I could only venture a guess. Alzheimer's dementia is insidious. The early clues are subtle, insubstantial, but always, if you look back, you will find them. And when I looked back at Mom, I often found myself looking back at Fred, too. Had Fred survived, would Martha have looked back one day—remembering those phone calls and tangential conversations and unshoveled snow—and concluded: Yes, that was all part of it but, in hindsight, that wasn't the beginning. Had Fred survived—and had his own worst fears about losing his marbles come true—would Martha or Mark or Margaret have realized, as I did with my mother, that Fred's dementia had really begun long before then?

A few years later, Margaret wrote to me again. Martha had died, peacefully at home, surrounded by family. Margaret wanted me to know that Martha had missed me, loved me, even to the end. About Fred, she wanted me to know how "all of us close to him felt tremendous guilt [about his death]; yours perhaps more profound because you were 'supposed to know more.' I have spent a lot of energy trying to sort it all out: reading, therapy, talking with Steve [her husband] and others. My conclusion, which I am now comfortable with, is that Dad was responsible, himself." She enclosed new photos, these from the recent wedding of her son. Everyone was there, except Fred and Martha. It was, Margaret wrote, "one of the happiest times of our lives and very sweet for our family, since many of our gatherings have been sad times." She wished me well.

I didn't write back. What could I say? After all these years, Margaret had finally found some peace. Who was I to turn it upside down again? Sharing my own personal sense of uncertainty and guilt could only hurt her. Was Fred's death caused by medical error, a tragic drug reaction that never should have happened? Or, did he take his life knowingly, to spare himself (and his family) from a long, sad slide into dementia? I would never know.

Still, from time to time, I wondered, fretted, hypothesized. Fred became my cold case: unsolved, new clues less likely to surface with each passing year, and yet . . .

When the Internet was born in the early 1990s, I discovered a memorial tribute to Fred published by the National Academy of Science (Engineering). There I learned about his time at MIT, General Motors, the U.S. Army Air Corps, and Ford. Fred, his eulogist had written:

> . . . had fun with engineering; he built paper and balsa wood airplanes for his children and for the child he kept alive within himself. Some of these planes were propelled with carbon dioxide cartridges and were perhaps the first jet-propelled model airplanes. He built a binary counter as a toy to amuse his grandchildren. . . .
>
> While in his seventies, Fred . . . continued his innovative work in the areas of prosthetic orthopedic bone replacements, music synthesizers, lightweight autos and computerized medical diagnoses.

This last part caught my eye, struck a chord, but at the time I didn't know why.

Then, just a few years ago, I Googled Scott Richardson, a doctor I had known at the University of Rochester. Then at Wright State University, Scott had become an international authority on "evidence-based medicine," the long-overdue idea that doctors' and patients' decisions should be grounded in valid, reliable scientific evidence. In our efforts to upgrade Chicago's public health system, we had embraced "EBM" as a way to analyze and improve our doctors' diagnoses and treatments, understand our mistakes, use medical technology more wisely. I wanted to invite Scott to come to Chicago as a visiting professor, teach us more about these things. I Googled Wright State to find Scott's new address.

By whatever magic Google mixes and matches its finds, there on page one, together with the Wright State University websites, was an entry from the *Dayton Daily News* in 1952 whose author was one Fred Coover. When he was fifteen years old, Fred and his boyhood pals had built a plane.

> Orville Wright was one of the trustees of the school we went to, and it seemed the natural thing to go ask his advice about our plans and ideas. . . . He was kind and natural with us, and talked for hours about aeronautics, the things he and Wilbur did, and the problems they ran into and how they solved them.

Fred never forgot how encouraging and accessible Wright had been, inviting him and his friends on many occasions to talk aeronautics and test their airplane models in the wind tunnel in Wright's personal laboratory. Fred wrote:

> As my family began to grow up, I wanted to ask [Wright] to come over to have Sunday night supper with us. But I was afraid to risk being changed from the boy who was always so welcome without reserve into one of those adults who might want to use him for something. . . .
>
> One night, I drove up to a stop light and waited. Another car drove up beside me. A horn made a little tattoo, and I looked over. It was Orville Wright, and we waved and smiled. I got a thrill out of that, and felt a little remorseful, because I hadn't been to see him for a long time, and he had been sick. "By gosh, I'm going to ask him over to Sunday night supper. . . ."
>
> But two days later, he was dead.

It was Fred's voice, come back to life. I wanted to hear more. And there, on Google's magic carpet ride through cyberspace, was a link to the Smithsonian National Air and Space Museum Library, where Fred's actual voice (and a video clip) has been preserved. There,

Fred's report describes in painstaking detail the tragic series of miscalculations and miscommunications by all involved in Amelia Earhart's historic, doomed attempt to fly around the world in 1937. He began this way:

> Before Miss Earhart took off on her Round-the-World flight she removed from her plane a modern radio compass that had been installed and replaced it with an older, lighter-weight model of much less capability. I am the engineer who had invented and developed the radio compass that was removed, and I discussed its features with Miss Earhart before the installation was made. I have reason to believe that it was the failure of her radio direction-finder to do what the more modern model could have done that caused her to be lost. The story is told herein, and it is plain to see why I have been so very much interested in the subject. . . .
>
> Too much time has elapsed for me to remember when it was that I learned that my device was not on the Earhart plane when it was lost, or even whether it was before or after the takeoff that I learned. But I have been possessed by the desire to know what did happen, and by the wish that things had happened differently.

Just as Fred had been my cold case, Amelia Earhart had been his. For decades, Fred had doggedly pursued the cause of her death. They had grown up in similar circumstances, in the Midwest, a few years apart. Both became pioneers in aviation. Fred knew her, liked her.

> Although she moved in a man's world, and wore men's trousers and wore a short haircut, there was nothing masculine about Miss Earhart. Every inch a lady, she was gracious and quiet-spoken, thoroughly feminine and attractive.

Fred's account of Earhart is a story about ambition and what drives it; the weighing of harms and benefits, risk and reward; failed teamwork; the power and perils of technology; fatal errors, denied and covered up. Amelia Earhart's loss at sea, still unexplained today, haunted Fred for almost fifty years.

As I read Fred's report—his voice so distinctive, risen from the grave—an eerie feeling came over me. At first, I assumed it was because Fred's voice had resurrected Martha's voice, too, drunk with delirium in her hospital room years ago.

Fred, I told you! It's not your fault! It's her own damn fault! Who does she think she is, flying around in men's pants? It's her own damn fault!

But, no, it was something else. When I finished reading Fred's report—sitting in my office, the magnificent Chicago skyline spread out before me—my gaze wandered to a small urn I have kept on my desk for years. It's about the size of a beer stein, dark green in color, its mouth topped with a removable cork plug. Written across the front of the urn, in large inlaid letters, are the words "Lost Marbles." Visitors to my office chuckled when they saw it, assuming it was a joke about the demented Cook County bureaucracy (which I, as its chief of medicine, represented). But the urn had nothing to do with Chicago politics. I had kept it all these years as a reminder of Fred.

Seeing it now, my heart leapt. Urgently, I read Fred's report about Amelia Earhart again. It was written not long before he died, shortly before I met him. If Fred was beginning to lose his marbles when I knew him, surely I would detect signs of it here.

Even after all these years, I wanted desperately to find those inconsistent facts and unsupported allegations, the overwrought reasoning, the telltale lapses in logic. Then, at last, I would know that Fred, even before he met me, had begun his decline. I would know that Fred would have pulled that trigger anyway, digitalis or not.

But no such signs were evident. Fred's report was brilliant, impeccable in every way—his prose style, scientific skepticism, nuanced judgments, even his wise recounting of Pacific Rim geopolitics in the years leading up to Pearl Harbor. A person with incipient dementia can't do this. No way. Fred was getting old, but he certainly hadn't lost any marbles. He concluded his report this way:

Whatever is finally learned about Miss Earhart's last flight, one certainty will always remain, that it was a needless tragedy. . . .

We hope that one day records will be found or released that will reveal the truth about [Miss Earhart's] fate. Meanwhile the memory of a brave and gracious lady remains bright after forty-five years.

In the end, Fred never found out what happened to Amelia Earhart. He never solved his cold case. But he solved mine.

His son Mark had been right all along.

After all my years of wondering, this discovery brought me more relief than anguish. Deep down, I suppose I'd always known it to be true. I had learned a lot from Fred and Martha, lessons that had made me a better doctor, teacher, researcher—maybe even a better man. Martha had trusted me, believed in me, comforted me. Milk spills sometimes no matter what you do. Knowing this had helped me long after I left her. But Fred would have seen it differently, and not just because he had lost the most. Had Fred been saved, had all our errors resulted in a "near miss" rather than a tragedy, Fred would have wanted to fix it, make the "system" safer, better for others. He would have known that you can't perfect medical care today any more than you could guarantee safe passage of a twin-engine monoplane across the Pacific Ocean in 1937. But, if Fred had had the chance, he would have made it better.

And, in his own remarkable way, that's exactly what Fred did.

That day in Chicago, after learning about Fred and Amelia Earhart, I wondered what had become of Mark. A Google link took me to one Mark Coover, an engineer in Ohio, but his photo showed a handsome, smiling guy much younger than the Mark I had known. This was Fred's grandson, the son of John. This Mark is a successful inventor and entrepreneur, the holder of many U.S. patents and the CEO of a big medical device company. One of his inventions is a new technology to treat atrial fibrillation, the heart rhythm abnormality that caused Fred to be treated with digitalis so long ago. Mark's new treatment, which has cured tens of thousands of patients around the world, uses radio waves instead of drugs. Slowly but surely, Mark's efforts are making digitalis obsolete.

Digitalis killed Fred. Now Fred's grandson is killing digitalis.

Part III

NOW

To tear down . . . a system is to attack effects rather than causes; as long as the attack is upon effects only, no change is possible. . . . If a revolution destroys a systematic government, but the systematic patterns of thought that produced that government are left intact, then those patterns will repeat themselves in the succeeding government. There's so much talk about the system. And so little understanding.

—Robert M. Pirsig, *Zen and the Art of Motorcycle Maintenance* (1974)

Part III

NOW

Chapter 8

NEVER SAY NEVER

Practice variations pose a special challenge to medical science. . . . America's medical schools do not teach the skills required to understand patient preferences, evaluate medical practice, assess clinical evidence, design and test clinical pathways, improve quality, and understand the effect of systems of care on clinical practice.

—John E. Wennberg, *Tracking Medicine* (2010)

January 2010. Thursday, 9:50 a.m.

Some people say doctors should keep their professional lives separate from their personal lives. Whoever says so either never practiced medicine or forgets what it's like. Doctors don't live two separate lives. It all comes together, whether we think that's a good idea or not.

I'm in the morgue, not my favorite place. Heads loll, limp and ghoulish, as their bodies are hefted on and off the long chrome dissection tables. Big slabs of human beef, darkening by the minute, glisten under hot white lights. Right now, I'm looking at Ms. Dubois, our elderly Alzheimer's patient whose giant heart clot we had seen on her echocardiogram last week in the ED. Now, here, her heart has been cut out of her chest and put on a small examining table. My team and I gather around with the pathologist. The rest of Ms. Dubois lies next to us, her body respectfully covered with sheets, her face only a little more vacant than it was yesterday before she died. It wasn't her dementia that killed her. Alzheimer's disease empties you out, leaving behind a husk where the person used to be, but it doesn't kill you. Something else—a heart attack, a stroke, pneumonia—does that. We've come down to the morgue to see what got Ms. Dubois.

But instead of seeing Ms. Dubois under these sheets, I'm seeing my own mother. It's like the pathologist is holding Mom's heart in his hand.

As I was leaving the hospital last night, Ruth called from Shelter Island to tell me that Mom had just been taken to the hospital again. Another fainting spell, much like that first one just ten days ago. Again, she had seemed unhurt after regaining consciousness on the bathroom floor, but Ruth did the right thing, called the island's rescue team to ferry Mom across the bay to the little hospital in Greenport. The ED doc there said she looked fine, her examination and initial heart tests all normal, but he had called in a cardiologist. Because this second fainting spell sounded suspiciously like the first one, the ED doc wondered if she needed a cardiac pacemaker. Ruth said Dad was very worried and refusing to take his pain medicine until he knew Mom would be all right. So I got in my car and made the two-hour drive to Greenport to see Mom and the cardiologist.

When I examined Mom myself at the hospital, her blood pressure dropped when I stood her up from her bed and she said her head felt heavy. This meant she may have fainted simply because she was so "deconditioned." (She rarely got up from her bed or chair at home.) The cardiologist, a young guy who seemed thoughtful and competent, wasn't so sure. He hadn't seen Mom the last time she'd fainted but he shook his head when he heard that, back then, we had decided to ignore her seven-second cardiac arrest, attributing it to the blood pressure drug Mom had received. He shook his head again when I told him what kind of shape Dad was in and that I wasn't sure Mom would want a pacemaker even if she needed one. He wished me luck when I told him I would try to discuss the situation with Dad.

As it turned out, when I got over to the island on the midnight ferry, Dad was in rough shape himself. There was no way to talk to him about Mom. He was grimacing, moaning in pain—this was highly unusual for him, a stoical, tight-lipped guy—and, though he said it was his hip (where his bladder cancer had spread), when I poked on him it was his lower abdomen that was sore to touch. Ruth confessed that Dad hadn't had a bowel movement in several days. We turned him gently on his side, but Dad shouted out—any movement of his hip was excruciating—and he groaned each time my gloved finger pulled out those rocks of stool from his rectum, something I had done a hundred times before but never for my own father. When it was done and we rolled him back, he grunted hard again but was better after the morphine kicked in. Soon he was sleeping, a welcome sight except for that dark red blood streaming out of his bladder catheter, flecks of clot swimming in the big plastic drainage bag hanging off his hospital bed rail. For months now I had asked myself, How long can he go on like this? One thing was certain: Dad couldn't help much with the decision about Mom. I would have to do that alone.

After a few hours of restless sleep, I got up, checked to see if Dad was still breathing, called the nurses' station at the hospital to check on Mom, and caught the first ferry off the island before dawn. On the highway in the dark, I thought long and hard about my parents as I sped back to Manhattan, beating most of the morning rush-hour traffic.

I arrived just in time to quickly eyeball my team's new admissions in the ED before rounds. I warned myself to be extra careful; at my age, I don't do well on three hours of sleep. But the adrenaline kept me sharp enough as we rounded on our twenty patients, examining them, answering their questions, figuring out what to do next. I forgot about Mom and Dad, temporarily. But then we saw Mr. Mukaj, out of bed, walking down the hall and laughing with his beautiful granddaughter, planning their flight home to Croatia. I couldn't help wondering: Should I have pushed Dad harder to have an operation? Both men have an incurable bleeding bladder cancer that has metastasized to the right hip bone, but they're headed in opposite directions. Thanks to very aggressive treatment and more than a little luck, Mr. Mukaj is on the upswing, at least for a while.

And now, here in the morgue with Ms. Dubois, it's Mom I'm thinking about.

With a twist of his wrist, the pathologist flips open Ms. Dubois's disembodied heart, filleted along a plane that best shows her mitral valve. Tina gasps when she sees Ms. Dubois's artificial heart valve. The rest of us, including myself, are dumbstruck.

I haven't seen a valve like Ms. Dubois's since I was a medical student, observing open-heart surgery for the first time. Then, forty years ago, C. Walton Lillehei had stepped back from a gaping chest cavity on his operating table, pointed down at his patient's beating heart, and asked the crowd of observers all around him, "Have you ever seen anything more beautiful?" Considered by many the "father of open-heart surgery," Lillehei meant what he said. After doing thousands of these operations, he remained genuinely awed by what he did. That day, he had held up the old-fashioned prosthetic valve for all to see—it looks like a miniature metal birdcage with a Ping-Pong ball inside—and then threw it scornfully at his scrub nurse. Reaching for the new floating-disc valve that he had invented himself, Lillehei intoned, "Behold the future . . . until a better one comes along." A few hours later, the patient had a crisp metal wafer where his floppy mitral valve used to be—and a new life.

But it's not the antiquity of Ms. Dubois's heart valve that shocks us at the autopsy table. Until she wound up in the dementia unit of a local nursing home a few years ago, Ms. Dubois's old birdcage valve had served her well for decades.

Jeez, Tina says now, peering intently into Ms. Dubois's heart. The whole thing came off!

Hmmph, Dan says, unable to avert his eyes from the sight of it. I didn't know that could happen.

I didn't know it could happen either. The thrombus itself, a round red glob of congealed blood about two inches in diameter, is impressive enough, huge as heart clots go. But we'd known how big it was right from day one and we'd also known why it was there; by mistake, her blood-thinner medication had been underdosed for the past few weeks at her nursing home, putting her at risk for a stroke. Part of the clot could break off from her heart and travel through her circulation into her brain. On top of her advanced dementia, a stroke was the last thing Ms. Dubois needed. Treatment with an intravenous blood-thinner, as we had done these past several days, almost always helps to dissolve the clot and prevent such complications. No one had anticipated that the whole clot could break off. But there it is, the entire blood clot, dislodged from the wall of Ms. Dubois's heart, stuck in the struts of her old metal valve. It fills the old birdcage completely, obstructing any output of blood from her heart.

No wonder she couldn't be resuscitated yesterday after her cardiac arrest. There's no way to treat this; prevention is the only hope. That's why we'd needed to see Ms. Dubois's autopsy. Had she died without an autopsy, Tina and Dan and Ashley probably wouldn't remember her a few months from now, just another old lady whose time had come. But they'll remember her now. They'll remember that this is what can happen when mistakes are made, when meticulous care is not taken to manage risky medicines like blood-thinners. I don't know whether the nursing home will get sued for its error, but I make a mental note to call our hospital's legal counsel after I call Ms. Dubois's son to inform him about the autopsy findings. And I remind myself to tell Brian what we've seen.

Brian, our senior resident, isn't with us this morning, but he'll want to know. The schedule says he's on duty today, but Brian has a good excuse. He's up on the sixteenth floor, lying in a hospital bed himself.

Brian came to work very early yesterday, about 5:00 a.m., just as the code team was calling it quits on Ms. Dubois. She'd been doing fine, her blood thinned by the intravenous medication exactly as planned. We'd never been able to have a real conversation with her—she was very confused—but there was something charming about her nonetheless. Every day we'd seen her, I thought of Mom. (Is this how bad she'll get? Worse, maybe?) She reminded Brian of his grandma, and when he'd come in yesterday morning, he'd been shocked to find her suddenly gone. Had we done something wrong? he wondered. Could we have prevented this?

The code team couldn't say. She had been sleeping when the alarms went off at 4:00 a.m. Her cardiac monitor showed ventricular fibrillation, a chaotic heart rhythm of disorganized electrical activity incompatible with life. Not a bad way to go—peacefully, in her sleep.

But Ms. Dubois was a "full code." Despite her advanced age and severe dementia, the resuscitation team did the whole deal: They put a breathing tube down her throat to ventilate her lungs; they pumped hard on her chest for more than an hour (at autopsy, she had three broken ribs); they shocked her heart at least a dozen times with powerful electrical currents; they stabbed big-bore needles into her neck and groin; they gave her powerful drugs to try to restart her heart, get a pulse, make a blood pressure. None of it worked, not even briefly. They pronounced her dead just as Brian arrived.

Afterward, Brian and I talked to Ms. Dubois's son. We offered our condolences, we explained the cardiac arrest as best we could, and asked his permission to do the autopsy; then, maybe we could tell him for sure what had happened. He said he had to think about it, but, when he called us back later in the morning, he agreed to the autopsy on one condition: He wanted his mother's birdcage heart valve as a keepsake. *Can you do that?* he asked me.

I wasn't sure what to make of this. When Ms. Dubois was hospitalized last week, we learned that her son had been accused of elder abuse a year ago. Apparently, this was the reason his mother had been moved to a nursing home in the first place, some kind of legal compromise, but still the son retained his power of attorney for all her affairs. He was the one who had rejected our do-not-resuscitate suggestions last week; he had insisted that we do "everything" medically possible for his mother, even if her heart stopped. Everything, that is, except surgery. He had refused to allow even a consultation with the heart surgeons, to ask what they thought would be the best treatment for her giant clot. This was not a totally illogical combination of decisions but the whole story was odd. And now he wants his mother's heart valve as a souvenir?

Why, may I ask, do you want it, sir?

Why? Because it's a real antique! I don't think they even make that kind anymore, do they?

It took a good part of the day yesterday to straighten this out and, by the time Brian finally obtained official permission to get the autopsy done, he looked a little peaked himself. He said something about having a "GI bug," so I didn't make much of it when he went home a little early. But late last night Brian was back in the hospital, on an operating table himself, his appendix ready to burst. When I checked on him this morning, he looked fine. In fact, fresh out of general anesthesia, Brian was concerned about *me* (*You look tired, Dr. Reilly*), and he asked about Ms. Dubois.

Now, standing here with the rest of my team, looking directly into Ms. Dubois's heart, I'm not sure what to tell Brian. Because Dan, our intern with M.D. and Ph.D. degrees who does cancer research, has asked exactly the right question.

Does this happen?

At first, his question seems silly. The answer appears pretty obvious when you're standing there, seeing it with your own eyes, this big glob of clot filling that little birdcage. *Does it happen? There it is, Dan: It happened.*

But, like all good scientists, Dan knows that causation is the hardest thing to prove. He's not questioning what we see; he's questioning whether what we see is the *cause* of Ms. Dubois's death. He points to her heart, cradled now in the pathologist's hands, and lays out an alternative hypothesis. Fact: She had a bad heart. Fact: As bad hearts often do, hers went into ventricular fibrillation. Hypothesis: The code team, by pumping on her chest and shocking her with the defibrillator machine, dislodged the big clot in her heart. It happened *after* her cardiac arrest; it didn't *cause* her cardiac arrest. To Dan's way of thinking, what we're seeing now is an epiphenomenon, an artifact.

The pathologist admits he can't answer the question with certainty. But that's Dan's point: We have no reason to believe that our own treatment (the standard treatment in cases like this) was a mistake or that speedier removal of Ms. Dubois's heart clot would have made any difference. We did what we could. It wasn't enough. In the end, it never is.

We can't say for sure why Ms. Dubois died, but Brian needs to know that his hard work yesterday to obtain permission for the autopsy was worth the effort. Some mysteries in medicine remain unsolved even after you look under every rock. But if you don't lift the rocks, you don't learn. Maybe that clot did break off and kill Ms. Dubois. But we don't know this any more certainly than we know whether Brian's long day at work yesterday precipitated his appendicitis. Sometimes, the best we can say is: *Could be*. So often, as in this case, medicine is all about maybe. Biology isn't physics. Medicine isn't math.

When I call Ms. Dubois's son, I'll tell him he can come in and pick up his mother's antique heart valve whenever he likes. After we clean the clot out of it, of course.

Right now, though, Tina is putting her hand into Ms. Dubois's heart. With her gloved finger, Tina traces a line from the wall of its left atrium into the opening of the right pulmonary vein, the big blood vessel that brings oxygenated blood into the heart from the right lung.

Here, you see? Tina says excitedly. This is what I was talking about in Mr. Warner's case. It's a straight shot, see? If he's eroded his posterior valve leaflet, it's a straight shot into his right lung, straight back through the pulmonary vein. That's why it's unilateral!

Mr. Warner, our elderly guy with chronic HIV infection and acute bacterial endocarditis, had another rough night last night. Tina, on call for our team, finally was able to help him sleep, but she didn't sleep a wink herself. She'd had an idea about Mr. Warner. So, despite her busy night, she hunted down her idea.

Something was going on in Mr. Warner's right lung that we hadn't been able to figure out. He'd been intermittently short of breath for the last few nights. His chest X-ray showed something new in his right lung that seemed to wax and wane, coming and going. We'd done more tests, consulted more specialists. No one had a good answer yet. Last night, Tina began to wonder if it was his heart, even though his blood cultures had remained negative on antibiotics, typically a good sign in patients with bacterial endocarditis. Her idea was highly unlikely. Heart valve malfunctions can cause blood to regurgitate into the lungs, but when this occurs, it happens to *both* lungs, not just one. However, on rounds this morning, Tina showed us copies of two case reports from Belgium and Texas published years ago in obscure medical journals. (Google found them for her last night when she searched "unilateral pulmonary edema.") Both case reports described patients like Mr. Warner, patients with a leaky mitral valve that caused "eccentric" regurgitation of blood into only one lung, not both. This was so rare—I had never heard of it, much less seen it—that, almost certainly, it was not Mr. Warner's problem. But if Tina is right, we can't afford to miss it. If she's right, Mr. Warner will need surgery to replace his infected heart valve with a new valve, a dangerous operation. And he will need it soon.

We should know today, I thought. After seeing him this morning, we'd scheduled Mr. Warner to undergo another echocardiogram, his fourth in ten days. This would be a repeat of the "transesophageal" echo he had a week ago, the kind in which the cardiac ultrasound probe is snaked down the patient's throat into his esophagus to obtain ultrasound movies from *behind* his heart. (The esophagus, as it descends through the chest before connecting with the stomach, passes directly behind the heart.) If Tina is right, that's where the *Staphylococcus* bacteria have eaten a hole in Mr. Warner's heart, clear through the rear leaflet of his mitral valve. If the hole is there, the transesophageal echocardiogram will show it, a narrow jetstream of blood spurting from his heart into his right lung. In fact, that's what cardiologists call this phenomenon: a jet. On the ultrasound machine, it looks like the exhaust from an F-15 streaking across the sky, its plume of smoke a trail of blood.

As Tina explains her idea visually, pointing out the relevant anatomical landmarks in Ms. Dubois's dead heart, my own thoughts wander. I'm seeing Mr. Mukaj—and Dad. Just an hour ago on rounds, Mr. Mukaj had been up, walking, using a four-legged walker with wheels. None of us thought he would ever look this good—certainly not now, just ten days after his dilemma had seemed impossible. I still worry about his hip but the orthopods don't—and they know more about it than I do. The orthopods have changed their mind: They've decided that Mr. Mukaj's cancerous hip isn't unstable after all and the likelihood of its fracturing from simple weight-bearing is minimal. So far, Mr. Mukaj has proved them right. After the cardiologists stented his heart, he got up and walked and hasn't stopped yet. A physical therapist helps him every day. He is no longer delirious; he has refused all pain medicines.

This is my preference, doak-toor, he told me. *I choose a little pain over being much crazy, yes? Do you agree with me about this, doak-toor?*

It's not my business to agree or disagree; it's his hurt, not mine. But the bleeding is still a problem, so now the urologists have bitten the bullet and plan to do the big operation on his bladder, the kind usually reserved for people who *don't* have metastatic disease. They plan to remove his entire bladder and connect his kidneys to a small pouch of intestine that will function as a substitute urinary bladder. It's a big, complex operation but everyone here is delighted for Mr. Mukaj, and for his family. His granddaughter beamed when she saw us this morning. She reached into her pocketbook, showed us two plane tickets.

One way for Papa, she said, nodding at Mr. Mukaj. Nonstop to Dubrovnik! Round trip for me but I will stay with him for a while. We are very excited! Next week, we are hoping!

Mr. Mukaj is beaming, too.

Doak-toor, you must come and visit my village! We will be welcoming you! We will have a festival, yes?

Some call it creep, a good word to describe a complex phenomenon in modern medicine, one exemplified by Mr. Mukaj, Ms. Dubois, and Mr. Warner: Slow, creeping changes gradually transform the structure of our health care system—sometimes for the better, sometimes not.

When mechanical engineers talk about creep, they're alluding to phenomena like buckling, corrosion, and fatigue. In their world, creep refers to the deformation of structural materials, such as steel or concrete, under the pressure of extreme weight or temperature or other stresses. This kind of mechanical creep explains why the World Trade Center buildings in New York collapsed on 9/11 and why a section of Boston's Big Dig tunnel gave way. But creep can be a good thing, too, when structural materials deform just enough to settle into an altered, but stronger, position.

Medical creep happens when doctors practice "outside the box," performing procedures or prescribing treatments for patients in the absence of clear evidence that patients will benefit. For example, doctors often use drugs or devices approved by the Federal Drug Administration for treatment of one condition (based on strong scientific evidence) to treat patients with other conditions (lacking any scientific evidence). Not surprisingly, pharmaceutical companies and medical device manufacturers promote this kind of creep, sometimes called "off-label" usage. Government regulatory agencies and insurers tend to take the opposite view; creep blows budgets and, sometimes, harms patients. But, like mechanical creep in buildings and bridges, medical creep sometimes saves lives.

Cardiopulmonary resuscitation (CPR), the procedure used to treat Ms. Dubois and many other patients who suffer cardiac arrest, is an example of medical creep. Before 1960, the only way to treat cardiac arrest required surgical opening of the chest cavity and manual cardiac massage, whereby the surgeon holds the heart in his hands and squeezes it rhythmically to pump blood to the brain and other vital organs. Extraordinarily heroic, such "open-chest" cardiac massage was attempted rarely—and succeeded even more rarely. Then, in 1960, surgeons at Johns Hopkins reported their experience with twenty patients in whom they had used a new CPR technique called closed-chest cardiac massage. This team of surgeons, who had also developed the external cardiac defibrillator, had devised a way to pump the arrested heart without opening the chest surgically. They successfully resuscitated every one of the first twenty patients they treated, fourteen of whom (70 percent) survived without brain damage or other ill effects. They concluded that "the method . . . can be used wherever the emergency arises, whether that is in or out of the hospital."

And so the creep began. Six years later, the National Academy of Sciences issued its own report, including illustrative diagrams, instructing medical personnel in the proper performance of closed-chest cardiac massage and CPR. Soon thereafter, *all* cardiac arrests in U.S. hospitals were treated with these methods. Resurrecting the dead became medicine's obsession—and not just inside hospitals. Many U.S. communities funded "mobile intensive care units" that enabled ambulance personnel to deliver CPR *outside* the hospital, too. In other words, CPR became—and remains today—the "default" treatment for every person who dies. Unless you explicitly forbid it, you will leave this world the same way Ms. Dubois did: Doctors or ambulance personnel will pump on your chest, put a breathing tube down your throat, squeeze oxygen into your lungs, jab you with needles, and electrocute your heart.

Anyone who has watched these things done to a frail, demented, or terminally ill ninety-year-old person understands just how crazy, and creepy, this can be. How did the CPR technique pioneered by the Hopkins doctors (which continues to save many lives today) become an accepted final rite of passage for *everyone*?

Three things doctors and researchers didn't understand in 1960 contributed to CPR creep. First, the Hopkins researchers, in their initial study, treated a very narrow spectrum of patients; most were young, healthy people (including several children) whose hearts had stopped during elective surgery, victims of anesthesia mishaps. Their impressive success rate (70 percent) was much higher than the success rate for patients who suffer cardiac arrest in hospital today (5 to15 percent), most of whom are elderly people with advanced heart disease and other serious conditions. (Recent large studies involving *only* elderly patients have documented CPR survival rates as low as *zero* and as high as 18 percent, with up to one-quarter of all survivors suffering permanent brain damage.) We now know that many new treatments, studied initially in a narrow spectrum of patients, aren't nearly as successful when used in a broader patient population. Ignorance of this "spectrum bias" potentiates creep.

Second, CPR creep reflects our failure to understand the difference between efficacy and effectiveness. The *efficacy* of a medical treatment refers to whether it *can* achieve its desired effect when studied under the ideal conditions of a research study. In contrast, the *effectiveness* of a medical treatment measures how well it performs in the "real world," where conditions are far from ideal. For example, the first study of out-of-hospital CPR in 1967 found that 50 percent of cardiac arrest victims in Belfast were resuscitated successfully. But when doctors in New York tried to replicate these spectacular results on the streets of lower Manhattan, their "mobile ICU" ambulances were able to save only 6 percent of cardiac arrest victims. (Recent studies have shown that survival rates after out-of-hospital CPR range from 2 percent in urban Chicago to almost 20 percent in suburban Seattle.) Medical innovations that prove efficacious in one research setting often are ineffective elsewhere. Confusing efficacy with effectiveness promotes creep.

Mass media promote medical creep, too. Episodes of television "doctor shows" like *ER*, the popular weekly series based fictionally on Chicago's Cook County Hospital (where I worked at the time), perpetuated spectrum bias about CPR and grossly inflated its effectiveness. Researchers found that two-thirds of all (fictional) cardiac arrests portrayed on *ER* (and other doctor shows) involved young patients who had suffered rare events like drowning or lightning strikes, rather than old people with heart disease (who account for 90 percent of cardiac arrests in real-life settings, including Cook County Hospital). Not surprisingly, most of these fictional TV patients did well, unlike the vast majority of CPR recipients in real life. In addition, as the researchers noted:

> On television, the outcome of CPR was generally portrayed as either full recovery or death . . . [as] if CPR were a benign, risk-free procedure that offered a good hope of long-term survival in the face of otherwise certain death. . . . But CPR can lead to prolonged suffering, severe neurologic damage, and an undignified death. In these . . . medical dramas and reenactments, such outcomes were never portrayed.

Did Ms. Dubois's son, who insisted that his mother receive CPR, understand these things? So much depends on whether doctors explicitly debunk CPR creep when they discuss resuscitation with patients or their surrogate decision-makers. One geriatrician, who cared for elderly patients in a long-term care facility like the one where Ms. Dubois lived, wrote that thirty-six of his forty patients (whose average age was eighty-seven) told him that they wanted CPR. This confused him until he found that they did not understand the low likelihood of benefit and the potential downside of CPR. After he had discussed the realities with his patients, thirty-nine of the forty *opposed* resuscitation.

Both doctors and patients are susceptible to the notion that if a potentially beneficial treatment *can* be done, it *should* be done—even if we don't know how often the treatment succeeds in a particular clinical situation or how its potential benefits compare with its potential harms. When Ms. Dubois's case, for example, was presented at Cornell's weekly Morbidity and Mortality (M&M) Conference, there was little discussion about the wisdom of performing CPR for an hour on an elderly, demented woman with severe heart disease. Instead, people wanted to talk about why she hadn't been offered cardiac surgery to remove the blood clot in her heart. And the take-home message from that M&M Conference was that surgery *might* have saved Ms. Dubois's life. Of course, surgery wouldn't have improved her dementia or her pitiful quality of life; more likely, it would have made her worse. But I would take odds that some doctors in that audience will push for surgery the next time they encounter a patient like Ms. Dubois.

Nevertheless, creep can propel medical progress, too. For example, it was not so long ago that patients with bacterial endocarditis like Mr. Warner were never offered surgery. *Never.* Even when their hearts began to fail due to worsening function of their infected valve, surgical treatment was not considered, because it was assumed that a new valve, surgically sewn into infected tissue, would become infected, too. But, in 1965, a surgical team replaced the infected heart valve of one such patient, saving his life. (Why did they operate? Because they felt certain that the patient would die if they didn't operate.) Ten years later, 239 endocarditis patients worldwide had undergone similar surgery, most of whom (73 percent) survived. Since then, thousands more endocarditis patients have opted to undergo surgery despite the fact that 25 to 30 percent of them will die. These (highly selected) patients are offered such risky surgery because their mortality rate is twice as high (55 to 60 percent) without it.

Nowhere is medical creep more prevalent today than in the treatment of cancer patients. For example, the disease that probably will kill Mr. Mukaj and my father—bladder cancer metastatic to bone—has a median survival of about six months. Recent studies have shown that new chemotherapy treatments can extend this median survival to about twelve months. None of these studies included patients like my father, a blind, bedridden ninety-one-year-old man with poor "functional status." (Frail, elderly patients like Dad are typically excluded from research studies of new treatments.) And yet, lacking any evidence about patients *like him*, doctors offered Dad the new chemotherapy treatment (which he refused). Mr. Mukaj, younger than Dad and very similar to patients in the relevant research trials, experienced creep of a different kind. In order to make it possible for him to receive the new chemotherapy treatment (at home in Croatia), our doctors planned to remove his bleeding bladder and replumb his kidneys, a radical operation rarely done for patients whose cancer has already spread to distant sites. Is this kind of creep bad?

Precisely *because* every patient is different, creep in medicine will continue, for better and for worse. Statistical analyses of large groups of patients cannot predict outcomes for individual patients. The poster child for this idea is Stephen Jay Gould, a famous scientist himself. Quoting Mark Twain in an essay titled "The Median Isn't the Message," Gould identified "three species of mendacity, each worse than the one before—lies, damned lies, and statistics." A renowned paleontologist and evolutionary biologist at Harvard, Gould was diagnosed with abdominal mesothelioma, a rare and deadly cancer, at the age of forty. After a systematic search of the medical literature (in 1982), he learned that patients with this disease had a median survival of eight months. Gould realized that this prognosis was not as gloomy as many (less statistically savvy) people might think. Rather than "I will probably be dead in eight months," this median survival means that one-half of patients die within eight months but the other half live longer. Most important, because the mesothelioma survival curve has a very long "tail," a few lucky patients *will live a lot longer.*

An otherwise healthy young man, Gould thought he might be one of the lucky ones and signed up for an unproven, experimental treatment. When he died, twenty *years* later, he left behind not only a lesson in statistics but a legacy of hope for all cancer patients. Gould wrote:

All biologists know that variation itself is nature's only irreducible essence.

> Variation is the hard reality, not a set of imperfect measures [like] means and medians. . . . Therefore I looked at the . . . statistics quite differently—and not only because I am an optimist who tends to see the doughnut instead of the hole but primarily because I know that variation itself is the reality. I had to place myself amidst the variation.

This is the challenge all doctors face: trying to see each of their unique patients within the context of natural variation. Mr. Mukaj, for example, like Stephen Jay Gould, sees the doughnut instead of the hole. I'm hoping he'll get lucky, too.

11:20 a.m.

I don't make a habit of spying on my patients, but right now I'm hiding behind the curtain that separates the two beds in Mr. Barensky's semiprivate room. He's in the bed near the window. His roommate, whose bed is near the door, has been transported downstairs for tests. I've tiptoed into the room, closed the door quietly behind me, and peeked around the curtain to watch Mr. Barensky. I've come back, unannounced, because I want to watch him breathe. When he's all alone.

Yes, this is a little weird. If someone walked in on me right now, I'd have some explaining to do. But fifteen seconds is all I need.

He's a big guy, tall and hefty, his thinning white hair mussed against his pillows. The head of his bed has been cranked upright, to ninety degrees, but his eyes are closed. He lies quietly now, no sign of agitation or discomfort. His jowls tremble slightly each time he exhales.

Eight. I count eight breaths in fifteen seconds. His breathing doesn't appear labored, but it's definitely fast. Thirty-two breaths per minute, twice the normal respiratory rate. Not what I was hoping for. If his breathing were normal, I might relax. As it is, until proven otherwise, he's trouble.

This is the fourth time I've seen Mr. Barensky in the past four hours. I'm nervous because I don't know what's wrong with him. He's an old guy who had open-heart surgery here three weeks ago. He did well—even at age seventy-eight he made it out of the hospital in less than a week—but he came back to the ED last night saying he didn't feel well. Partly what gets my red flag flapping is that he can't explain *how* he doesn't feel well. He's Russian, his English halting and heavily accented, but even with the help of our professional interpreter the best he can do, in answer to many pointed questions, is: *I don't feel good.* This might not make me nervous if his blood count weren't so low (half the normal level) and if his blood coagulation weren't so screwed up. His blood-thinner pills (the same ones Ms. Dubois took) were not monitored after he left the hospital; now his blood clotting is so impaired that his risk of hemorrhage is dangerously high (exactly the opposite of Ms. Dubois's problem). The worry, then, is that he's bleeding somewhere, but so far we haven't found it. And now he's breathing fast, a worrisome sign.

I don't like it. We're missing something. And, in an old guy like this, that's trouble.

Tina saw him in the ED last night and, as usual, did all the right things, including carefully reviewing his history. One month ago, he'd been evaluated at another New York hospital for chest pain and shortness of breath and had come here for a second opinion. Our cardiologists discovered that all three of his coronary arteries were blocked and his aortic heart valve critically narrowed. The surgeons bypassed his blocked arteries and gave him a new aortic valve, put him on a blood-thinner pill, and then sent him to a rehabilitation facility to complete his postoperative recovery.

He'd been home from rehab for a week now and, two days ago, saw his regular doctor for the first time since his surgery. After doing a routine blood test to check his blood-thinner medicine, his doctor called the next day to tell him that his blood test was so out of whack that he should go to the hospital right away. When Tina saw him in the ED, he looked anxious and pale but otherwise okay. He was anemic but this was not a dramatic change—he had been anemic when he left the hospital—so Tina wasn't convinced that this was his only problem. He described a vague discomfort in the back of his chest, below his shoulder blade. Tina wasn't sure what to make of this either because he'd had this same feeling even before his surgery.

His heart looked larger on chest X-ray than it had two weeks ago and Tina wondered if he might have a pericardial effusion (a fluid collection around the heart), a common complication after cardiac surgery (sometimes a serious one). She discussed this idea with the ED docs—she also told them about Ms. Fuchs, one of our patients upstairs who has a large pericardial effusion—so they brought out their new, handheld portable echo machine and obtained ultrasound images of Mr. Barensky's heart. It looked normal, no sign of a pericardial effusion or any other acute cardiac condition. Tina checked the oxygen level in his blood; this was normal, too. These findings, taken together, reassured Tina about his heart and lungs. Still, she was nervous. She wasn't sure what was going on. As a precaution, she gave Mr. Barensky intravenous infusions of Vitamin K and blood plasma to begin correcting his blood-clotting deficiency.

After all this, Mr. Barensky was exhausted. He tried to sleep—it was the middle of the night—but still he couldn't get comfortable. *I don't feel good.*

When I saw him in the ED a few hours later, before making rounds with Tina and the team, that was the best I could get out of him, too—*I don't feel good*—even with his daughter translating English to Russian and back again in response to my questions. He looked very tired. He said he hadn't been sleeping well ever since his surgery. He couldn't explain why. *I don't know,* he shrugged brusquely. His breathing (twenty-two breaths per minute) and his pulse (ninety beats per minute) were slightly fast but these could be explained by his anemia, anxiety, and exhaustion. He admitted he had felt light-headed and sweaty since yesterday but this had begun after his doctor called to tell him to come back to the hospital. *Yes, of course, I am concerned,* he answered me through his daughter. *Depressed? No, I am not depressed.* He admitted to some "numbness" in his right arm for the past few hours but I could find nothing wrong with it. And I couldn't make much of his vague shoulder blade discomfort either. He shrugged it off. *I don't know,* he said, waving me away, tired of all the questions. *I told you: I don't feel good.*

When we saw Mr. Barensky together as a team, we went through it all again, this time with a Russian interpreter, not his daughter. We agreed to get him upstairs to the Cardiology floor and watch him closely while we gave him more transfusions to correct his blood clotting and anemia. We came back to see him again after we had finished rounds on the rest of our patients and visited Ms. Dubois in the morgue. Dan thought Mr. Barensky's neck veins looked engorged (sometimes a sign of heart or lung problems), but it was hard to be sure. Anyway, Tina reminded Dan, the tests done in the ED on his heart and lungs had looked good. Ashley, assigned to be Mr. Barensky's intern, was more concerned about his anemia and wondered if he was bleeding internally in a location we couldn't see. This seemed unlikely, Tina thought, because his blood count, although low, hadn't dropped very much since he left the hospital a few weeks ago. Still, Ashley ordered a CT scan of his abdomen to make sure he wasn't bleeding into his retroperitoneum, the large space in the rear of the abdominal cavity where patients who take blood-thinners sometimes bleed. We explained all this to Mr. Barensky as best we could.

He shrugged. I asked him if he had any questions.

He looked at each of us in turn—Tina and Dan and Ashley, then me. He stared at me. As he did, his breathing seemed to get faster. He looked as if he wanted to know something. I asked again.

Any questions, Mr. Barensky?

You, he said, gesturing to me.

Yes?

You . . . you are . . . Jewish?

No.

He nodded, said nothing.

This is a problem? I asked.

He shook his head, shrugged again. As he did, I wondered if his breathing speeded up.

I told him we would return again after his CT scan and repeat blood tests were done. He seemed to understand. Outside his room, we all agreed to check on him often today. Along with Mr. Warner, our guy with endocarditis, this is the guy who worries us most. Tina, who'd been up all night, left the hospital to get some sleep. Dan and Ashley went off to work on our other patients. I've come back now, to spy on Mr. Barensky from behind the curtain.

I would like it to be true. My current hypothesis—that Mr. Barensky is anxious, not seriously ill—has much to recommend it. Open-heart surgery, especially at an elderly age, can be terrifying and debilitating. Perioperative anxiety and depression are common. After undergoing heart surgery, many elderly patients seem different—they don't think as clearly, their personalities change—for reasons that are poorly understood. Maybe it's because suddenly their whole life seems to hang on a suture, a stitch. But, whatever the reason, Mr. Barensky hasn't slept well since he left the hospital and his physical complaints are vague and suspiciously diverse. His symptoms—shortness of breath, lightheadedness, chest discomfort, subjective numbness—are classic somatic symptoms of psychological distress. And, despite all our tests, we haven't found anything "objective" to explain these symptoms.

But just because my hypothesis makes sense doesn't mean it's true. There's no test I can do to *prove* that Mr. Barensky's current problem is psychosomatic. So, I've come back to spy, hoping that when he's unobserved and all alone his breathing will be normal. If it were normal, it wouldn't prove a thing, but it would make me less nervous that I'm missing something bad.

No such luck. Even in his sleep, he's breathing fast. His heart monitor is bleeping faster than what's healthy, too. Can anxiety do that? Can it make your heart and lungs speed up nervously even when you're asleep? I don't know and I think of Paul, who taught me about psychosomatic symptoms at Dartmouth, long ago. Paul might know.

I slip around the curtain, walk to the side of Mr. Barensky's bed. His eyes remain closed, his head slumped, his arms limp. Now, for the first time, I notice the small row of numbers on the inside of his left forearm. How did I not see this before? (What else have I missed?) Six numbers, etched in black, midway between his wrist and his elbow. Not ink. A tattoo.

He senses my presence, stirs, opens his eyes. He sees where I am looking.

You . . . know it? he asks, gesturing at the numbers.

Yes, I think so. Where were you?

He shrugs.
Birkenau. Then, Bergen-Belsen.
How long?
Four years.
Your family?
Yes.
I'm sorry.
He shrugs. His breathing, his bleeping heart don't change.

Two orderlies arrive with a stretcher. They're here to transport him to Radiology for his abdominal CT scan. They wheel him away.

I page Ashley, his intern. She's busy. Even so, I suggest she go to Radiology with Mr. Barensky, watch him closely, view the CT images right away with the radiologist. Chances are good we'll see nothing. But, right now, I'm not liking my psychosomatic hypothesis one bit. Postsurgical angst? In this guy? I don't know him but I'm thinking that maybe open-heart surgery for this guy is like a stroll in the park.

Out in the corridor, a group of medical students gathers around the chief resident. Karen sees me and waves, gestures for me to join them. They're standing outside the room of Ms. Fuchs, our lady with the big pericardial effusion. She's scheduled for surgery today. She's had all the tests; the underlying cause of her pericarditis remains unknown. ("Idiopathic," doctors call it, a ten-cent word meaning, literally, "of unknown cause.") And, despite the powerful drugs we've used, the inflammation of the lining around her heart has worsened, exuding so much fluid there that the pressure of its accumulation has begun to compromise her heart function. So, today, the surgeons will open her up, drain the fluid out, and then strip off the pericardial lining of her heart to prevent any future recurrence. When we saw Ms. Fuchs on rounds earlier this morning, she was anxious but raring to go. *Let's do this,* she said, *I got things to do, places to go.* At age fifty-five, she does four triathlons per year.

Karen, the chief resident, is taking the opportunity to teach the medical students about Ms. Fuchs's problem. I join them for a few minutes. Karen shows the students all the important things about diagnosing pericardial effusions, how to understand the telltale findings in Ms. Fuchs's neck veins and blood pressure and heart examination. Equally important, Karen shows the students how to calm an anxious patient, even one about to have heart surgery. As she teaches, Karen joshes playfully with Ms. Fuchs, who, grateful for the diversion, clearly enjoys joshing her back. It's fine work by a gifted young teacher. But, as I watch, I begin to feel . . . unnerved. Like I've forgotten something really important. What is it? I can't put my finger on it. I know I'm tired. Still, I can't shake the feeling, a powerful sense of foreboding. *What is this?*

My pager buzzes on my belt. I leave Ms. Fuchs with Karen and the students and grab a phone at the nursing station. Dan, our intern, is calling from the echocardiography lab.

Mr. Warner, he says.

I tune out Ms. Fuchs and her pericardium and my strange feeling. This is more important. Does Warner's echocardiogram show the jet Tina was worried about? Has the guy's infected heart valve failed to the point where he needs urgent surgery?

They can't do the echo, Dan says.

My own heart sinks.

Why not?

They're not sure, Dan says. Mr. Warner's cooperating as best he can. But the Cards guys can't get the echo probe down his throat. It's like there's a blockage of some kind in his esophagus. They've called the GI guys to come over, scope his esophagus, see what's down there.

Shit!

Talking to Dan, I wonder out loud whether an obstruction in Mr. Warner's esophagus might explain his reduced food intake the past few days. I had assumed it was just the hospital food. But now I'm kicking myself. I haven't asked him the obvious question, the one you always ask: *Are you having any problem swallowing?* Then there's the mystery about his right lung, the haziness on his chest X-ray that waxes and wanes, coming and going. Tina's hypothesis about this, unilateral pulmonary edema from heart valve leakage, is rare as hell. But, if something's blocking the guy's esophagus, maybe he's been aspirating bits of food into his lung. (The right lung is where aspirated stuff typically goes.) Worst of all, obstruction of the esophagus in an old guy usually means cancer. Damn!

Hmmph, Dan says, listening to my rant. HIV *and* bacterial endocarditis *and* cancer of the esophagus? Some trifecta.

Dan tells me he'll page me back after the GI guys are done. I'm
thinking ahead. Then what? I'm not sure. But it would make one
decision a whole lot easier. We wouldn't have to anguish anymore
about whether Mr. Warner needs heart surgery. The surgeons won't
touch him if he's got cancer, too.

Now my strange, unsettled feeling returns. Something is eating
at the back of my brain, something I can't identify. *I'm missing something.* But what is it? And which one of my patients is it about? Ms.
Fuchs? Have we forgotten to do something important before the
surgeons strip her pericardium? Mr. Barensky? Is he just anxious
or is he bleeding somewhere, maybe even critically ill? What am I
missing there? And now Warner, too?

Ay-yi-yi.

After all these years, I've learned to pay attention to my *Ay-yi-
yis.* Especially when I'm sleep-deprived. I need a time-out to figure
out what the hell is bugging me. I need to take a breath, get my act
together, think this through.

As usual, most of the computer terminals on the ward are occu-
pied, all the nurses and doctors and clerks scrolling and clicking and
typing away. There must be fifty terminals here on the fourth floor
alone but finding an open one can be a challenge. Everyone in the
hospital these days seems to spend more time interacting with the
damn computer than with the patients. It's unavoidable. *Everything*
is in the computer: orders, lists of medicines, nurses' and doctors'
notes, lab results, radiology reports, even the X-ray images themselves. Everything except the patient, that is.

I find an unoccupied terminal in the back corridor. A couple of
clicks, my password entered, and I'm in. There's my list, all twenty
patients currently on my team. But where do I start? Which one of
them is bugging me?

Ms. Fuchs looks as good in the computer as she does in person,
joshing with Karen and the students. Her lab numbers are perfect,
her preop meds ordered for her trip to the OR. The Anesthesia and
Cardiology guys are on board. She's good to go. So, unless we're

all clueless about something, she's not the one who's bugging me. Mr. Barensky's numbers look good, too. His blood tests are much improved; he's responding well to the transfusions Tina gave him overnight. When I click on his Radiology tab, I'm surprised to see an entry for his abdominal CT scan already. There's no report yet—the radiologist hasn't typed in his formal interpretation—but the CT scan images are all there, hundreds of them. From the bottom of his chest down to the tops of his legs, the CT scanner has cut Mr. Barensky's abdomen like a loaf of thin-sliced bread, each cut just a few millimeters thick, his internal organs displayed on the computer screen in hundreds of cross-sections, one after another. When I push a button, these cross-sectional images appear in sequence and very fast, rolling through his abdominal cavity from top to bottom like an old-fashioned, black-and-white movie in a kinetoscope. It's hypnotic to watch, fun to use. As the images scan, up and down, I look at all the places in the abdomen where occult bleeding can hide: around his liver and spleen, behind his kidneys and bladder, in the muscles of his spine, along the top of his pelvis and thighs.

I see no signs of bleeding. I can't say I'm surprised. I'm betting now that, like a lot of old people, he'll follow Hickam's Dictum, not Occam's razor: in his case, one diagnosis won't explain everything. Yes, his blood was thinned too much and his blood count is low and he's breathing fast, but we've found no sign of bleeding or any other "unifying" diagnosis to tie all of these things into one neat little package. I make a mental note to talk to his daughter again, find out more about how Mr. Barensky handled the psychological stress of his heart surgery.

Next I click on Mr. Warner, our guy with endocarditis. His labs look okay, too, his kidney function borderline but his blood cultures still negative, a good sign. I check his Radiology reports, review his chest X-rays again, flip through his previous ones to compare with today's. There it is again, that haziness in his right lung. I click on his consultants' reports. The Pulmonary specialists aren't sure yet what's going on. And there's nothing new from Cardiology except a brief note about their aborted transesophageal echocardiography procedure today and their request for help from the GI guys. I quickly check several other patients, then log off.

I don't like it. I'm still missing something. Maybe it's Mom. She did fine overnight in the hospital in Greenport, but got agitated this morning, didn't know where she was, made a fuss about going home. Maybe I shouldn't have let them discharge her from the hospital. Maybe that's what's bugging me.

I reenter the main corridor on 4 North and see Ashley outside Ms. Fuchs's room, speaking excitedly to Karen about something. As I walk toward them, Ashley sees me, breaks away from the group, and hurries in my direction.

It's the pericardium! Ashley says, her voice a loud whisper, urgent like a shout. All along the corridor, heads turn.

It's the pericardium! Ashley says again, thrilled and incredulous.

I look at her, then at Karen, who has joined us.

Right. We talked about her on rounds, remember? She's going to the OR soon.

Huh? Ashley says. Karen grins from ear to ear.

What? I say to Karen. Ms. Fuchs is fine, right? You were just with her!

Fuchs? Ashley shouts. No, not Fuchs! The guy! The guy with the valve!

Now, all around us, people have stopped in their tracks. The head nurse stares crossly at Ashley from behind a counter, puts a finger to her lips. *Shush!*

I try to speak quietly. The guy with the valve? Warner? Dan just called me. Cards couldn't do Warner's echo, some technical problem. Why are you talking about his pericardium?

No, no, not Warner! The other guy! The new guy! Barensky! He's got a massive pericardial effusion on his CT scan! Must be where he's bleeding! Could be tamponade! I called Cards. They're coming up now to do a bedside echo!

What . . . ?

Two orderlies turn the corner into the main corridor, wheeling Mr. Barensky past us and back into his room. He looks ashen, sweaty, stuporous.

Karen, who has never seen Mr. Barensky before, shoots me a look.

Uh-oh, she says softly, then spins around and follows him into his room, Ashley at her heels.

Quickly, we help the orderlies transfer Mr. Barensky from the stretcher into his bed. He's breathing very fast now, maybe forty or fifty a minute. We crank up the head of his bed, put an oxygen mask on his face. Ashley grabs his left arm and wraps a blood pressure cuff around it, just above his tattoo. Fast, Karen listens to his lungs and heart, feels the pulse in his neck, then speaks to him loudly.

Sir! Can you hear me? Sir! Open your eyes, please! Sir?

Mr. Barensky groans, mumbles something unintelligible.

Heart rate 130, Karen says. Pulse is feeble, low pulse pressure. What's his BP? she asks Ashley.

It's . . . it's low . . . hard to tell . . . eighty, maybe . . . it comes and goes . . . he's breathing so fast . . .

A portable echocardiogram machine is wheeled into the room. Maria, one of the cardiology fellows, pushes it up close to Mr. Barensky's bed, plugs it into a wall socket, and motions Ashley away. Karen strips the hospital gown off Mr. Barensky's chest. The scar from his recent heart surgery looks like a giant zipper, a long raw track down the center of his chest. Maria squeezes a big glob of Vaseline out of a tube, slops it on the head of the echo machine's microphone, and positions the microphone under Mr. Barensky's left nipple. A racket of static erupts from the machine, its video monitor suddenly alive with motion.

Left parasternal, Maria murmurs. She moves the microphone to the center of his chest, near the bottom of his scar. Subcostal view, she says, more to herself than to us.

Now, on the screen, we can see the shadows of his heart. A healthy heart looks like a fistful of energy, jumping and pumping. This one barely moves at all.

Two guys in surgical scrub suits appear. One of them, an anesthesiologist, opens a metal case that looks like a carpenter's tool kit. The other one, a cardiac surgery fellow, carries two thin packages wrapped in sterile cellophane. Inside each package is a foot-long pericardial needle, the size you need to hit the heart. Maria directs his attention to the video screen.

There, she says to the surgeon, pointing to a thick rim of black shadow encircling Mr. Barensky's failing heart. Maria points at the ventricular septum, the wall of heart muscle that separates the right ventricle from the left.

Paradoxical septal motion, Maria says. No doubt about it. Tamponade physiology, for sure.

As she speaks, the surgeon is opening one of his sterile cellophane bags. The needle looks like something you'd see in a fencing match.

Get me some sterile drapes, he says to no one in particular. Let's get the head of his bed flat.

Karen shouts.

No respirations here!

Everyone looks at Mr. Barensky. He's not breathing.

Let's go! Let's go! Karen shouts.

We lift him, dead weight, off the bed and slide a hard board under his body. We move the bed, on wheels, away from the wall. The anesthesiologist moves quickly to get into position. He pulls a laryngoscope out of his metal case, snaps it open. From behind the head of the bed, he grabs Mr. Barensky's chin and lifts it up, hyperextending his neck. Then he slips the curved blade of the laryngoscope into Mr. Barensky's mouth, pushing the tongue out of his line of sight. Frowning, he peers down into the throat, searching for the windpipe.

No pulse! Kirana says now. No pulse! Start CPR! Now! Now! Let's go! Let's go!

Ashley puts her hands, one on top of the other, near the bottom of Mr. Barensky's chest scar. The Vaseline smeared there makes a gooey, sucking sound as she begins to pump on his heart.

Wait! Wait! says the anesthesiologist. Hold compressions! Wait!

Holding the laryngoscope in his left hand, he uses his right hand to slip a rubber endotracheal tube down into Mr. Barensky's windpipe, slick as a whistle. He inflates a little balloon attached to the bottom of the breathing tube, anchoring it in place inside Mr. Barensky's airway.

Okay! I'm in. Go! Go!

Ashley resumes pumping on Mr. Barensky's chest, rhythmically, up and down. The anesthesiologist squeezes oxygenated air down into his lungs, breathing for him. Maria, the cardiology fellow, presses her hand into Mr. Barensky's groin. She pokes here, then there, trying to find a pulse.

Barely palpable, she tells Ashley, who grimaces, then pumps even harder on his chest.

All of this takes less than a minute but, from where I'm standing, doing nothing, it seems a lot longer. The surgeon watches, warily fingering his long pericardial needle.

Maria puts her echo probe back on Mr. Barensky's torso, just below Ashley's pumping hands. On the viewing screen, his heart, surrounded by pericardial fluid, barely moves at all. Ashley's heart compressions are like trying to squeeze a ripe orange trapped inside a tense water balloon. No way.

Seeing this, the surgeon stuffs his needles into his pocket and leaps onto Mr. Barensky's bed.

Everybody off! he says, sweeping Ashley and Maria and Karen out of his way. He gets up on his knees, straddles Mr. Barensky's chest, and begins pumping himself.

Let's go! he says to the anesthesiologist, who is squeezing an air bag into Mr. Barensky's breathing tube. Somebody call the OR! Let's go! Push! Let's go!

Ashley and Karen grab the bed rails on each side and start pushing the big bed out of the room. I get out of the way. The anesthesiologist stumbles, then catches himself, keeping his hand on the breathing bag as they wheel out the door. In the corridor, everything stops. Everyone backs away, wide-eyed, as the bed is hustled down the hallway, the anesthesiologist scrambling to keep up, the surgeon sitting atop Mr. Barensky's horizontal, unconscious body, pumping his chest rhythmically, yelling at anyone in their way.

Comin' through! he yells ahead. Move! Move! Comin' through!

Useless, I follow from a distance. It's about a city block from 4 North to the operating rooms. Far ahead, I see the wide double doors swing open, sucking them all inside. Karen and Ashley peel away from the bed as the big doors close and a flurry of scrub suits converge around the young surgeon, still up high on the bed, rising and falling above Mr. Barensky.

Now, in the corridor, everything is deadly quiet. Nurses glance at me, then look away. An old lady, walking in the hallway with a physical therapist, has stopped, her hand at her throat. An intern approaches Ashley and Karen, both breathless, as they walk back down the corridor toward me.

What was that? he asks them.

Pericardial tamponade, Ashley answers. Hemopericardium, most likely. Warfarin overdose.

He makes a low whistle.

We couldn't figure out where he was bleeding, Ashley tells him. Didn't seem like he'd lost much blood, a liter at most. But now it all makes sense. The pericardium is pretty much the only place you can bleed so little yet look so bad. The echo in the ED last night missed it completely.

The intern whistles again.

As Ashley speaks, I'm mortified. After the fact, it seems so obvious. This is exactly what Tina had worried about last night in the ED. The echo in the ED missed it, sure, but it's not like I've never seen a false-negative echocardiogram before. (No, I don't tell Ashley about Fred.) And then there's Ms. Fuchs, right next door, with the exact same diagnosis! Worst of all is that CT scan. *I just looked at it* myself, for Crissakes. Mr. Barensky's heart was right there in front of me on that computer screen ten minutes ago. But I, thinking only about his *abdomen* for potential sites of bleeding, *never even looked at his heart!* A guy who had open-heart surgery just a few weeks ago! Talk about blinders. Out of mind, out of sight. A total whiff.

Ashley looks at me.

Lucky thing we did that CT scan, huh, Dr. Reilly?

That wasn't luck, Ashley. That was real smart. You did good.

Karen gives Ashley a high five, then turns to me.

Think he'll make it?

All I can do is shake my head.

It never should have happened.

I don't mean my own shortsightedness, missing what was right in front of my nose. I mean it never should have happened in the first place. The guy makes it through lifesaving heart surgery and then no one monitors his risky anticoagulant medicines after he leaves the hospital? This is like crash-landing a plane safely and then forgetting to disembark the passengers before the fuel tank explodes. It's crazy, utterly irresponsible. And yet, in Mr. Barensky's case, it's not immediately obvious *who* was irresponsible. The surgeons performed his heart operation flawlessly. Postoperatively, in consultation with our cardiologists, they started him on warfarin, in his case an essential blood-thinner drug. Then, before discharging him from the hospital, they made sure that Mr. Barensky had appointments with his own primary care physician and cardiologist, both of whom planned to follow him, monitor his medicines, adjust them as needed. What, then, went wrong?

Mr. Barensky didn't go home from the hospital after his heart surgery. An old guy who'd been through a lot, he needed physical therapy and temporary nursing care to help him get back on his feet again. So, as an interim step, he went to a skilled nursing home for ten days of postoperative rehabilitation. But Mr. Barensky's primary care physician and cardiologist had no relationship with the nursing home. (Neither did the surgeons or cardiologists who had cared for him in the hospital.) As a result, during the ten days when Mr. Barensky was in the nursing home, he was "between doctors." It was assumed that the nursing home staff would monitor his blood-thinner medicine. But they didn't. It fell through the cracks. So, Mr. Barensky fell through the cracks, too.

He's not alone. Thousands of people in the United States—perhaps hundreds of thousands—fall through the cracks every year. Like the creep in our health care system, where doctors extemporize to provide *more* care than scientific evidence supports, cracks in our health care system often cause patients to receive *less* than the standard of care. It's one hell of a problem. And, as in Mr. Barensky's case, the devil's in the details.

Everyone in medicine, including the staff at Mr. Barensky's nursing home, knows that blood-thinners like warfarin are powerful, potentially dangerous drugs. In fact, among elderly patients, warfarin is the most common cause of medication-related emergency hospitalizations. More than twenty thousand elderly people in the United States are hospitalized annually for life-threatening hemorrhages due to warfarin. (The abdomen is the most frequent site of bleeding, but catastrophic hemorrhages in the brain happen, too. Mr. Barensky's problem—bleeding into the pericardium—is very rare.) The most precarious time for the patient is when warfarin treatment is first begun, because finding the right dose of warfarin—the amount of drug that thins the patient's blood enough to prevent blood clots (like Ms. Dubois's) but not enough to cause bleeding (like Mr. Barensky's)—is a trial-and-error proposition. *Every patient is different.* The effective dose for Ms. Dubois may be ten times larger than the effective dose for Mr. Barensky. For this reason, a generation ago, patients like Mr. Barensky often remained in hospital until their correct warfarin dose had been established. But this doesn't happen today. Hospitals can't afford to keep patients simply to adjust the dose of one pill each day.

"Someone else" has to do it.

Like shift work in hospitals—where patients can get hurt if the hand-off from the day shift to the night shift isn't compulsive and complete—transitions of care between the hospital and home (or nursing home) are fraught with hazard. After Mr. Barensky had his heart surgery, there was an awful lot to tell the nursing home staff about him. Ninety-nine percent of this complex "information transfer" was perfectly done. But lost in the shuffle was the fact that Mr. Barensky *had just been started* on warfarin and so needed careful, daily monitoring with blood tests. The nursing home staff didn't know this. Mr. Barensky's life was endangered because this one "minor" detail fell through the cracks when he was most vulnerable to such an oversight.

Bad luck? Sure. But, in hindsight, entirely preventable, a "systems" problem. Harmful transitions of care usually have nothing to do with bad luck.

Some aspects of this problem are subtle. If Mr. Warner, for example, survives his bacterial endocarditis to go home, his own doctor (who has not visited him in hospital once) will have seen none of what Mr. Warner has been through. This is not a big deal if, when

Mr. Warner leaves the hospital, I can bring his doctor up to speed on what he's missed. But, as in any serial drama, missing entire episodes makes it harder to understand the story line. How much harm patients experience as a result of these "doctor discontinuities" is poorly understood, but there can be no doubt that they add redundancy, expense, and "occasion for error" to our health care system.

In fact, these cracks raise questions about whether the United States has a health care "system" at all. At the policy level—the view from sixty thousand feet—the most gaping cracks in U.S. health care are three continental divides: the uninsured, 50 million people and counting; the lack of a universal electronic medical record accessible in all settings where patients receive their care; and the administrative morass created by our smorgasbord of different health insurers, each with its own bureaucracy and rules. Repairing these giant fault lines will require societal consensus and political courage, neither of which is easy to find today. But at ground level—the view from the trenches of daily patient care—two smaller cracks in our health care system can (and must) be repaired now: perverse financial incentives for health care institutions and our loss of focus on the *patient* as the "unit" of care.

Consider the financial incentives in Mr. Barensky's case. Medicare, which pays lower rates than most commercial insurers, reimburses hospitals about forty thousand dollars for a patient who undergoes the kind of heart surgery Mr. Barensky had. The hospital will receive its forty thousand dollars no matter how long Mr. Barensky stays in the hospital (because U.S. hospitals are reimbursed a fixed fee for each "episode" of patient care). It is only smart business, then, for the hospital to discharge Mr. Barensky as soon as possible after surgery. This is doubly true because, if the patient requires readmission to the hospital soon thereafter, as Mr. Barensky did, the hospital will be reimbursed *again*, for another "episode" of care—even when, as in Mr. Barensky's case, the second hospitalization is *caused directly* by a preventable complication of the first hospitalization. This is like selling cars without lemon laws, or even a thirty-*day* warranty. Under such perverse reimbursement rules, hospitals have had no incentive to dismantle their revolving door of readmissions, a lucrative "line of business." In fact, in 25 percent of U.S. hospitals today, *one-quarter of all admissions* are thirty-day readmissions!

One big part of this problem is the revolving door between hospitals and nursing homes. It is not widely known that "post-acute-care" patients today account for more than 70 percent of all new patient admissions to Medicare/Medicaid-certified nursing homes. (In other words, only a minority of these nursing home admissions are "residential" patients like Ms. Dubois.) One-quarter of these "acute rehabilitation" patients wind up back in the hospital within thirty days, just like Mr. Barensky. This revolving door is speeding up, not slowing down. Hospitals "feed" nursing homes, which then return the favor. And both the hospital and the nursing home get paid every time, for each "episode" of care. The result is that everyone wins. Except the patients. Bounced from one setting to another, patients get caught in the middle—and sometimes lost in the cracks.

This is not the result of some vast, nefarious conspiracy. The simple reality is that, because insurers reimburse hospitals and skilled nursing homes on a fee-for-service, per-episode basis, no financial incentives slow the revolving doors of cost-shifting and discontinuous care. As Jack Wennberg and his Dartmouth colleagues have shown, this phenomenon is highly variable in different regions of the United States. For example, the thirty-day hospital readmission rate for patients with congestive heart failure in Bend, Oregon (14.5 percent), is less than half the rate in Oxford, Mississippi (36.6 percent). Patients in Utah who are discharged from hospitals to post-acute-care nursing homes are only half as likely to require readmission to hospital as patients in Louisiana (15.1 percent versus 28.2 percent). Various interventions designed specifically to address this problem—to reduce hospital readmissions and improve "transitions of care" for high-risk patients like Mr. Barensky—have been shown to make a big difference. But these interventions have been done piecemeal—here or there, this or that—and not in any coordinated, "systemwide" way.

In response to these concerns and variations, the federal Affordable Care Act of 2010 includes the National Pilot Program on Payment Bundling. In this program, a single health provider (for example, a hospital or physician group) will receive one "bundled" payment for a prolonged episode of care, typically defined as starting three days before hospital admission and ending thirty days (or more) after hospital discharge. It provides strong financial incentives for institutions and doctors to work together, to coordinate care across all settings while reducing total costs, by holding all care providers (hospitals, physicians, nursing homes) *jointly* accountable, through *shared* payment, for the total cost and quality of patients' care. Bundling will not be easy to do well, and it may not work as planned. But perhaps, by forcing doctors and health care institutions to work together, these innovations will refocus our "system" on a greater goal: doing what's best for patients—not just for thirty days but continuously, over a lifetime of care.

The irony is that, not so long ago, no one had to force U.S. health care providers to think this way. It was part of the job. Indeed, for many doctors, it *was* the job.

7:20 p.m.

It's dark outside the Step-Down Unit, an open, eight-bed ward adjacent to the medical ICU. Red and yellow lights blink in the tall wet windowpanes, snow-blurred reflections from the street traffic below. For most patients, moving to Step-Down is an encouraging development, a step in the right direction. Most of them have been deathly ill in the ICU; moving here usually means that they've turned a corner, improved enough to no longer need life-support machines and critical care docs. But when I moved Mr. Warner in here yesterday it was a step in the wrong direction. He's not so sick that he needs the ICU, but I'm worried that he's headed that way. If I'm right, he could crash fast, so fast that maybe not even the ICU guys could save him. So, as a precaution, I've stepped him up to Step-Down.

Mr. Warner can see for himself that this is not a hopeful sign. The patient in the bed next to him is a young guy who's brain-dead. Mr. Hernandez has been here for weeks, transferred in after an even longer stint in the ICU. I've seen his pretty young wife sitting by his bed every day, her head bowed, pink rosary beads dangling from her fingers. She knows that her husband won't wake up, but she can't let go. They have little kids at home. So, his breathing machine and feeding tube keep him alive. Sort of. The hospital has nowhere to send him, an uninsured illegal alien. Barring some new catastrophe or his wife's change of heart, Mr. Hernandez will be here for a long time.

None of this is lost on Mr. Warner, whose confusion has resolved, a good sign. He is what the nurses call a "good" patient—quiet, cooperative, grateful for their help. He knows where he is, what's happening to him, and why. He's still blind in his left visual field, the result of one of his strokes, but he even made light of that yesterday morning. Then, gesturing at poor Mr. Hernandez in the bed to his left, he said, Maybe half blind isn't half bad.

Tina told him we hoped his vision would improve over the coming weeks.

Weeks? he asked Tina. Will I still be around then?

Uh, well, remember, Mr. Warner, six weeks of IV antibiotics is the standard course of treatment for bacterial endocarditis.

Yes, I know, Dr. Johansen. That's not what I mean. I mean, will I still be alive in a few weeks?

Tina, caught off guard, stammered her reply.

Well . . . of course . . . you . . . do you . . . ? Why do you ask?

My heart. It's getting worse, right? Makes you wonder, you know?

He had seen my frown two days ago when I listened to his heart, when I told the others that they needed to listen more carefully, too. Since day one, his heart murmur—a soft musical *Whew!*—had sounded like a small tropical bird, cooing at dawn. But the day before yesterday, day ten, his heart sounded like a lion in heat, a loud carnivorous roar. This change was trouble. We repeated his cardiac echo, which showed that his mitral valve was leaking more. Worse, unlike his two previous echocardiograms, it also showed a vegetation on the valve. That's where the *Staph* bacteria are growing, and eating. It's a small vegetation—in itself, not a worrisome thing—but the fact that we hadn't seen it on either of his two previous echoes suggests that, despite our powerful antibiotic drugs, the bacteria may be winning.

His right lung has been the confusing part. He's had all the tests—chest X-rays, a CT scan of his lungs, tests for blood clots and other things—and yet I and the lung specialists and cardiologists and infectious disease consultants still aren't sure what's going on. Last night, after we moved him to Step-Down, he developed shortness of breath again. Tina tried different treatments to help him, then finally gave him an intravenous diuretic, telling him that maybe his heart was the cause of his breathing problem. After he peed out a liter of urine and felt a whole lot better, he began to think Tina must be right. And so, while Tina was Googling her brainstorm about "unilateral pulmonary edema" last night, Mr. Warner was ruminating about his heart.

On rounds this morning, after Tina told us what she had found to support her theory, we told Mr. Warner we would need still another echocardiogram today (his fourth), to define more clearly the condition of his infected heart valve. He asked us if he would need heart surgery.

Yes, I answered him, you might. But, if you do, timing is everything. In most cases, it's best to clear the infection before trying to repair the damage it's done to the heart valve. We've called the surgeons. They'll look at your new echo today with the cardiologists. We'll know a lot more then.

Mr. Warner nodded, slowly. Then his Caribbean-blue eyes locked into mine.

Sounds like it might be time to throw in the towel, he said.

This caught me off guard. It's an expression my father uses sometimes. Just a few weeks ago, when we talked about hospice, Dad talked about throwing in the towel. (I didn't argue with him. In his condition, I'd throw in the towel, too.) But it was more than Mr. Warner's turn of phrase that gave me pause. Over the years, I've learned that when sick people begin to think that death is near they're often right, whether their doctor realizes it or not. Mr. Warner thinks he's dying.

This morning, I had said what I could to encourage him. I emphasized how much he has improved. I could tell he was unconvinced. We've seen a lot of each other these past twelve days, but that doesn't mean he knows me or trusts me. And, even if he does, I'm not sure if I can trust *him*. He's had strokes in several areas of his brain. Has this impaired his cognitive function? Can he handle complex, life-or-death decisions?

He's had a long day today. After the cardiologists couldn't get down his throat with their echo probe this morning, the GI guys found the reason: a rip-roaring fungal infection in his esophagus, all swollen and red, those ugly raw erosions everywhere in his swallowing tract, from top to bottom. No wonder he's not eating. Afterward, lots of other people came to see him and everyone suspected that his heart was getting worse. The question now wasn't whether he would need heart surgery. The question now was when.

The surgeons asked for the neurologists' help. They posed one very specific question: If we operate on his heart, will we destroy his brain?

To perform this kind of valve repair, the heart surgeons must first stop the patient's heart from beating. Then, while the surgeons cut and sew, a heart-lung machine is used to pump the patient's blood, maintaining circulation to his brain and other vital organs. But this can be done only if the patient is given large doses of powerful blood-thinner drugs that prevent the patient's blood from clotting in the heart-lung machine. We have scrupulously avoided giving Mr. Warner even small amounts of these drugs because they greatly increase his risk of bleeding into the areas of his brain damaged by his strokes. (His CT scan had shown bleeding in his brain on day one, even *without* these drugs.) Dare we give him anticoagulant drugs now? The surgeons are asking the neurologists: What's his risk of bleeding into his brain *now*, twelve days after his strokes? Has his brain healed sufficiently to operate safely on his heart?

The neurologists can't answer this question. The risk of bleeding in Mr. Warner's situation is high. This risk decreases with time, as the strokes heal. But no one knows if twelve days is enough time. (In general, strokes take months to heal.) Some rare patients with bleeding strokes caused by bacterial endocarditis have been reported to survive open-heart surgery, but these rare cases tell us little about Mr. Warner's chances. What can I tell *him*?

Nancy, Mr. Warner's niece, is with him tonight, holding his hand. She has visited before but this is her first time in the Step-Down Unit. Fiftyish, well-dressed, and fashionably slim, Nancy is Mr. Warner's closest living relative, the married daughter of his deceased sister. Well aware of her uncle's strokes and visual deficit, she sits on his right side so he can see her comfortably. Unfortunately for Nancy, this means she is constantly viewing Mr. Hernandez, the brain-dead man in the bed to Mr. Warner's left. Seeing this, as I approach, I draw closed the curtain between their beds.

Oh, Nancy says softly. Thank you.

I go to her side of the bed so Mr. Warner can see me, too.

Nancy thinks she is here tonight to help her uncle decide whether to risk the heart surgery. She's nervous about this; Mr. Warner has been like a second father to her. It takes a few minutes for her to comprehend the news I'm delivering now: There is no decision to be made. A repeat MRI of Mr. Warner's brain, completed just an hour ago, shows three *new* strokes. Now there are at least five strokes that involve both sides of his brain, front and back. They're all relatively small. But they're all bleeding. There's no way we can put him on a heart-lung machine and operate now.

It's a remarkable thing, the fact that Mr. Warner looks so good when the MRI of his brain looks so bad. It's one more reminder of the fallibility of my old-fashioned physical examination, so valuable in some cases and yet so inadequate in others. Our high-tech, expensive tests really do make all the difference sometimes. Like now.

I'm not sure I understand, Nancy says.

Mr. Warner, holding her hand, says nothing.

May I have your hand, Mr. Warner?

Uncertainly, Nancy draws her own hand away. I take Mr. Warner's right hand in my own and turn his palm up. There, on the tips of three of his fingers and on the thumb side of his palm, are a half-dozen dark red blotches and violet bumps, angry-looking things. Most are smaller than a dime; one is the size of a nickel. He has more of them, just like these, on both feet. During the past week, half the medical students in the hospital, always graciously received by Mr. Warner, have come by to see these blotches and bumps. Called Janeway lesions and Osler nodes, they are visible proof that tiny pieces of his heart valve vegetation have broken off, traveled through Mr. Warner's circulation, and lodged in the little blood vessels of his hands and feet. Their red and purple colors mean that they are bleeding.

I explain to Mr. Warner and Nancy that this same phenomenon is what we are seeing in his brain. The neurologists and surgeons can't know whether he will bleed even more into his brain if he is put on the heart-lung machine and receives the blood-thinners to undergo the heart surgery. But it seems highly likely, especially in the three areas of his brain where the strokes are *new*.

Nancy sees immediately the damned-if-you-do-damned-if-you-don't side of this.

But the heart valve infection is the *cause* of these strokes, right?

Right.

Then Uncle could develop even more strokes if you *don't* do the surgery?

It's possible, yes.

Nancy pauses, thinking, as she cradles Mr. Warner's hand in hers.

Then what's the worst thing that could happen if he went for the surgery? Why not take the chance?

I turn to Mr. Warner.

You could die.

He looks at Nancy, then shrugs at me.

Feels like that's what's happening anyway, Dr. Reilly. I'd rather die trying than just lie here waiting.

Nancy squeezes his hand and gives him a smile, tears in her eyes.

There's my guy, she says.

I walk around the foot of Mr. Warner's bed and pull back the curtain to reveal Mr. Hernandez. Neat sheets cover him, all tucked in. Only his head and neck are visible. An older woman—his mother, I think—is sitting by the side of his bed now. She doesn't look up. She seems to be praying. The mechanical ventilator whooshes air into Mr. Hernandez's lungs, makes a metallic clicking noise, then wheezes the air out. His chest rises, then falls, with each ventilation. *Whoosh-click-wheeze*. And again.

Mr. Warner has turned his head far to his left so that he can see what Nancy and I can see. I close the curtain and walk back to his good side.

I speak to them both, very softly. I don't know if Mr. Hernandez's mother speaks English, but I don't want her to hear me.

Mr. Warner, that's what the surgeons and neurologists are afraid will happen to you if you have the surgery now. The surgeons are confident they can fix your heart. But they don't want you to end up like that.

Mr. Warner looks down, doesn't speak. Nancy does the same. All is quiet now, except Mr. Hernandez's ventilator. *Whoosh-click-wheeze. Whoosh* . . .

Now Mr. Warner looks up.

No, he says. No. Anything but that.

He's looking at me hard now. He's clear as a bell, I'm sure of it, clicking on all cylinders. No matter what the MRI of his brain looks like, Mr. Warner knows what he wants.

Anything but that, he says again.

Before I leave them, I explain again what we're doing. The different drugs, how they help. The fact that the great majority of patients with bacterial endocarditis are cured with antibiotics, without surgery. I know that hope helps—and sometimes, like now, I can offer it precisely because we *can't* predict his outcome with any certainty.

The odds are with you, Mr. Warner. Try to think positive. I think you're gonna be okay.

Nancy gives him a playful tap on his arm.

Yeah, she says to him, wiping away her tears.

I wish them a good evening. I tell Mr. Warner to call the nurse if he's concerned about anything. Dan is here for our team all night. I tell him Dan can reach me anytime.

He looks at me hard again before I go. He doesn't say anything. Then I'm gone.

As I walk out into the corridor, I feel more tired than I've felt in a long time. At my age, this can't be good. But I have one more stop to make before I get out of here tonight. Ashley paged me a while ago, thrilled that her guy had made it. Mr. Barensky's in the recovery room, a big open space adjacent to the operating rooms. His breathing tube is out. He's awake. From across the room, he looks damned good.

I type my password into a computer at the nursing station. What did they find? What did they do? There it is: the surgeon's brief operative note.

> I was called emergently to the operating room. . . . When I arrived at the OR, the patient was getting chest compressions and had no pulse. . . . Left pleural cavity was entered. Pericardium was identified. The first attempt to open was anteriorly. There was no significant return of fluid. We then opened it a bit further posteriorly. Approximately 900 mL of bloody fluid came out under pressure. Once the fluid was drained the patient's hemodynamics improved immediately. . . . The patient left the operating room in good condition.

He makes it sound so easy, so matter-of-fact. I couldn't do what he did if you gave me a hundred tries.

I sign off the computer and walk to Mr. Barensky's bedside. His daughter is with him, the one who speaks Russian. They are surrounded by monitors and machines. Pink fluid oozes into two drainage bags taped to his chest. His eyes are open. He sees me, seems to recognize me. We don't need his daughter to translate.

You're looking good, sir.

He shrugs. He lifts his arm, the one with the number tattoo, and waves me off.

I've been worse, he says hoarsely.

You're a lucky guy.

He shrugs again, grimacing.

I've been better, he says.

Chapter 9

TO THE LIMIT

> Art has something to do with the achievement of stillness
> in the midst of chaos. A stillness which characterizes prayer,
> too, and the eye of the storm . . . an arrest of attention in the
> midst of distraction.
>
> —Saul Bellow, *The Paris Review* (1966)

Friday, 5:45 a.m.

I don't believe in ghosts. But that's what comes to mind when I see him coming toward me: Is it a ghost? It's like those hallucinatory movie scenes in spaghetti westerns where at first you're not sure what you're seeing as the lone rider emerges slowly out of a shimmering horizon on a high mesa. I can't see his face from this distance—the hospital corridor, eerily empty and silent now, is the length of a city block—but there's something about him that makes me stop and watch and wait. If his crumpled white suit and running shoes are any indication, he's a surgical intern. I don't know any surgical interns. And yet, there's something about the way he walks, tired but effortless, an elite athlete heading for the locker room after a long, tough game. I've seen this walk before.

I'm on my game this morning, after collapsing into bed early last night and sleeping straight through the night. Before I did, though, I called in to check on Mr. Warner—he looks good, Dan said—and then called out to Shelter Island to check on Mom and Dad. Mom was resting comfortably, Ruth said, but she was exhausted from her hospital stay the night before. Dad was flying. Twenty-four hours ago, when I had been out there myself, he had looked as if he could die at any moment. But last night, he was jabbering away, telling old stories, jiving with Ruth and making her laugh. It's the morphine, Ruth said, he loves his morphine. This was true, I knew—Ruth put Dad on the phone and, pleasantly delirious, he made me laugh, too. But he also made me wonder: Hospice nurses, who know a lot about such things, say that the dying often revive transiently, just before the end. Like the embers of a banked fire, some of us pop and flame just before we go cold. We spark, laugh, take a curtain call. Briefly, we flare up, ourselves again, for a few hours or days. I wonder if that's what's happening now to Dad. Either way, I'm glad he had some fun last night.

As the young intern approaches, he can't help noticing my interest. He shoots me a benign but wary look. He's the spitting image of his father. He even moves like him. It's been decades since I've seen Phil, a respected surgeon in Connecticut who was my medical school classmate here forty years ago. The only memory I have of Peter, Phil's youngest son, is watching a towheaded two-year-old whack golf balls like Tiger Woods in his parents' backyard. His golf club was taller than he was but no one was surprised by Peter's precocious skills. His dad had been a great athlete, too. Years later, I heard through the grapevine that Peter had become an All-American golfer at Princeton. I hadn't known that he'd followed in his dad's footsteps to become a surgeon as well. He's got the genes, that's for sure.

I stop Peter in the corridor, introduce myself. I can see from his reaction that I'm not the first to do this. Peter's dad was a surgical resident here long ago; clearly, some other old-timers have seen the ghost, too. Peter's in a hurry now, lots to do, but he's polite and respectful, glad to remember me to his parents. As we head off, we find ourselves approaching the same private room. We've come to see the same patient, Mr. Principo.

I've read the ED doc's overnight admitting note about Mr. Principo and I've looked at the X-rays and CT scan of his chest. So I know some important things about him before I meet him. But there are other things I don't know, things I can know only by doing what I'm about to do now. In the old days, Peter and I might have examined the patient together, the young doctor watching the older one and vice versa, each of us learning from the other. But there's no time for this now. Peter has two other preoperative patients to see before he makes rounds with his Thoracic Surgery team at 6:30 and I have to meet my own team at 7:00. Peter says he'll circle back after I'm done. Before he leaves, I tell him what I'm concerned about. Putting a big tube into Mr. Principo's chest, which Peter's surgical team has been asked to do, may not be the right way to go. Briefly, I explain why. For an internist, even an experienced one like me, it's a subtle point, but Peter, less than a year out of med school, is way ahead of me.

Yeah, I saw the pictures, too, Dr. Reilly. Not a problem. In cases like these, we just do VATS. I'll discuss it with my seniors but it shouldn't be an issue, assuming the patient consents.

VATS is video-assisted thoracic surgery, a "minimally invasive" surgical technique that allows the surgeon to perform major chest operations through very small incisions between the ribs, using instruments equipped with miniature movie cameras. It's easier and safer for the patient, especially an elderly one like Mr. Principo, because the surgeon can work inside the chest without cutting it wide open. VATS is fairly new, something I don't know a lot about. As Peter leaves, I josh him a little, suggest that maybe we should call his dad to come in and help.

Peter chuckles, shakes his head. Yeah, well, in the old days, maybe. But, today, even Dad would admit this one's out of his league. He doesn't do this stuff.

I don't mention that I don't do it either. Peter is used to doing newfangled things that the old farts like me know little about. In medical centers that do cutting-edge stuff, it's a given that I and other doctors of my generation are being left behind. Peter's dad is a general surgeon, trained decades ago to operate on almost anything, the surgical equivalent of an old-fashioned internist like me. (Back then, it was often joked that great general surgeons like Phil are good internists who, unlike internists, also can fix things.) Today, just as I'm being replaced by subspecialists in medicine—cardiologists, oncologists, gastroenterologists—general surgeons like Phil are competing with surgical subspecialists, elite technicians who operate *only* on the neck or the breast or the colon. I can almost hear the conversations around the holiday dinner table at the McWhorter house, Phil needling Peter about the decline of "real surgeons," Peter noodging him back about the cool new surgical technique he's learning every day.

If I were Mr. Principo, based on what I've just seen on his CT scan, I'd want the superspecialized technician who does these new VATS procedures every day, not an old-fashioned general surgeon (who doesn't). But Mr. Principo shouldn't have to choose between cutting-edge technical skills and old-fashioned clinical expertise. It's my job to make sure he gets the benefit of both. To do this, though, I have to know more about him than what his CT scan shows.

As I enter his room, his wife is hovering at his bedside. There's nothing unusual about this except the time of day—it's very early—and Ms. Principo herself. She looks like someone who used to be in the movies, an actress whose name you can't quite recall. As it turns out, that's exactly who she is. Mr. Principo is a retired film director. His wife started out as an actress, then became a successful editor. She's about my age, at least twenty years younger than her husband but no spring chicken. Still, despite her lack of sleep, makeup, or reason to smile, she'll turn heads even here in the hospital.

I introduce myself. She seems relieved to see me.

I was beginning to think all of the doctors in this hospital are thirty years old, she says.

Yeah, well, on the night shift, that's not far off.

Isn't this still the night shift?

Technically, yes.

So?

At my age, I need a head start to keep up with the young ones.

I know what you mean, doc, her husband says.

I like him right away. He reminds me of my father. Like Dad, he's tall, his sheeted feet extending to the bottom of the big hospital bed. The same white hair, brainy forehead, strong jaw. And the resemblance is more than physical. As we talk, I get the sense that this is a guy you can trust. It seems silly to describe an eighty-four-year-old man as mature, but that's the feeling I get: Like Dad, this guy's an *adult*. There's something about him that tells you he's been around the block—he's had his fun but taken his hits, too—and he's learned a few things along the way. In just a few minutes, I can see that he knows what he's up against. And yet, his equanimity is almost palpable. I've marveled at this phenomenon before: There really is something to this "Greatest Generation" stuff. Whatever your battle, you'd want Mr. Principo on your side. Somehow, you can just tell that he'd have your back.

The pain and shortness of breath began about a month ago when he fell out of a tree. At the time, he was pruning branches in his apple orchard in New Jersey. Unfortunately, from the look of him now, I doubt that's when all this really began. He's a lean, muscular guy—men half his age would envy his physique—but his cheeks and temples look more hollow than healthy. When he fell out of the tree, they took him to the local hospital, where the doctors told him he had two broken ribs and some bleeding in the space around his left lung. It should get better on its own, they told him, though it would take several weeks. Instead, it got worse, not only the pain and the breathing trouble but also Mr. Principo's sense that something bad was happening. He returned to his local hospital yesterday; he was told that there was more blood in his left chest than before, not less, and that he should stay in the hospital to have more tests. Instead, he and his wife got into their car, made the four-hour drive to Manhattan, and plunked themselves down in our emergency department together with a couple of hundred other people. His entire left chest is filled with fluid—blood, probably—so you can't see his left lung at all, not even on the CT scan. Despite this, he can walk and talk and get around all right, so the ED guys admitted him to us after talking to the surgeons. Dan, who saw him during the night, hasn't typed his own assessment into the computer yet, but I can see that he decided to wait until morning before removing any fluid from Mr. Principo's chest. Now that I see what I've come to see, I'm glad Dan waited.

At first, I don't find what I'm looking for. I don't feel any abnormal lymph nodes in his neck or behind his collarbones. His voice isn't hoarse, though his Adam's apple deviates to the right, pushed to one side by all the fluid in his left chest. His liver isn't enlarged or hard and his neurological exam is normal. When I tap on his chest with my fingers—it's like playing a bongo drum—the percussion note over his air-filled right lung is tympanic, as it should be, but the sound on the left is deadly dull. When I listen with my stethoscope, I'm surprised to hear breath sounds on this dull left side but then, thinking as I listen, I'm pretty sure that the breath sounds I hear on the left are being transmitted from the right. His left lung isn't breathing at all. If that's what Dan thought, too—and if that's the reason he didn't put a tube in there yet to drain the fluid—then Dan's even smarter than I thought. Putting a chest tube in there could make Mr. Principo worse, not better.

Still, after finishing my examination, I'm not sure about any of this until I sit him up to help him put his shirt on. I didn't see his drooping left eyelid while he was lying down. But I see it now.

His wife has been watching me, waiting patiently. Now she begins to ask questions. She has heard that we'll be putting in the chest tube this morning. When? she asks.

I hold up a finger, ask her to wait one more minute. I look at him again.

His left eyelid droops by only a few millimeters, so subtly that in someone else I would pay no attention. But, in his case, it means everything. I press my thumbs above his eyebrows so he can't use his forehead muscles to help lift his eyelids. No doubt about it, then, his left eyelid is weak. I also see that his left pupil is slightly smaller than his right. Just a few minutes ago, when I wasn't specifically looking for this, I missed it completely. And now, when I shine my penlight into his eyes, both pupils constrict normally, just as they did before. But, this time, I keep looking after I pull my penlight away. Only the right pupil relaxes, dilating back to its resting size. The left one doesn't; it remains constricted, as if my light were still there.

Such a minor thing. It doesn't bother Mr. Principo a bit. He doesn't even know it's there. But, together with his hollow temples and fifteen-pound weight loss, it means that his fluid-filled chest probably has nothing to do with his falling out of an apple tree. To try to confirm this, I feel behind his collarbones again, digging deep, so deep that he grimaces a little. Nothing there. Too bad, in a way. It would have made things easier for him if I'd found the cancer there, too.

You're about the sixth doctor who's examined me here, Dr. Reilly. I don't recall any of them being so interested in my eyes. Or my collarbones. What's it about?

His wife watches us silently.

Mr. Principo, your left eye has a slight abnormality called Horner's syndrome. In itself, it's nothing to be concerned about. But it's a sign that something in your chest is pressing on an important nerve bundle.

The fluid in my lung is pressing on a nerve?

No, sir. What I see in your eye means that there's another problem in your chest. In addition to the fluid. Most likely, there are swollen glands in your chest, outside the lung itself, that are pressing on the nerve.

Swollen glands?

Most likely, yes. Usually we would see this on the CT scan. But there is so much fluid in your chest, it's hard to say for sure.

So, after you drain the fluid with the tube, we will know?

That's the question, Mr. Principo. Based on what I see, I don't think draining the fluid with a tube is the best way to go. I will speak with the surgeons in a little while. They know more about this than I do, but I think that they will want to put you to sleep and deal with this in the operating room.

His wife inhales audibly. Mr. Principo nods calmly and takes his wife's hand. But his eyes never leave mine.

My wife and I have talked about this, Dr. Reilly. That's why we came here. I don't think my lung problem is from my accident at all.

As he speaks, he watches me, gauging my reaction.

I don't tell Mr. Principo that I think he has a cancer obstructing the bronchial tube to his left lung, a cancer that has already spread to the lymph nodes in his chest and to the lining around his lung. I don't tell him that this kind of cancer is inoperable and incurable, almost certain to kill him in the next few months no matter what we do. I don't tell him any of this because I don't know it for sure yet. But he doesn't need me to tell him. I'm a lousy poker player. Mr. Principo can see what I think without my saying a word.

If I've got cancer, Mr. Principo continues, I know what I want. I don't want chemo and radiation and machines. I'm eighty-four years old. I've lived a damned lucky life. If it's my time to go, I want to go fast. For my own sake, and for Helen's.

I've seen death watches, doc. No thanks. Not for me.

His wife inhales deeply again. They exchange a brief, intimate look.

I tell them that they will want to know for sure before making any final decisions. I tell them that he may be right—he may have cancer—but there are different kinds of cancer, some of which are treatable, even curable.

Ms. Principo inhales again. She looks like she could kiss me. Her husband squints.

What I've just told them is true. Curable cancers—Hodgkin's lymphoma and a few others—can cause similar findings. I don't think that's what's wrong with Mr. Principo but it doesn't matter what I think. What matters is that we need to find out for sure.

Mr. Principo is still squinting.

And after the surgery? Then what?

Then we'll be able to tell you for sure what this is, what the treatment options are. At that point, it's your call about what to do.

Mmm.

He looks at his wife, a stern conspiratorial look. She shakes her head in disbelief.

Wow, she whispers to him.

She looks at me, then at her husband.

Okay? she asks him, gesturing at me. Okay?

He looks at me for a moment, then nods again and looks away.

She takes another deep breath.

Dr. Reilly, Nick's first wife died of lung cancer twenty years ago. They told her they could remove it. She had the surgery. The cancer was too advanced to cure. There were complications. She stayed on the breathing machine for months, one thing after another. She refused to quit even when the cancer was terminal. It was awful . . . for . . . for everyone.

Yes, I see. I'm sorry.

Mr. Principo nods at his wife. She's crying quietly. Now he looks at me.

It was . . . very hard, Dr. Reilly. For . . . everyone. When Jane got sick, Helen and I were already . . . friends. So . . . it was hard . . . for . . . everyone.

Yes, I see.

I ask them to think more about what we've discussed so far. I tell them I'll be back in an hour with Dan, whom they've met, and the rest of my team. I tell them that a surgical intern will see them soon and then brief the senior surgeons this morning.

Mr. Principo says he understands. Then he says he wants assurances about two things.

First, if we go ahead with the surgery, I want a clear plan. If the surgery shows that I have cancer—the bad kind, the untreatable kind—I want everything stopped. I don't want treatment that might buy me a few extra weeks. I want out. Can you do that? Can you assure me that you will stop everything, just keep me comfortable, and let me die in peace? Can you do that?

I don't tell him about Dad.

Yes, Mr. Principo, I can do that.

He pauses, searches my face for something, then continues.

One more thing. I'll be on a breathing machine for the operation, right?

Yes.

After the operation, if they can't get me off the machine, I want out. I won't live on a machine, like my wife did. Do you understand? Even if you find something in my chest that you can treat, maybe even cure, I won't live on a machine. Can you do that? Can you stop the machine if it looks like I can't live without it?

Yes. If we are all agreed, yes, I can do that.

I look at his wife. She looks at her husband, then at me.

Yes, she says, biting her lip. Whatever Nick wants.

An hour later, after I've seen my other new admissions and talked to the chest surgeons, I'm back with my team in Mr. Principo's room. He's tired. His eyes are closed as Dan recounts his findings—Mr. Principo's history, physical examination, and test results—to Tina and Ashley. Ms. Principo listens intently as Dan tells the story of her husband's accident, his fall from the apple tree, and subsequent events. She can see Tina's and Ashley's frowns, their growing perplexity and doubt, as Dan describes Mr. Principo's progressive worsening ever since, the weight loss, the apparent collapse of his entire left lung. Dan doesn't say anything about Mr. Principo's sagging eyelid or constricted pupil. He hadn't noticed these things himself. Nor does he describe the subtle difference in breath sounds when listening to Mr. Principo's lungs. But Dan has come to the same conclusion I did. He didn't get there using my old-fashioned methods. For Dan it was high-tech all the way.

I reviewed the chest CT with the radiologist last night, Dan tells us. There's so much fluid in the left hemithorax, it's hard to be sure, but the left mainstem bronchus isn't visible, likely obstructed.

Tina and Ashley begin to nod. It is beginning to make sense to them, now.

So, Dan continues, we did a head CT. It shows multiple, enhancing lesions in both cerebral hemispheres.

Tina and Ashley nod again, averting their eyes from the Principos. They know now that the apple tree is a red herring. This is inoperable lung cancer with multiple metastases to the brain. It's not Hodgkin's lymphoma or any other curable kind of cancer. It's fatal. Always. Mr. Principo has only weeks to live.

Mr. Principo's eyes remain closed as Dan finishes his story, but his wife steps forward, looks at me anxiously.

His head? There's something wrong with his head?

I look at Dan. This is news to me, too. I found nothing on Mr. Principo's neurological examination to suggest brain metastases. Neither did Dan. But, based on what he saw in the chest, Dan did the right thing. Strongly suspecting cancer, he looked to see whether it had spread outside the chest, the crucial clinical question. In response to Ms. Principo, I motion to Dan to explain. He does it well.

There are several spots on the brain scan that look abnormal, ma'am. We can't be sure what these mean yet, but they're probably related to your husband's chest problem. We'll know more after the surgeons drain out the fluid and give us tissue specimens to examine in the laboratory.

She looks at Dan, then at me. She doesn't speak. Now she looks at her husband, his eyes closed peacefully.

I see, she says. She steps back, says nothing more.

Mr. Principo opens his eyes. In response to my question, he says, Yes, he's heard everything we've said, including Dan's report about the brain scan. I ask him if we can briefly listen to his lungs again. He agrees, and now Dan and the others hear the subtle difference I had heard before. I show them Mr. Principo's eye, the sign that his cancer has invaded the mediastinum, the central chest compartment where lung cancers typically spread first. Finally, we repeat his neurological examination. It's normal, cold normal, no sign of the cancer in his brain. All of this takes only a few minutes. When we're done, we don't need to articulate the obvious. My generation's old-fashioned physical examination can tell doctors important things. But the new generation's high-tech approach works well, too. Sometimes better.

None of this is lost on the Principos, who watch and listen as we go through our paces. When we're done, Ms. Principo thanks us and speaks softly to her husband.

You were right, hon. You were right to come here.

He nods at her, then turns to us all.

Doctors, you don't know my wife but she has very good taste. In everything. Clothes . . . hospitals . . . husbands.

We laugh.

Mr. Principo reaches out and shakes Dan's hand.

Looks to me like you did pretty good, young man.

Dan, not the blushing type, blushes.

Thank you, sir.

I tell the Principos that Dan is a scientist as well as a doctor, both a Ph.D. and an M.D., a cancer researcher with a special interest in "solid tumors" such as lung cancer. I tell them that Dan's generation of researchers will find ways to cure these kinds of cancer.

Mr. Principo is not a sour grapes kind of guy.

I hope you will, he says to Dan. Good luck, son.

Here, in the room, I don't tell Dan and the others about Mr. Principo's wishes. About not wanting treatment, or life support machines, once the diagnosis is proved. We'll talk about it after we've left his room. Then they will all understand why Mr. Principo says what he says now.

So, Dr. Reilly, the surgeons will come to get me around midday today?

Yes, sir, that's what they tell me.

And they might have answers to my questions right away, in the operating room, is that right?

It's hard to say for sure, sir. But it's possible, yes.

He nods, looks at his wife, then looks at all of us.

Then, doctors, please excuse us. We'd like a little privacy now, if you don't mind.

Medical decision-making can be difficult for many reasons, but two of these stand out. First, there is always more than one way to manage any given medical problem; which approach to take depends, in large part, on the patient's goals. Second, no matter which approach is taken, the outcome of every medical decision is uncertain and the possible outcomes always include harms as well as benefits. Patients typically focus more on the benefits than the harms, not always a good idea.

For these reasons, active engagement by the patient is essential to the decision-making process. Mr. Principo is most unusual in this regard. His own goals, when facing serious illness, are well informed and clearly articulated. He is well aware of the uncertainties involved; in his case, a definitive diagnosis has not yet been made. Even so, he is sufficiently self-aware to know that, *for him*, the worst possible outcome of his exploratory surgery is not a devastating diagnosis, but a protracted downhill course, utterly dependent on mechanical life support, with no hope of recovery. He is taking great pains to ensure that this outcome *cannot* happen to him. In so doing, Mr. Principo is not acting purely out of self-interest. Like many ill and elderly people, he dreads becoming a burden to his loved ones even more than he fears death itself. For his wife's sake as well as his own, he is drawing a line in the sand. He is saying: This is as far as I go.

He is specifying precise, strict *limits* to the types and amount of care he will allow.

Equally remarkable, Mr. Principo has done these things with no advice from me or, as far as I know, any other doctor. The limits he has drawn—their specification, timing, and contingencies—are entirely his own idea. If his goals and wishes didn't make sense to me, I, as his doctor, would explore them more, maybe push him to reconsider. But the limits he has set make perfect sense.

Other patients might choose differently: undergo the surgical procedure—both to confirm the diagnosis and to gain some temporary symptomatic relief—and then perhaps agree to receive radiation therapy to the brain. Radiation cannot cure the metastatic brain cancers but it can shrink them and, perhaps, buy patients more time. If they survived the surgery and radiation therapy, many of these patients would then agree to undergo chemotherapy treatments to try to retard further spread of the cancer. Although the median survival of patients like Mr. Principo is only a few months *despite treatment*, some will survive longer (as Stephen Jay Gould reminded us). Thus, for every patient like Mr. Principo who declines treatment, there is another (like his first wife) who will embrace it. Each individual patient must decide for himself.

Today, aggressive treatment of incurable, end-stage disease in elderly patients is highly controversial. Such decisions raise many concerns about the appropriate limits of medical care that is only marginally beneficial yet extremely expensive, especially now when millions of other Americans can't get even basic medical care. Like many other controversies about health care today, this one ostensibly is about money and budgets. How, given finite resources, can we optimize the "value" of medical care (its benefit-per-dollar-spent) equitably for all citizens? But the deeper controversy here is about *values*: What makes a life worth living? What makes a day or week or month of additional life worth fighting for? This is why, when doctors and patients make medical decisions, clarifying the patient's values is the most essential step of all.

On a national scale, then, we must consider *societal* values when considering how, if at all, to limit medical care in the United States today. Daniel Callahan has reminded us that several deeply ingrained values in U.S. society *work against* any notion of systematically imposing limits on doctors' and patients' clinical decisions.

> First, we prize autonomy and freedom of choice and want everyone to have them. . . . Second, we cherish the idea of limitless medical progress, which has come to mean that every disease should be cured, every disability rehabilitated, every health need met, and every evidence of mortality, especially aging, vigorously challenged. . . . Finally, we long for quality in medicine and health care, which in practice we define as the presence of high-class amenities . . . and a level of technology that is . . . better today than yesterday and will be even better tomorrow. . . .
> Yet . . . the unrestrained embodiment of these values . . . is precisely what creates contradictions and renders meaningful reform so hard. . . . Setting limits means we cannot have everything we want or dream of . . . unlimited medical progress, maximal choice, perfect health, and profits and income.

Unlike Callahan, many people believe that "meaningful reform" of U.S. medical care does not require imposition of *any* systematic limits on patients' choices, doctors' decisions, or medical progress. Personally, I wish they were right about this. Leaving private medical decisions *entirely* in the hands of patients and their doctors is, and always will be, preferable. In fact, imposing limits on patient choice or medical progress feels downright un-American.

But time is running out for those who disagree with Callahan about the need for limits. More than twenty years ago, when the United States spent 11.4 percent of its gross domestic product (GDP) on health care (and 6.8 percent on education), Callahan warned that health, although hugely important, is not society's *only* priority. But today, we spend 18 percent of GDP on health care (and only 5 percent on education). By 2040, health care is projected to consume 33 percent of GDP. Even if you believe that health is society's single most important priority, these trends are unsustainable.

Most doctors believe that the "system" is beyond their control. Many believe that the call for limits can be circumvented if the government would reform medical malpractice laws (which promote costly defensive medicine); restrain insurance companies' profit margins and administrative overhead (or eliminate them entirely with a single-payer national health insurance system); and rein in the bountiful perks of the pharmaceutical and medical device industries. No doubt these systemic changes could substantially reduce the rate of rise of health care costs. But they could also *decrease* the quality of care, medical innovation, and patient autonomy.

There is no simple prescription to resolve this dilemma. However, the "real money" in health care—almost two-thirds of *all* health care expenditures in the United States— is spent on just 10 percent of the population: patients with chronic medical conditions such as diabetes, emphysema, and heart disease. Ezekiel Emanuel and other experts have argued that only physicians can lead the effort to redesign care delivery for *these* patients and thereby create a more cost-efficient system. But this effort would require substantial societal investment in a new kind of health care delivery system, one with universal electronic medical records, nonphysician "care coordinators," and less reliance on expensive subspecialist physicians. It would require "thinking outside the box" about new technologies (such as home medical monitoring systems), essential "nonmedical" services (such as transportation to doctors' offices), and even some old-fashioned practices (such as house calls). Why has this not happened yet? Because the cost savings made possible by such system redesign can occur only if they substantially reduce unnecessary hospitalizations, emergency department visits, and referrals to specialist physicians. What do you think lobbyists for the hospital industry and physicians' special interest groups say about such reductions?

Emanuel is right about the need for physicians to lead the effort to change the system. But which physicians, exactly, does he have in mind? Who will do this?

7:00 a.m.

It happens fast, as I had worried it might.

Mr. Warner did well overnight, Dan says, standing in the corridor outside the Step-Down Unit, no shortness of breath like the past few nights.

Good news, I'm thinking. Maybe we can buy him some time, get him through the next few weeks, eradicate his infection, let his strokes heal. Then his surgical risk might be acceptable. Maybe then the surgeons can repair his damaged heart valve, make a new man of him.

A nurse bustles out of the Step-Down Unit into the corridor, wheeling her vital signs machine behind her. She looks worried. She approaches us hopefully.

Is Mr. Warner yours?

She's already turned up his oxygen and cranked up the head of his bed. But when we get in there he's breathing fast and hard and beginning to fidget, agitated and restless from insufficient oxygen. Sweat glistens on his forehead and neck. His blood pressure is holding but, even with the extra oxygen streaming through his plastic nasal cannula, the oxygen reading in his blood is low. Tina runs to get a face mask and call Respiratory Therapy while the rest of us surround his bed. It's hard to hear his heart sounds well because his breathing is so noisy and fast. His hands and feet are clammy cold. He resists the oxygen mask that Tina brings him, a "nonrebreather" that covers his face from the top of his nose to below his chin, a claustrophobic thing even if you're not gasping for air. We hold him down, give the mask a chance to help, and in a few minutes he settles back against his pillow and closes his eyes. His breathing slows a little. His gown is drenched in sweat. The nurse clips the oxygen sensor on his finger again. The machine beeps a few times, then reads 82 percent in bright red flashing digits. We're giving him as much oxygen as we can without putting him on a breathing machine but it's not enough. Tina runs out to STAT-page Anesthesia and grab the ICU guys next door. Ashley rolls in the cardiac arrest cart, just in case. Dan and I try again to listen to his breathing. Loud rhonchorous noises fill his lungs wherever we put our stethoscopes.

A few minutes later, Dave, one of the ICU fellows, has intubated Mr. Warner's windpipe after sedating him with an IV injection. He lies limp in his bed now, unconscious. Copious bloody secretions are suctioned out of the endotracheal tube, now streaming pure oxygen directly into his lungs. Still, his blood oxygen level remains low, only 84 percent.

Damn! Dave says, and checks the breathing tube for leaks. Quickly, he puts his stethoscope on Mr. Warner's left chest, then his right.

Shit! he says, and pulls the tube back an inch or two out of Mr. Warner's mouth, repositioning it. Now he listens again to both lungs, one then the other.

Okay, okay, Dave mutters to himself, as the oxygen sensor beeps, then flashes 96 percent in bright green digits. Carefully, Dave tapes the tube around Mr. Warner's mouth, securing it in place. A respiratory therapist wheels a ventilator machine into the room. It's a cabinet the size and shape of a street-corner mailbox, its surface panel covered with dials and gauges. Dave connects the machine to Mr. Warner's endotracheal tube. Now the machine is breathing for him.

Whoosh-click-wheeze!

There are two of them now, side by side, each connected to his own breathing machine, their whooshes and wheezes like questions and answers. Mr. Warner and Mr. Hernandez, his young brain-dead roommate, are having a mechanical conversation. And what I'm hearing are Mr. Warner's final words last night to his niece and me: *Anything but that.*

As usual, there are no empty beds in the ICU. They will need to move someone out to move Mr. Warner in. The ICU guys do this every day, make judgments about which patients need their life-saving treatments most. Some days they can't move anyone; then, they horse-trade with the other ICUs in the hospital—like the Cardiac ICU or the Burn Unit or the Neurosurgical ICU. They figure it out. Somehow, they always figure it out. In what seems like only a few minutes, the ICU guys are wheeling Mr. Warner's bed and breathing machine and IV poles out the big door of the Step-Down Unit and down the corridor to the ICU. Now Mr. Warner has stepped up as high as he can go. If he can't make it in the ICU, he can't make it anywhere. Tina goes with him to do a proper hand-off, tell the ICU team what they need to know about him. There's a lot to tell.

Dan and Ashley and I stay behind. We exit the Step-Down Unit and the strangely empty space just vacated by Mr. Warner's bed. We have people to see—more of Dan's new overnight admissions and all of our other patients. We have to keep our eye on the ball, even as Mr. Warner disappears down the corridor. He belongs to the ICU guys now.

Down in the ED, it's been one of those nights when one theme seems to repeat itself. It's random chance, of course, no real pattern to it, but sometimes it seems like the ED is running a special—on heart attacks or cancer or trauma. Last night's special was pus. Three of our ED admissions need pus drained. One of them, a young woman nine months pregnant with her first child, has a high fever and a hot red arm, swollen from her hand to her shoulder. She received antibiotics two days ago in another hospital's emergency department but when she got worse she came here. Dan started her on stronger IV antibiotics last night but one look at her arm this morning shows that she needs more than that. When you've seen one of these you never forget it, and I've seen many more than one, so it's fun to walk Dan through the procedure of draining the pus out of her elbow, which, if we didn't drain, would make her and her baby a lot sicker soon. Dan numbs the elbow with an injection of anesthetic before inserting his big drainage needle but Tina is the anesthetic that makes all the difference. As Dan and I work on the elbow, Tina canoodles with the frightened young woman about childbirth and babies—the patient's (a girl, any day now) and Tina's (a boy, four months to go). As the barrel of Dan's big syringe fills with thick yellow-green pus, the young woman giggles and sighs with Tina about their latest ultrasounds and nursery preparations. Then, over the course of the next hour, Dan does the same thing to an old man's knee—after draining what pus we can get out, we call the Orthopedics guys because he'll need even more drainage in the OR—and then Ashley does the honors for a young guy screaming and yelling about the "royal pain in my ass." The top of his buttock is red and sore but the ED guys have used their echo machine to see if there's a pocket of pus in there and it doesn't look like it, so they started him on antibiotics and admitted him to us. But now when we put a finger on his swollen butt, one particular spot hurts more than any other and it bounces when you poke your finger on it. So we numb him up and Ashley says Wow! when the pus starts to flow into her syringe, too, and the guy says Aaah! so relieved he wants to hug her even when we tell him he'll need to go to the operating room, too. It's one of those mornings when time seems to fly. When we're done, Dan goes home to get some sleep and Ashley heads over to the surgical ICU—she's thrilled that Mr. Barensky survived his pericardial tamponade yesterday—and Tina and I go back up to the medical ICU to check on Mr. Warner.

When we get there, his room is crowded with doctors and nurses, not a good sign. There are twenty critically ill patients in this ICU but most of the staff right now is working on Mr. Warner. From outside his glass-enclosed room, I peer in at the visual display of vital signs on his monitors. His oxygen level is holding steady at 96 percent on the mechanical ventilator but the digital readout shows his heart rate is in the high twenties, only one blip every two or three seconds. His blood pressure barely registers at all.

Jeez, Tina says.

I stand on tiptoes and crane my neck to see over the crowd. It looks like a scene from a movie about extraterrestrial germ warfare. Everyone is covered, head to toe, in blue floor-length gowns, some of them spattered with blood. All faces are masked, even their eyes shielded behind plastic see-through visors, splash-proofed against Mr. Warner's HIV-infected blood. One nurse is applying round sticky pads to Mr. Warner's bare chest. Two others are dialing up the infusion machines to pump powerful drugs into his veins to try to raise his heart rate and blood pressure. Dave, the ICU fellow who intubated Mr. Warner in the Step-Down Unit, is standing at the head of the bed, rapidly swabbing Mr. Warner's neck and shoulder area with an orange-colored disinfectant. Josh, a senior medical resident, stands on the opposite side of the bed, pushing a syringe filled with drug into one of Mr. Warner's IVs, his eyes glued to the vital signs monitor to assess its effect. Oren Friedman, the ICU attending, stands at the foot of the bed, surveying the scene, calmly calling out numbers, ordering this then that, everyone hopping to his commands. From where I'm standing, looking at those shrinking

numbers on the vital signs monitor, it's a disaster. Mr. Warner is trying hard to die. But Friedman's team, gowned and masked, hushed
and grim, has other ideas. They move and mesh like one multilimbed
organism. They've done this before.

No response to atropine times two, Friedman announces to the
room. Dopamine is at twenty mikes, right, Sue?

Right, someone says.

Kristen, Friedman says, set the external pacer at ninety. Sue, start
the Levophed. Dave, you ready to go with the eye-jay?

Yeah, someone says.

Now Friedman addresses the senior resident, whose eyes are
glued to the vital signs monitor.

What do you see there, Josh?

Looks like complete heart block with a slow junctional escape
rhythm, Josh says. We need a twelve-lead but there's ST-elevation
in lead two, maybe he's having an inferior MI.

Right. And what do you make of that?

Friedman, in the heat of the battle, is teaching.

Maybe he's embolized his right coronary, Josh's voice answers.

Right. Might just be spasm from his hypotension but I agree,
that's the worry. So what do we do?

Nothing we *can* do if we don't get his heart rate and pressure up.
So?

Gotta have that pacemaker.

Good, Josh. Dave?

I'm in the eye-jay, someone says. Balloon is up, advancing the
pacing catheter now.

Dave, the ICU fellow at the head of the bed, has inserted a big
needle into the internal jugular ("eye-jay") vein in Mr. Warner's neck,
spilling rivulets of blood on the sterile drapes covering Mr. Warner's neck and shoulder. Through the needle Dave has threaded a
metal wire into the vein and then, after removing the needle, he has
passed a yard-long rubber catheter, like a long piece of spaghetti, over
the metal wire and down through the vein into Mr. Warner's heart.
Embedded in this special catheter is a cardiac pacemaker wire that,
if Dave can position it properly in the right ventricle of the heart,

can begin to spark Mr. Warner's heart, stimulating it electrically to pump faster and raise Mr. Warner's blood pressure. No one survives a heart rate of twenty or a blood pressure this low for very long. It's now or never.

Tina and I squeeze into the room at the foot of the bed near Friedman. Except for the *whoosh-click-wheeze* of Mr. Warner's ventilator and the scary-slow tinny blips on his heart monitor, the room is dead quiet now. Mr. Warner himself is invisible, unconscious beneath all the sheets and sterile drapes. Can he feel any of this? Does he somehow know what's happening?

The blips accelerate. On the monitor, spikes of heartbeat go faster now, ninety per minute.

I've got pacing, Dave says calmly from the head of the bed.

Yeah, Tina whispers.

Friedman says nothing. He looks at the vital signs monitor, where the pulse registers ninety but the blood pressure is still only sixty. Friedman sticks his gloved hand into Mr. Warner's groin, feeling for a pulse.

Barely palpable, he says. Levophed on?

Just running now, someone says.

Silence again. They're doing everything they can do.

Now the blood pressure tracing on the monitor begins to bump. What had looked like a slow feeble wave is now a sharp spike, higher and faster. Friedman sticks his hand in Mr. Warner's groin again.

We got pressure here. Let's move, everyone, let's move!

Yeah, Tina whispers again.

Now, the many limbs of the organism do their thing, all of them perfectly coordinated. Dave sews the pacing wire into Mr. Warner's neck and sets the dials on the pacemaker power box. Two of the nurses fuss with the IV pumps, adjusting the doses of the antishock pressor drugs. Another begins to clean up the mess around Mr. Warner, careful to put the blood-spattered drapes in special infection control containers. Josh wheels in an electrocardiogram machine to take another heart tracing, look for the heart attack he thinks may have just occurred. Friedman watches all of this, then nods and steps out of the room with me and Tina.

Not sure yet, Friedman says calmly in answer to my question.

He fills us in on what has happened these past few hours. The ICU team has been able to oxygenate Mr. Warner with the mechanical ventilator, but not without difficulty. His new chest X-ray shows a dense infiltrate throughout his right lung, much more suggestive of pneumonia than heart failure.

But your idea of unilateral pulmonary edema is still possible, Friedman says, and nods admiringly at Tina. Really good idea. We've been trying to stabilize him enough to find out for sure.

They've started additional antibiotics and blood pressure drugs to treat Mr. Warner for pneumonia and septic shock—he's now receiving nine different antibiotics, including his HIV drugs—but his diagnosis is still no more than an educated guess. Friedman was planning to put a bronchoscope down into Mr. Warner's lungs to sample the bloody fluid there, test it for infections, but that was before Mr. Warner crashed and needed the emergency cardiac pacemaker. Otherwise, Friedman has done all he can to treat Mr. Warner's respiratory failure and to prevent kidney failure, but it may be too late; Mr. Warner hasn't made a drop of urine since coming to the ICU. We don't know yet whether a failing heart is the primary cause of Mr. Warner's failing lungs and kidneys, or whether everything is failing for multiple different reasons. Either way, Friedman will need help.

A Cardiology fellow arrives, wheeling his portable echocardiogram machine.

Friedman did his own bedside cardiac echo an hour ago but he doesn't trust the results. His echo machine is not as accurate as the cardiologist's transesophageal echo device. This is the test Mr. Warner couldn't tolerate yesterday. But, unconscious and intubated, he'll tolerate it now. We need to know.

The echo probe slides down his esophagus quick as a wink. On the vital signs monitor, Mr. Warner's numbers hold their own: His oxygen level is adequate (thanks to the ventilator); his heart rate is ninety (thanks to the pacemaker); and his blood pressure has come up (thanks to the powerful "pressor" drugs). But now, even before Friedman or the Cardiology fellow says a word, I can see the echo jet on their video monitor, right where Tina said it would be. Mr.

Warner may have pneumonia and kidney failure, too. But if he does, they're the least of his problems. It's his blown heart valve that's killing him.

There's only one chance to save him now. Friedman and the Cardiology fellow confer quickly. The fellow runs off to alert the senior cardiologists and to free up one of the operating rooms in the cardiac catheterization lab. There, the interventional cardiologists can insert a catheter into the big artery in Mr. Warner's groin, snake the catheter up into his heart, and inject dye to see whether he's had a heart attack, treat it, and also visualize his damaged heart valve even better. Then, they can float a big balloon up into Mr. Warner's aorta, near his heart, and start up the intra-aortic balloon counter-pulsation pump. This is a machine that sucks blood out of the failing heart into the circulation, perfusing the body's vital organs while limiting leakage back into the lungs. The balloon pump is only a "bridge therapy"—it can't be used for very long, typically no more than several days—but it can temporarily support the heart through a transient, treatable stress. Can the balloon pump buy him some time? Time enough for his lung to clear and his strokes to heal? Barring other catastrophes, then could the surgeons make a go at fixing his valve? It's a long shot, but it's the only one he's got.

Mr. Warner's niece, Nancy, arrives at the ICU nursing station. She looks scared. Her eyes dart from mine to Tina's and back again. We find a place to sit and talk in the waiting room just outside the ICU. I tell her what we know. She's a quick study. As she assimilates the new information, she becomes increasingly distressed.

I don't know . . . if he would want this, Nancy says. He . . . he seemed . . . ready . . . he seemed . . . like maybe he'd had enough. I don't know . . .

She asks if she can see him. We take her there.

As we reenter the ICU, alarm bells are sounding somewhere. A monitor is ringing. Someone's in trouble. Down the corridor, we see a nurse and a resident and then Friedman run into Mr. Warner's room.

Bing-bing-bing-bing-bing-bing-bing!

Mr. Warner's heart—so slow, so close to stopping just a few minutes ago—is now banging like a trip-hammer on a fire bell. The nurse checks the monitor and his blood pressure.

Sixty systolic, she says.

Bing-bing-bing-bing-bing-bing-bing!

Josh, the resident, reads the heart tracing on the monitor.

One-eighty, irregularly irregular, narrow complex. Ay-fib, he says to Friedman.

Bing-bing-bing-bing-bing-bing-bing!

Cool as ice, Friedman speaks calmly to one of the nurses.

Get the paddles, please. Fentanyl and Versed, too.

Mr. Warner's niece has entered the room behind us. Wide-eyed, she surveys the scene. She hasn't seen her uncle since last night. Unconscious, plugged into monitors and IV pumps and the breathing machine, he looks like Mr. Hernandez, the brain-dead guy in the Step-Down Unit.

Bing-bing-bing-bing-bing-bing-bing!

Oh, God! Nancy exclaims out loud.

Friedman sees her, and shoots a disapproving look at me and Tina.

We'll need to ask you to excuse us for a few minutes, ma'am, Friedman says.

What . . . ?

A nurse pushes past Nancy with the fire-engine-red code cart.

Ma'am? Friedman says again, then nods at Tina, his eyes wide. Tina takes Nancy's elbow and ushers her out of the room.

Bing-bing-bing-bing-bing-bing-bing!

Versed two, Fentanyl one hundred, Friedman tells the nurse. He motions for Josh to grab the defibrillator paddles, grease them up with goo.

Settings? Friedman quizzes Josh.

Uh, synchronized, Josh says. A hundred joules?

Start with seventy, Friedman says. Then, we'll see.

Josh waits just long enough for the nurse to push the two sedative drugs into Mr. Warner's IV. Then he yells, Charge! Everybody off? Everybody off!

Bing-bing-bing-bing-bing-bing-bing!

Josh presses the buttons on the cardioversion paddles. Mr. Warner's whole body jumps with the shock.

Then everything is quiet.

BP ninety, the nurse reports.

Sinus rhythm, one-ten, Josh says.

Friedman turns to the head nurse.

Marsha, stop the dopamine, restart the Levophed. Remember, we're shooting for one hundred. Some urine output would be nice, too, if you could arrange that, please.

Marsha rolls her eyes. I'll see what I can do, she says.

Friedman remains for a few minutes, reviewing the cardioversion procedure with Josh.

Outside the room, Nancy is wringing her hands. Her right eyelid twitches nervously.

I don't know, she says, I don't . . . I don't think he would want . . .

Nancy looks at Tina, then at me.

Dr. Friedman, she says, he looks very . . . young.

Friedman *does* look young, not much older than Tina, but he's been a critical care attending here for several years. I tell Nancy this—and more.

Maybe you saw him on the news a few months ago, ma'am. He was on all the TV shows. He's the one who saved that guy who arrested on the subway. The one who had no pulse for more than an hour? Friedman used the new resuscitation techniques—body cooling, they call it, post–cardiac arrest hypothermia—to bring the guy back. A week later, the guy walked out of the hospital smiling, healthier than ever. The TV people called the patient Lazarus, Friedman a miracle worker. Oren told the TV people he was just doing his job.

Oh, Nancy says, as Friedman comes out of Mr. Warner's room toward us.

Oren tells us that the immediate crisis is over. Mr. Warner is sleeping now. He's very unstable. Yes, ma'am, he could die. Our only hope is to buy him some time, as we just discussed.

Nancy thanks him. Then she says her uncle told her last night that he didn't want any "heroics." That's what he told me, she says.

A look of doubt flits across Oren's face. He turns to me.

He was willing to have the surgery, right?

Oh, yes, Nancy answers. He was very disappointed when he heard it couldn't be done. He wanted to try.

Friedman explains that what we're contemplating now is not nearly as risky as the surgery.

He may not make it, ma'am, Friedman says. But I recommend that you let us try. If it looks like it's not going to help, or if you think he is suffering more than he would have wanted, we can stop. We can always stop.

Nancy looks at Friedman, then me, then Tina. She looks past us toward the room where her uncle lies. Her eye twitches. Then she nods, looks away.

A short time later, the caravan is moving, taking Mr. Warner to the cardiac cath lab, where the cardiologists will install the balloon pump. All told, he needs seven people just to transport him there. Two orderlies push the big bed. A nurse and a respiratory therapist push the ventilator machine while holding Mr. Warner's breathing tube in place. Josh, the senior resident, and another nurse wheel the IV poles and temporary pacemaker machine. A third nurse takes up the rear, pushing the red cardiac arrest "crash cart," just in case. Slowly, the caravan exits the glass-enclosed ICU room, rolls down the center hall, then heads out the big double doors into the main hospital corridor. Inching along, it looks like a giant mechanical spider, its many legs stepping tentatively in tandem. At its center, Mr. Warner's unconscious head is visible above crisply tucked sheets, his white hair neatly combed by the nurses for the trip. When he starts to move in his bed, Josh thinks he's waking up, his sedatives wearing off, and Josh gently tries to restrain him, all those life-support wires and IVs so precarious, so easy to disconnect. But then Mr. Warner is arching his back, his torso lifted violently off the bed, as if possessed by demons. He begins shaking, rattling the whole bed, his eyes open wide and look up to his left, staring, terror-stricken by something there, over there. The seizure lasts about thirty seconds; it seems a lot longer. Patients and visitors in the corridor stop and back away, physically repelled, their hands held up to their faces. Still, they can't stop watching as Mr. Warner's body seizes up, unconscious, fighting off Josh and the respiratory therapist as they try to keep breathing for him. Only a short way down the corridor, it looks like a long way to go to the cath lab, so Josh yells Stop! Stop! and then the giant spider is scrambling in reverse, scuttling back to the ICU. The portable monitor shows a heart rate of thirty and no blood pressure and Josh hopes this is just an artifact from the seizure but, when they get Mr. Warner back into his room and Friedman rushes in, the heart rate is still thirty and Mr. Warner has no blood pressure and he's limp, post-ictal, drooling around his breathing tube. Luckily, only one of his lines has been disconnected and the external pacemaker pads are still taped to his chest and in a flash the pacer is activated and the Levophed is running into his big IV line again and soon the spikes reappear on his pulse monitor, one hundred beats per minute. But Friedman can't feel any pulse in his groin and neither can Josh in his neck. They dial up the Levophed to try to raise blood pressure and then the cardiologists arrive and reposition his pacemaker wire and then it captures just the way it should but still there is no blood pressure and then the monitor rings ventricular fibrillation—*bing-bing-bing-bing-bing-bing-bing-bing-bing-bing!*—and they shock him once and then again and they give the epinephrine and calcium and everything else and then they shock him again but nothing happens and then they shut off the pacemaker to see what they can see and all there is now is a long, flat line and they turn the pacer on again and it captures as it should, one hundred beats per minute, but still Friedman can feel nothing in his groin. The cardiologists put their echocardiogram probe on Mr. Warner's chest and there it is on the video screen, his heart not moving, not beating at all, even as the pacemaker fires.

Now everything is quiet, all but the *whoosh-click-wheeze!* of the ventilator and the low dull drone of a long flat line on the heart monitor.

Friedman addresses the room.

I've got asystole with paced pulseless electrical activity.

No one speaks.

Any questions?

Friedman looks at the monitor again, then at his wristwatch.
Time of death is 1:33 p.m., Oren says. Thank you, all.

Rationing? Few people would use the "R word" when reflecting on Mr. Warner's illness and treatment. For years, he received expensive, lifesaving antiretroviral drugs for his HIV disease. During the final two weeks of his life, he received state-of-the-art hospital care. True, his doctors didn't do "everything"; Mr. Warner did not undergo open-heart surgery to replace his infected heart valve, but this decision had nothing to do with rationing; it was made because Mr. Warner's doctors believed that surgery would do more harm than good. And yet, if Mr. Warner was *not* a victim of medical rationing, doesn't this mean that someone else was? Medical rationing happens every day in the U.S. health care system. And, yes, this means that some people get what they need only because others get less.

Medical insurance—and, indirectly, the price of medical services—is the principal means used to ration health care in the United States today. The well-known fact that the medically uninsured are medically underserved is only one (egregious) aspect of this phenomenon. Another is that medical insurance has its own "rationing function." In order to limit *overuse* of health care services, all medical insurance policies refuse coverage for particular services in particular situations. Unless the patient is willing to pay out of pocket for these uncovered services, it is the insurer who decides "which patient will receive which services when." Thus, all medical insurers ration health care in two ways: They decide which patients they will (and won't) insure; and, for the patients they insure, they decide which services they will (and won't) pay for.

Rationing by private insurers is unique because they inject profit motives into these calculations. This distorts insurance-mediated rationing so irrationally that Lester Thurow, a noted economist, questioned whether "insurance" has any place in a rational health care system.

Insurance is an appropriate remedy in situations where there is a small probability of a disaster that will incur large fixed losses. Fire insurance is the best example. Only a few of us will be unfortunate enough to have our house burn down, and the maximal loss is fixed by the value of our house. We therefore pool our risks and compensate those who suffer losses. . . .

But the probability that each of us will incur large health expenditures before death is becoming almost universal. In this circumstance insurance becomes not a pooling of small risks but . . . a pass-through system in which the insurance companies [take] a management fee that depends on total expenditures. . . .

The result, not surprisingly, is a system with exploding expenditures.

Mr. Warner's care was not rationed by his medical insurance; he was covered by a "Cadillac" private policy that supplemented his Medicare benefits. He was a man of means; if he had any outstanding medical bills after his death, his heirs had little difficulty paying them. In addition, Mr. Warner was a well-educated, Caucasian, English-speaking American citizen who received attentive, preventive medical care in a geographical region (Manhattan) where the overall use (and cost) of health care services is very high. In other words, Mr. Warner's care was not constrained by any of the other (noninsurance) "mechanisms" that irrationally ration health care in the United States today: racial and class prejudices; cultural, language, and ethnic barriers; low levels of health literacy; lack of primary and preventive care; and unscientific medical practice variations that (unintentionally but systematically) underserve many patients, including some with insurance. In all of these respects, Mr. Warner was on the lucky end of the rationing seesaw.

But make no mistake: Mr. Warner received "enough" medical care in part *because* others received less. For example, the level of hyperacute, sophisticated care he received on his last day of life can be provided only in an intensive care unit. Mr. Warner received this care only because Dr. Friedman and his team, under duress, made room for him in their fully packed ICU *by moving another patient out*. This kind of rationing—the real thing, in which doctors' decisions weigh one patient's need for intensive care *against* another's—happens every day in U.S. hospitals. And, although many hospitals are building many more (very expensive) ICU beds, all experts agree that the increasing number of sick, elderly patients will continue to outstrip our expanding ICU capacity—and make this kind of rationing even more frequent in the future.

Rationing is not restricted to intensive care units, nor is it a new phenomenon. Thirty years ago, for example, doctors never would have entertained even the possibility of open-heart surgery for Mr. Warner, an unthinkable treatment for a patient with (then universally fatal) HIV infection. In fact, in those days it was generally agreed that *otherwise healthy* elderly patients were not "candidates" for open-heart surgery either. Why? Because they were *old*. Today, thousands of elderly people safely undergo open-heart surgery every year (as do many patients with HIV disease). Medical progress, then, may decrease the "irrational rationing" of some clinical services (such as heart surgery for old people) but simultaneously increase the need for "rational rationing" of other services (all of those elderly heart surgery patients need ICU beds).

It seems obvious, then, that we need authoritative, rational, transparent methods to ration finite resources. But, with the notable exception of solid organ transplantation, this has been easier said than done. Neither health care payers nor providers have led the way. As a result, today's doctors are stymied, trapped like Homer's Odysseus between Scylla and Charybdis. Our Scylla has been described thus:

> In caring for an individual patient, the doctor must act solely as that patient's advocate, *against the apparent interests of society as a whole, if necessary* [my italics].
>
> When practicing medicine, doctors cannot serve two masters. The doctor's master must be the patient.

According to this view, when doctors "serve" their patients, how much it costs (and who pays for it) is not the doctor's problem.

In some cases, this attitude is self-serving. Under current fee-for-service reimbursement rules, doctors make more money by providing more services, even when the marginal benefit to patients is vanishingly small or very unlikely. But why would doctors behave otherwise when we can easily convince ourselves that our patient *might* benefit from such services—and might sue us if we don't provide them? More important, individual doctors have no reason to believe that rational rationing (practicing high-quality, cost-effective medicine) for *their own* patients will make the U.S. health care system more equitable or cost-effective *overall*. In the U.S. health care system, uncontrolled by a central budgetary authority, there is no mechanism whereby one doctor's wise rationing of resources will help fund more or better care for other doctors' patients. In such an "open-ended" system, why *not* offer (probably futile) cancer treatments to Mr. Principo—or my father? Why *not* offer (probably futile) heart surgery to Mr. Warner?

In contrast, doctors' Charybdis has been described this way:

> It will be far better if American doctors begin to build up a social ethic and behavioral practices that help them . . . disseminate better information on the cost-effectiveness of alternative medical techniques for treating different ailments. . . .
>
> Like it or not, Americans are going to have to come to some social consensus concerning the trade-off between costs of medical services and the life-extending benefits that result.
>
> Health care costs are being treated as if they were largely an economic problem, but they are not. To be solved, they will have to be treated as an *ethical* problem [my italics].

Ethicists have suggested that doctors can best navigate between our Scylla (serve each patient as best we can, regardless of cost) and Charybdis (ration finite resources cost-effectively) by first clarifying our central obligation to patients. In this view, our job is *not* to do everything that *might* benefit our patients; our job is to partner with patients to help them decide (and receive) the care that is best for them. But to fulfill this daunting obligation requires a meaningful, *value-sharing* doctor-patient relationship, a loss leader in today's business-driven health care system. And, even if we could resuscitate these relationships, *systemic* demand for more medical care will continue to grow inexorably, apace with new scientific discoveries and our aging population. What to do, then?

Daniel Callahan, who recognized the inevitability of rationing decades ago, proposed a radical solution. Rather than ration health care as U.S. society does now—irrationally, inequitably, and ineffectively—ration health care for the elderly. Explicitly and systematically, deny expensive curative medical treatment to those who have completed their "natural life span." For patients who are very elderly (above age eighty-five), restrict use of health care resources to caring, not curing: Relieve their suffering and support their quality of life as best we can while letting nature take its course. No heart surgery, no intensive care units, no cancer treatments for old folks.

Callahan's proposal, of course, was dead on arrival. Everyone shoveled dirt on its grave: politicians, geriatricians, medical researchers, even feminists (because women, on average, live longer than men). Many of them believed that health care rationing is not inevitable (even though it's been a fact of life for decades). Others protested that age-based rationing would be inequitable because wealthy old people would find ways to get around it (which they do). Still others insisted that life-prolonging medical care should be rationed according to the likelihood that a patient will benefit, not the patient's age (though this is what doctors do now, with mixed results). Finally, some worried that Callahan's proposal—so concrete, so easy to administer—might be *too easy*, a slippery slope leading to even more draconian exclusions as societal medical costs continue to rise.

But Callahan, well aware of these objections, proposed that U.S. citizens, young and old alike, consider his idea seriously and enact it democratically. Why would sane people choose to do this? Because, in Callahan's view, it is the most *ethical* way to ration health care, an essential step to preserve the medical commons and achieve other societal priorities (such as education, national defense, and a living wage). In Callahan's view, we can't have it all. Limits must be set; why not use our natural limits, our mortality, to set them?

I suspect that Callahan's ideas might have gained more traction had he presented them satirically, along the lines of *A Modest Proposal*, the famous essay by Jonathan Swift, author of *Gulliver's Travels*.

Tongue in cheek, Swift had proposed in 1729 an "easy solution" to the abject poverty of his native Ireland: Poor Irish peasants could sell their infant children as "a most delicious, nourishing and wholesome food" to their rapacious landlords, "who, as they have already devoured most of the parents, seem to have the best title to the children." Like Callahan, Swift's proposal had appealed to intergenerational justice in pursuit of a shared societal goal. But, unlike Callahan, Swift also made people laugh. And that's what got them talking.

Americans need to start talking, too, and a little levity might help. Age-based rationing of health care won't happen anytime soon—nor should it, in my view. But if we don't find a rational, ethical, democratic way to set limits on medical care, we will have no choice but to enforce partisan budgetary fixes for a problem that budgets (and partisanship) can't fix. As our society struggles, painfully, to find that better way, laughter may be our best medicine.

6:10 p.m.

She holds sheaves of paper in both hands. She's not crying. She doesn't look angry. She just wants to do the right thing. She promised her husband she would.

The papers in Helen Principo's left hand are the notarized advance directive documents that her husband brought with him from home. They say he doesn't want cardiopulmonary resuscitation or treatment with a mechanical breathing machine or lifesaving interventions of any kind, under any circumstances. It's an unusually explicit, absolute, and unambiguous statement of his wishes, lacking any contingent provisos about "terminal" diseases or "futile" treatments so often found in living wills and other such documents. The papers in Ms. Principo's right hand are the medical power-of-attorney documents designating her as her husband's sole legal decision-maker in the event he becomes incapacitated to make medical decisions for himself. Right now, she is extending her hands toward me, holding up these papers with an anxious, skeptical look: I don't get it, she says without speaking, what is going on here?

Whoosh–click–wheeze.

We're in the CTICU, the Cardiothoracic Surgical Intensive Care Unit, several hours after Mr. Principo came out of the operating room. He did well during his video-assisted thoracic surgery. The surgeons drained the fluid from his chest, biopsied various tissues in and around his lung, and brought him to the recovery room in good shape. Two hours later, he looked so good they removed his breathing tube and helped him wake up, cough, take deep breaths, visit briefly with his wife. But soon they saw that he was struggling, unable to cough up the phlegm in his throat, still too weak to breathe on his own. So, the Anesthesia folks put him to sleep again, reinserted his breathing tube, hooked him up to the ventilator, and brought him here, to the CTICU.

Whoosh-click-wheeze.

Helen shakes her head as she watches the machine inflate her husband's lungs. His eyes are closed. He looks comfortable. Narrow strips of white tape tether the clear plastic breathing tube to his mouth. Electronic infusion pumps drip intravenous fluid into his veins. Wide swaths of tape cover his torso, a big drainage tube bubbling fluid and air from his chest cavity into round plastic containers. His heart monitor bleeps softly, his pulse rate reassuringly normal. As these things go, he looks good. Helen doesn't think so.

I thought we weren't going to do this, she says.

This morning, as part of the informed consent process for his surgery, Mr. Principo agreed to temporarily "suspend" his advance directive for the perioperative period. You can't do this kind of chest surgery without a breathing machine. And you can't ask the surgeons to operate but simultaneously tie their hands, tell them they're not allowed to rescue the patient if he crumps on the operating table or in the recovery room. If you're serious about wanting the surgery, you have to agree to let the surgeons do whatever it takes to get you through it. Then, after you've come through it, you can "reinstitute" your directive that no further lifesaving interventions be done. In other words, right now Mr. Principo is in limbo, out of surgery but not "through" it, still recovering from the effects of anesthesia.

We discuss this. I tell Helen that her husband may need another twelve to twenty-four hours on the machine before we can remove his breathing tube again.

And then?

Then, we'll see how he does without it.

And if he's still too weak? You won't let them put him back on the machine again, right?

I hesitate for a moment. Officially, I am no longer Mr. Principo's attending physician. Here, in the CTICU, the surgical critical care specialist is the attending-of-record for all patients. I wrote the official order to suspend Mr. Principo's advance directive this morning. But, as long as he's here in the CTICU, legally I can't write the order to reinstate it. Does Helen Principo need to know, want to know, these arcane matters of hospital policy and law? I don't think so.

Ma'am, I will make sure that we do what your husband asked us to do. Right now, as you know, we don't have a definitive diagnosis yet. The fluid from the lung shows abnormal cells. Almost certainly, as we discussed earlier, this is cancer. But we haven't proved it yet for sure. More tests will be done on the fluid and the tissue biopsies. While we wait, let's let him rest, recover from the anesthesia. We'll support his breathing overnight. We'll keep him comfortable. We'll know more tomorrow.

Whoosh-click-wheeze.

Helen looks at her husband, shakes her head, then looks at me.

This is exactly what he was afraid of, Dr. Reilly. If he were watching us right now, he would be furious. This is what Jane looked like—his first wife—for all those weeks and months while he waited for her to die. He wouldn't believe it if he could see himself now.

It won't be like that, ma'am. I promise. We will honor his wishes, as we said we would.

Biting her lip, she looks at her husband. Then she nods, says nothing.

Whoosh-click-wheeze.

Chapter 10

GO GENTLE

> On the last night . . . I went over and looked at that huge
> incoherent failure of a house once more. On the white steps
> an obscene word, scrawled by some boy with a piece of brick,
> stood out clearly in the moonlight, and I erased it. . . . Most
> of the big shore places were closed now and there were
> hardly any lights except the shadowy, moving glow of a fer-
> ryboat across the Sound.

—F. Scott Fitzgerald, *The Great Gatsby* (1925)

Saturday, 2:00 p.m.

Meant to be? Was it *meant* to be? What kind of question is that?
Considering what I do, all that I've seen, it may seem odd that the
question had never occurred to me before. Meant to be? Before
today, the idea would have seemed to me preposterous, the stuff of
fairy tales and wistful widows. It doesn't work that way. Not from
what I've seen, anyway. Fate? Come on.

It hits me in the Pine Barrens, the narrow strip of thick evergreen
forest that lines the Long Island Expressway for a few miles near its
eastern end, a strange stretch of uninhabited land unchanged since
I was a kid. An hour into my drive, these woods are a welcome relief
from the malls and the mess they've made of everything else out here.
It's the hawks, I guess, that turn my thoughts back to Mom and Dad.
Two of them, their wings wide high above the Pine Barrens, drift

south, side by side, toward the ocean where the low winter sun has begun its afternoon commute back to the city. In July, on a Saturday like today, this stretch of highway just west of the Hamptons is a parking lot. Now, in the dead of January, it's a cold lonely ride into the past. Back then, when Mom was still Mom, she would have answered my question with another question. Was it meant to be? Well, Bren, she would have said, with that hey-you-never-know twinkle in her eye, what are the odds?

Odds. Like Mom, who holds a master's degree in economics, I'm good with numbers. Now, as the exits fly by on the expressway, I count the days. They were fifteen when they met, at a summer camp in Maine. They've been a couple ever since: seventy-seven years. Almost thirty thousand days. The Roaring Twenties, when Mom's mother was a star. The Depression, when Dad's family lost everything. The war. Eight pregnancies, five children. Dad damned-near dead of the booze and, years later, Mom in trouble, too. Teen-age kids in the sixties. The family illness—all that lithium, all those hospital stays, all that worry. The death of a son—their firstborn, their favorite—and the splintering of their family. The move to Shelter Island on a hope and a prayer, resentments largely unspoken. Détente eventually, even some happiness, or so it seemed. Then, Mom's slow fade. Dad's cancers. So, after all that, what *are* the odds? After those tens of thousands of days—their careers and their kids, the heartbreaks, the lucky breaks—what are the odds that these two people, still together in their nineties, will synchronize their biological clocks to stop, dead and done, on the very same day?

Do such things happen? How? By chance alone?

Past the Pine Barrens, I look for Exit 71, easy to remember, the year my son was born. When I first moved back to New York from Chicago eighteen months ago and started making these house calls to Shelter Island, I didn't know the back roads, how to bypass the traffic circles and the mall sprawl around Riverhead. Now I'm making good time, only an hour since I left the city. When the call came from the hospice nurse this morning, I knew I'd be driving out here today but not at eighty miles per hour. You might want to visit today, Dad's nurse had suggested gently on the phone, he's in and out now, comfortable on the morphine, but I'm beginning to get that feeling, you know, Dr. Reilly? She didn't say anything about Mom, who was still sleeping when she called, so none of this crossed my mind until a few hours later when the operator paged me in the hospital. Ruth, one of our home health aides, had just shipped Mom off to the hospital again in an ambulance. She hadn't been able to get Mom out of bed. Mom was conscious but very weak and Ruth checked her pulse and it was only thirty-two, or maybe twenty-eight, so Ruth had called me but got no answer and Ruth didn't know what else to do, so she called 911 and the island ambulance guys came right away and stretchered Mom down the stairs and headed for the ferry and the hospital across the bay. When Ruth finally reached me, I knew I had to get out here fast.

Not that I could do anything myself. Besides, my head is full of what's happening right now to Mr. Principo in the surgical ICU and what I've just seen of Mr. Warner in the morgue. None of that makes it easy to see what I could do for Mom, except maybe make the call about what *not* to do. I mean, really, who am I to get in the way if Mom's heart decides to slow down and stop on the very day Dad decides to stop breathing, too?

Halfway to Riverhead, I was able to reach the docs in the Greenport hospital ED. They said Mom looked okay, her heart rate sixty-four and her blood pressure fine. Still, if Ruth had been right about that pulse rate of twenty-eight, it could happen again fast, so I kept my foot heavy on the gas. Until I get there, I know the docs will do what they were trained to do and now I'm not so sure they should. If today is Dad's day, could it be Mom's day, too? *Should* it be Mom's day, too? It's a preposterous question, but, somehow, what I've just gone through with the Principo family—and Mr. Warner's morgue scene—makes it seem not so crazy. Somehow, all of this has come together in my head, my patients conflated with my parents, their doctor-son conflicted with himself and wondering seriously whether some things are meant to be.

After exiting the expressway, I turn north at the fork, cross the railroad tracks, and make a beeline for the back road. When I was young I never came this way. Then, in the sixties, it was always south at the fork, never north. Who wanted to see endless fields of potato farms, stretching from the bay to the Sound, when you could be in paradise instead? That's what the South Fork—the Hamptons—was fifty years ago, before the new money and the crowds drove the old money away. For people like me, invisible to the bluebloods in their mansions on the dunes, it was enough just to share the air, working nights in a pizza parlor to support a habit more addictive than any drug: the surf at Georgica, the golden light of late afternoon, the giant elms, the gray salt-air-shingled houses built before Bunker Hill, the timeless understated grandeur of the place. Had they known about it, Daisy and Gatsby would have come here, not West Egg.

But not today. Now the Hamptons is Manhattan East, tolerable if you have your own hedge fund, your own helicopter, and one of those sprawling places on the dunes. Were they still alive today, Pollock and de Kooning would have left long ago, despite the light.

Luckily, time and money have been kinder to the North Fork, so far anyway, the potato fields replaced by lush green sod farms and fine vineyards, their perfectly combed rows marching to the sea. Oh, it's coming, all right—the helicopters and the traffic, the houses with tree-high privet hedges and twelve bathrooms for two people—but, here on the back road of the North Fork, I can still talk myself into long ago as the pale winter sun lengthens my car's shadow, pointing my way eastward.

My destination, Shelter Island, sits in the mouth of the Peconic Bay between the tines of Long Island's North and South Forks where they reach out east into the Atlantic. Shelter Island has always been an in-between kind of place, demographically as well as geographically. A British earl built Sylvester Manor there in the 1600s, amid the huts of the Manhasset Indians. Today, the mega rich on Big Ram and Dering Harbor cohabit with the working class in the island center and with city folks like my parents lucky enough to have bought waterfront cottages here decades ago, before the craziness began. Mom bought her house in 1975 for sixty thousand dollars, most of which she mortgaged with her teacher's pension. Today, it's worth a few million, and Mom, even now, gets a kick out of this. She can't remember much but she knows enough to say sometimes, as she looks out the window at her private sandy beach, This was a pretty good deal, don't you think?

Now their house is their retirement fund, their bank account. I haven't had to get them a reverse mortgage yet but that time is fast approaching. Their pensions and Social Security barely cover the taxes and the oil bills, and their modest savings won't last long, not with two live-in caregivers. I pay their bills now—their mail is sent to me—but the part of Mom who's still here occasionally asks me about their finances. You're a rich old lady, I tell her, because it makes her laugh and because that's what she always wanted to be. (Dad never cared about money; Mom didn't know this when she married him.) She can't remember what she had for breakfast and she can't subtract seven from ten but still it happens sometimes that Mom, sitting in her recliner, eyes half closed, will giggle when some talking head on CNN opines about federal estate law or pending congressional legislation to raise the inheritance tax. Hah, Mom will say to no one in particular, sounds like this would be a good year for Dad and me to get dead, huh?

As a matter of fact, yes, it would, I tell her, and she giggles again. Dad, who can't see TV and is confined to bed, laughs, too, when later I repeat the conversation for him. Well, maybe that can be arranged, Bren, he says with a chuckle, and he's only half kidding.

The shaded single-lane road widens briefly as it approaches the town of Mattituck. To my left, the Old Mill Inn looks north to the Sound, proud of its shingle announcing its continuous operation since 1821. Long before then, it had been a grist mill, owned by a Dickerson, my wife's father's family. Janice grew up here, her family part of the original expedition that sailed south from Connecticut in 1640, the first colonists to settle eastern Long Island. The place they landed, called Founders Landing ever since, is a pretty cove on the bay side of Southold, the township they named in memory of Southwold, their erstwhile English home. The vast tracts of land once owned here by the Dickersons have long since been sold for a halfpenny on the dollar, but, like the other founding families here, their name lives on quietly in the cemeteries and local maps, where places like Tuthill Road and Dickerson Creek dot the landscape.

Here now, to my right, is another such name: Wickham, a founding family whose deep roots include the big old farm just up the road and the old-fashioned single-story law office on Main Street that I first visited with Mom and Dad years ago. Ten years? Fifteen, maybe. Back then, Dad was losing his sight and maybe he knew already that Mom was losing more than that. He asked me to fly in from Chicago, drive them here, to Gail Wickham's law office on a Saturday morning in the fall. There are things we should do, Dad had said to me on the phone, things we should get straight, while we still can.

They didn't own much except their house, so their will and estate plan were simple. The health care stuff was boilerplate, too, the living wills stipulating no "heroic" or "futile" treatments when their medical conditions became "hopeless," whatever that meant, their powers of attorney signed over to me. Now, as I remember these things on the back road near Mattituck, I'm wishing we had spent more time, fleshed out the bones of what "heroic" meant—in their minds, not mine. So, Dad, what if you get cancer that can't be cured? What if you lose your marbles, Mom? Okay, no machines or CPR. But how about intensive care units? Blood transfusions? Feeding tubes? How about a pacemaker, if you need one? I think I know what their answers would be, but I'm not sure. If only we'd spent more time.

Would that have helped? I wonder, as I speed east. All that planning hasn't helped the Principos. Not yet, anyway. I'll call her when I get to Greenport. I promised her I would.

Ms. Principo was beside herself, more angry than dejected, when I arrived in the Cardiothoracic Surgery ICU this morning. She'd been there all night, pacing restlessly in the ICU waiting room, and Mr. Principo had had a rocky time. His blood pressure had plummeted when his heart started to race but the electric shocks with the cardioverter had stabilized him, at least for now. The ICU docs had had to snow him with sedatives, then paralyze his muscles so he couldn't fight the breathing machine. This had improved his oxygen level but now he needed the mechanical ventilator even more. The ICU staff said her husband was "improving," but Helen didn't see it that way. She couldn't feel his hand respond to hers. She couldn't explain to him what was happening. At first, all she could say to me was: *It's a*

good thing he's not here to see this himself. Dr. Reilly, you promised him.
This is not what he wants.

It didn't help that today is Saturday, the weekend shift. This morning, the surgical attending in charge of the CTICU is different from the one in charge yesterday when we had all agreed on our plan. Dr. Itrasca, covering for the weekend, is thoughtful and diligent but that's part of the problem. Surgeons like Dr. Itrasca, who repair and revive hearts and lungs, aren't in the habit of pulling the plug on life-support machines when their patient is getting better. Under the circumstances, Dr. Itrasca tells Helen and me, withdrawal of life support at this time is "medically inappropriate." Mr. Principo is still in his postoperative limbo, not even twenty-four hours out of surgery. We need to wait and see, Dr. Itrasca says.

This is not an argument I can win. Strictly speaking, Dr. Itrasca is correct. It takes a while to explain this to Helen. I don't tell her that surgeons tend to see the world differently, their perspective on such things unique. Nor do I tell her that few physicians, when "covering" their colleagues' patients on weekends or holidays, make decisions that rock the boat or change its course. Instead, I tell Helen that I agree with Dr. Itrasca's view: It *is* too early to know whether we should withdraw life support.

How long, then? Helen asks, exhausted and angry.

Monday.

Two more days? Why Monday? What will you know on Monday that you won't know today or tomorrow?

We'll know that your husband has incurable cancer. That's when we'll have the final pathology report from his lung tissue.

Oh.

And then we can stop all this, as he asked us to do.

When I returned a few hours later to tell Helen that I was leaving town to deal with my own family emergency, her two sons and their wives had joined her. They were all standing around Mr. Principo's bed. It was quiet now except for the *whoosh-click-wheeeze!* of his ventilator and the soft, metallic bleeps from his monitor. Motionless and comatose, Mr. Principo looked peaceful. Helen was bleary-eyed but, surrounded by her family, she seemed at peace now, too. Dr. Itrasca had agreed that, if Mr. Principo's heart fails, we won't treat it. If that happens, we couldn't blame it on his lung surgery. Given the patient's prior wishes, and having discussed them with me and his family, Dr. Itrasca agreed that she needn't do "everything." Either way, then, Mr. Principo would be like this—asleep, anesthetized, not suffering at all—for, at most, only another day or two.

Okay, Helen said. He could live with that.

I didn't tell her anything about Mom and Dad, why I was leaving. Still, despite everything, she put her hand on my arm and thanked me.

Dr. Reilly, I hope things go smoothly for your family, too.

Smoothly. What would that feel like? I wonder, as my car speeds into the town of Southold.

I pass the old country road where my wife grew up, a quiet lane near the center of town where all those Dickerson headstones grace the graveyard of the First Presbyterian Church. As always when I pass here, I remember Lloyd, Janice's father. For decades, he had run a marina in this seaside town, selling and repairing boats back in the days when you could troll a short way out into the Sound or the bay, drop a rake, and drag up buckets of blue-point clams and soft-shelled crabs, a fine easy dinner on a summer's night. Everyone here liked Lloyd, admired him. When he died, the church was packed. Not many African-American families lived in Southold but they were all there, too. After the funeral service, outside the church, old Ms. Jackson had reminisced about how sometimes her folks couldn't afford to get their boats serviced. But we could always count on your dad, she said to Janice, who remembered Ms. Jackson's husband well. A hardworking, handsome man, he would appear from time to time on a summer evening in the Dickersons' driveway, carrying tubs of fine fish and lobster and crab to pay back her dad for how he'd helped him. And there, on the front porch, the two men would sit and talk about the town and the tides and where the fish were running, and reminisce sometimes about the old days when they played semipro ball with the young Yastrzemski, then just a kid who couldn't hit the curveball. Outside the church, Janice told Ms. Jackson that her dad had always said just to do what you think is right and it will all turn out in the end and Ms. Jackson had nodded and clucked and said, That's right, that's right, and then she shook her head and held Janice's hands and said, He will be missed, God bless his soul, he will be missed.

Now, remembering, driving out of Southold, I wonder who will miss Mom and Dad. Most of their relatives are long gone and they never had many friends, not really. Dad was a loner, something he never talked about and didn't seem to mind. Mom attributed this to his drinking. Dad lived two lives, she said: the first as a party boy, his charm and humor unlocked by the booze; the second as a recluse, shunning former friends who wouldn't get on the wagon with him. Mom didn't really have friends, either. After they moved to Shelter Island, they kept largely to themselves, as they had done in the city. Once, sitting on the big porch at sunset in the days before she quit drinking herself, Mom had clicked her ice cubes, gulped her Canadian Club, shrugged, and said: I've always liked things more than people anyway. Whenever their children and grandchildren visited, they would put on a good show but Dad stayed in his room a lot and took long walks on the beach, usually alone, while Mom worried constantly about the kids spilling stuff on her rugs or furniture. Truth be told, both of them were relieved when it was time for all of us to go home. Mom liked to say that she had bought the house on Shelter Island so her family would always be able to be together, and I think she meant it. She just never knew how to make it happen.

Now it's too late for all that. As the road skirts the shore just west of Greenport, the beach deserted, the Sound colorless and calm, I know I will miss them. I miss them already. But who else will miss them? Should we even have a funeral service? Will anyone come?

I turn onto the road toward the hospital, prepare myself for what I have to do there. But now, in my mind's eye, it's not Mom I'm seeing. It's Mr. Warner, in the morgue this morning. A broad flap of scalp, its underside raw and oozing, has been peeled forward over his face, covering his eyes and nose. The brain has been removed, his cranium now an empty bowl of bone. When the pathologist opens his heart, the hole in his mitral valve—located exactly where Tina said it would be—seems too small, too neat, too perfectly round to have killed him. But kill him it did. Before they cut the brain, slicing it in neat coronal sections like a melon at a picnic, we could see the bleeding on its surface, dull and red where the shine should be. Deep inside, the hemorrhages were small but everywhere—too numerous to count, many more than even the MRI had shown. The surgeons had been right: Almost certainly, he wouldn't have made it if they'd operated on his heart. Save his heart to lose his brain? What sense does that make?

That's what I told Mr. Warner's niece, Nancy, on the phone this morning after I left the morgue: He never would have made it. I didn't tell her the "almost certainly" part. No, I'll keep that part to myself. It can't do her any good to wonder, after he's gone, "If only . . ." Why give her cause for regret?

Doctors know about regret. But we don't talk about it. Ever.

Even today, when the medical profession is beginning to deal more openly with medical error, regret remains locked in the closet. Occasionally, when reflecting about our personal lives, doctors will express regret about having worked too many hours, too many Saturdays, missing the more important things in life (like our kids' childhood). But in more than forty years of working with doctors, I can't recall a single instance when I've heard one express regret about a clinical decision. Guilt? Yes, rarely, when a doctor has made a bad mistake. Disappointment? Sure, doctors often feel disappointed when their patients don't do well. But regret? It's as if the word has been expunged from the medical dictionary. Regret is the feeling that happens when you feel personally responsible for a decision that turns out badly and you wish you had a second chance, a do-over. Different from guilt (when you've done something "wrong") or disappointment (when you don't feel personally responsible for the bad outcome), regret happens when you wish you could take back what you did and do it differently. If only . . .

How can doctors avoid regret? (After all, *what doctors do* is make fateful decisions, some of which turn out badly even when we do everything right.) We avoid regret by purposefully defending ourselves against it, both consciously and subconsciously. Our regret avoidance is not the same thing as "defensive medicine," actions doctors take to avoid lawsuits. No, regret avoidance runs deeper than that. It's personal, very personal.

Regret, researchers tell us, requires two things: agency and imagination. Agency? We regret what we *do*: decisions we make, actions we take. Importantly, we regret what we do *ourselves*, not what others do. Doctors' agency is complicated because the ideal model of medical decision-making is "patient-centered" yet "shared": The patient decides, but in collaboration with his doctor. (The reality, of course, varies widely from this ideal. Mr. Principo, for example, made his decisions with *no* help from his doctors; the opposite happened in Mr. Warner's case.) Doctors' imagination is complicated, too. Psychologists call it "counterfactual thinking," the ability (and propensity) to conjure up possible outcomes different from the actual outcome. Regret's critical question, then, is: If only . . . *what?* After Mr. Warner died, I imagined that he might have survived if only we had taken him to surgery before it was too late. Had we been smarter, more prescient, we *might* have acted differently—against the odds, and contrary to the conventional wisdom that the risk of surgery was unacceptable. Even when I was convinced—after the fact, in the morgue—that we had made the right decision, I could still "see" Mr. Warner recovering from surgery (in the same ICU where I saw Mr. Principo this morning), he and his niece chuckling at how lucky he'd been. This is the essence of regret: The fact that my wished-for, alternative outcome is "counterfactual" doesn't mean it *couldn't* come true. Oh, yes, it could. *If only . . .*

The simplest way to avoid regret, then, is not to act at all. No agency, no regret. This may explain, at least in part, why doctors who "cross-cover" patients for other doctors (on weekends or holidays) typically defer important decisions until the patient's "real" doctor returns. Often this passivity is wise, when an important decision can wait, but sometimes it is irresponsible. Worse, in rare cases, a doctor may disengage completely: Faced with a difficult decision (or a difficult patient), the doctor eschews all responsibility and insists that the patient *alone* decide. This is reprehensible, unprofessional behavior; it is patient abandonment, plain and simple.

When doctors *must* act, we often "dilute" potential regret by sharing our agency with others. We ask consultants—subspecialists in various fields—to opine about our patients, thereby sharing the responsibility (and potential regret) for decisions made. Often helpful to patients and their families, this common practice also can be overdone. Jack Wennberg's researchers at Dartmouth have documented that greater use of subspecialist consultants doesn't always result in higher quality of care for sick patients. (In fact, in some parts of the United States, this practice correlates with *lower* quality of care.)

When doctors can't deny or dilute their agency, we often deflect it by invoking the "standard of care." There are several types of such standards, and their differences are important. *Evidence-based standards* reflect state-of-the-art scientific evidence about the "right" thing to do. For example, my (unregretted) acquiescence to Mr. Principo's and my father's decision to forgo treatment for their cancers reflected not only their preferences but also the prevailing scientific evidence that the likely harms of such treatment outweigh its likely benefits. In such cases, the decisive agent is not one doctor but, rather, a scientifically validated standard of practice. Other types of standards of care, however, are not based on strong evidence. For example, the scientific evidence opposing surgical treatment for patients like Mr. Warner is weak. To address such problems, international panels of experts often publish *consensus standards*; after reviewing whatever (inconclusive) evidence is available, they articulate a consensus expert opinion about what to do. Less scientific still are *local institutional standards*, which vary from one hospital (or community or state) to another. Mr. Principo's request to discontinue ventilator support postoperatively, for example, did not conform with our hospital's *local* standard of care; the ICU attending surgeon cited this standard to deny the "appropriateness" of Mr. Principo's request. Such local standards of care, no less than standards based on strong evidence or expert consensus, serve many useful purposes. But one of these purposes is to "institutionalize" doctors' decisions—and thus "depersonalize" any one doctor's agency—in difficult clinical situations.

Finally, when doctors cannot finesse their agency to avoid regret—when we can't deny, dilute, or deflect it—we finesse our imagination instead. When we do this, most doctors fall into one of two groups. Some of us—a minority, in my experience—avoid regret by making decisions in a strictly rational, logical manner. Like many economists and scientists, these doctors adhere to "expected utility theory" and rely on quantitative decision analyses to justify their actions. These "quant" doctors assign a value (called a utility) to every possible outcome of a decision. Typically, these utilities are given a numerical value on a decimal scale (ranging from zero to one), based on input from the patient. Then, when faced with a set of risky alternative options, each with its own probability of success, quants recommend the decision that yields the highest "expected utility" for the patient. For example, my father would assign a lower value to one possible outcome (living a month or two longer by suffering through cancer treatment) than to another outcome (dying sooner without suffering the treatment). Knowing this, a quant would multiply—literally, *mathematically*, multiply—the statistical probability of each possible clinical outcome by the utility value my father had assigned to it. The preferred decision, which incorporates both the patient's values (utilities) and the doctor's knowledge of statistical probabilities, would be the one with the higher numerical "score."

This approach avoids regret because, if the patient's outcome is unfortunate, quant doctors think like hedge fund managers: You win some and you lose some. The goal is to win more than you lose. Quant doctors argue that, if they consistently implement the logically preferable decision, they will win more often than they lose. *And, when they lose, they don't look back and second-guess their decision.* In an inherently probabilistic, always uncertain business—a description that fits medicine no less than finance—the best you can do is make your most rational bet, accept your "gain" or your "loss," and then move on. Counterfactual thinking doesn't happen, so neither does regret. (Disappointment, maybe, but not regret.) Like Edith Piaf, then, quants tend to sing: *Je ne regrette rien.*

Most doctors, however, are not quants. Their thinking is more qualitative than quantitative. (They may concede that expected utility theory is the most *rational* decision-making process but they also know that most patients don't think this way.) When making clinical decisions, then, most doctors *anticipate* the outcome that, *if it occurred*, would cause the most regret; then, consciously or subconsciously, they avoid decisions that *could* lead to that outcome. For example, they might ask which would be the worse outcome: an aggressive treatment that does more harm than good or a purely palliative treatment that leaves open the door to (retrospective) criticism that "nothing was done"? But anticipating regret is tricky. Not only are patients' clinical outcomes uncertain and their probabilities imprecise, decisions about them often revolve around murky existential issues like *time*. For example, regret avoidance about a risky surgical operation may involve a choice between death in the near but unpredictable future (if the operation is *not* done) versus an even earlier death if the operation *is* done (but kills the patient). When anticipating outcomes like these, one doctor's recommendation may be another's worst regret.

It's no mystery, then, why doctors don't talk about regret. Needing a buffer, most of us do the job but protect our *selves* in the process. Critics claim that these defense mechanisms tend to "dehumanize" doctors, make us unfeeling. (Maybe so, but it is doctors' humanity that necessitates these self-protective adaptations in the first place.) Avoiding regret may hurt doctors in other ways, too. For one, we lose an unparalleled opportunity to learn, to become better doctors. For another, we foreclose chances to feel *good* about ourselves because, in suppressing regret, we tend to suppress positive emotions, too: joy, when our patients do well, and the sense of privilege we feel because patients allow us into their lives. This is no small thing. Feelings matter in medicine. Not just patients' feelings.

But most doctors avoid regret so successfully that we don't even recognize it when it happens. After the fact, for example, I can easily convince myself that we did the right thing for Mr. Warner. Surely, the quants would agree. Save his heart to lose his brain? By any rational calculus, this makes no sense. No regrets, then, right?

And yet, there it is: *Je regrette*. If only . . . *what*?

Just past the town beach, the Connecticut coast invisible in the haze across the Sound, the road begins its rise into the back streets of

Greenport. Here, some of the older cottages and fishing shacks, their paint peeling and porches listing, have resisted the gentrification spreading relentlessly north of the railroad tracks. Greenport has always reminded me of Mom, or at least what I know of her life. She grew up on both sides of the tracks, simultaneously.

Mom's mother, the youngest child of a penniless Irish family, had hit it big as the Great War was winding down. Still in her twenties, she was the "It-girl" of costume design for the Broadway stage, outfitting the Ziegfeld Follies, the flappers, and all the rest. She died in childbirth when Mom was two. Mom's father was a dashing, fast-talking guy who liked fancy cars, Cuban cigars, and expensive whiskey, but his principal means of support died with his wife and stillborn son. He didn't know much about raising kids, so Mom was shipped up to the Bronx to live with her maternal grandmother, who cleaned other people's houses to support her own family. (Mom's maternal grandfather, a "mathematical genius" according to family lore, was confined in a state mental hospital for most of his adult life.) From time to time, Mom's father would show up in the Bronx, his fine car piled high with gift boxes, each engraved with the rich maroon logo of the Patricia Shop, a high-end children's boutique he had opened on Madison Avenue (and named for Mom after her mother died). The velvety tasseled boxes he brought to that four-flat in the Bronx were filled with silk dresses and Italian shoes for a little girl who slept on a cot in a kitchen pantry and went to school with the children of cabbies and blacksmiths and maids. When Mom's father remarried, a decade later, he arranged a "tryout" visit for Mom with his new wife. Eileen, a stylish chain-smoking executive secretary to a famous Wall Street tycoon, had a worldly way but a heart of gold. Long afterward, she admitted that her "tryout" had been a flop and Mom an enigma, a spoiled brat who had grown up poor. But they made a go of it; Mom moved in and learned some things about love. Still, despite her many accomplishments in life, Mom never developed the self-esteem needed to make real friends—or even to know who the good people are. Like Greenport, Mom had never been sure who she was or wanted to be.

Right now, she looks tiny and frail in her big hospital bed. Eyes closed, Mom lies by a window that looks out over the winter harbor, empty now but for a few fishing boats. I can see Shelter Island in the distance, across the bay. Mom opens her eyes, hesitates for a moment when she sees me, then smiles.

Oh! Hi, Bren! she says, perking up. I didn't expect to see you today!

Physically, her ninety-two years have been more than kind, her thick hair still more chestnut than gray, her Elizabeth Taylor eyes clear and twinkling. She's awfully cute, the nurse said at the front desk, as if she were talking about a three-year-old.

Now a puzzled look crosses Mom's face as she looks up at me from her bed. You're . . . very tall, aren't you? she says, as if meeting me for the first time.

In fact, I'm not very tall, just a few inches above average height, but Mom says this lately every time she sees me, even if, during a visit, I leave her for just a few minutes and then return. This phenomenon doesn't seem to be only about her memory, the fact that whatever she sees or talks about disappears in just a few minutes, lost forever. Instead, it seems to reflect a distortion of her brain's visual processing mechanisms, one of the countless ways in which Alzheimer's disease remakes its victims, decomposing them into shadows of themselves. My siblings don't understand any of this. To them, Mom, who still looks like Mom and talks like Mom, is merely forgetful, like a lot of old people. She's ninety-two, they say, what do you expect? I don't beat them over the head about this. They'll learn. But, for me, Mom's been gone for some time now. Whoever this adorable little old lady is, propped up primly in her hospital bed, she's not Mom.

Did you stop in Dad's room, Bren? I know how he loves to see you.

Uh, well, we're not at the house, Mom. I'll be going over to the house to see Dad later. Right now, we're in Greenport, at the hospital.

Oh.

She looks around the room, then out the window at the harbor.

Is it . . . ? Am I . . . sick?

It's a good question. Ever since they got Mom over here in the ambulance from across the bay, her heart monitor has looked fine, nothing abnormal. No sign of the life-threatening bradycardia, the pulse rate of twenty-eight, that Ruth thought she had detected at home.

No, Mom. You're not sick. The doctors here just want to monitor your heart for a little while.

Puzzlement crosses her face again. Then she smiles and cracks her joke.

They want to see if I've got one, right?

I laugh with her, then explain.

Your heartbeat seemed a little slow at home, Mom. The doctors are just being careful, in case you need a pacemaker for your heart.

A what?

A pacemaker.

She frowns, then shakes her head with great conviction.

Well, I don't want that!

Her head still shaking, she looks out at the harbor again, then back at me.

Do I?

I sign the do-not-resuscitate forms at the nursing station. I've done this a thousand times before, but always on the doctor's line, not the patient's. The nurse photocopies the notarized power-of-attorney form I've brought with me. Now it's official. If Mom's heart stops, we do nothing. Years ago, in that law office in Mattituck, it's what Mom and Dad both said they wanted.

But if her heart just slows down . . . ? Then what? What if it doesn't stop, not completely? What if it just slows down, so she can't hold her head up, or talk, or feel peaceful as she goes? How long could that go on? If she suffers, moaning and agitated, as her heart winds down, slowly, oh, so slowly . . . What then?

The doctor in me knows that's why God created morphine, the angel of death. But the son in me isn't so sure.

The light is fading fast into the bay as I drive onto the north ferry for the eight-minute trip to the island. To the east, the mansions on Dering Harbor, most of them empty in winter, glow orange in the sunset. Their color reminds me of the votive candles in church when

I was a kid, an altar boy every morning, praying hard that my father would "get well," whatever that meant, and come home. The priests and nuns knew me well, the second son of the "saint" of Stuyvesant Town.

Mom's "sainthood" was announced when I was in third grade. Sister Anne, the school principal, was visiting Sister Brigid's classroom, where, for some reason that day, Sister Brigid was going around the room asking each kid to stand up and tell the class what he or she had had for breakfast that morning. All of us wore uniforms—the girls blue jumpers and white blouses with puffed sleeves, the boys blue pants and ties with white shirts—and, as usual, Mom had ironed and starched my white shirt the night before, as she did every night for each of her four young sons, after she'd cooked the dinner and done the dishes and corrected most of her homework papers. (Mom taught social studies at a local public high school.) When Sister Brigid called my name that morning, I stood up from my desk in my starched white shirt and tie, my shoes shined shiny, and told her what she wanted to know. Breakfast had been no different that day than on any other day—orange juice and cereal with fresh bananas, then scrambled eggs with bacon and sausage and toast, no buttah, Sis-tah, I don't like buttah—so I just said it and shrugged and sat back down at my desk and waited for the next kid to get called and do the same.

Sister Brigid, who looked like Ingrid Bergman (and on whom I had a secret, sacrilegious crush), stared at me with a strange smile on her face. Then she turned demurely to her principal. Sister Anne, a tall, commanding presence with the graceful gait of an athlete, walked to the front of the classroom and clapped her hands once, authoritatively. (Later in life, I would learn that she had known all about my father's troubles and my mother's plight.) Sister Anne spoke with a deep, melodious voice.

Children, listen to me, please.

Obediently, all forty kids leaned forward in our desks, the kind you could hide under so the atom bomb wouldn't kill you.

Children, I want you all to know something.

You could hear a pin drop.

Children, I want you to know that Brendan's mother, Mrs. Reilly, is a saint. You all know about the saints in heaven, don't you?

Yes, Sister Anne! our forty voices sang out in perfect harmony.

Well, just like the saints in heaven, children, there are saints on earth, too. And Mrs. Reilly is a saint.

Then Sister Anne nodded to Sister Brigid and strode briskly out of the room.

That was the last I heard of it myself. The other kids said nothing to me. We all just went on about our business, whatever it was that nine-year-old kids did back then. But, years later, I learned that Sister Anne's extemporaneous canonization of my mother had spread quickly all around lower Manhattan. *There's a Mrs. Reilly in Stuyvesant Town who's a saint. The head nun said so.*

I also learned later that the other kids' mothers hadn't been entirely thrilled about this; after all, they made breakfast for their kids, too. But, as far as I know, none of them said boo when a few months later Mom won the five-hundred-dollar grand prize at the church's annual drawing, a sort of lottery for parishioners. Even Mom wondered if Sister Anne and old Father McCabe had cooked it so she'd win. Decades later, Mom would shake her head and say, I don't know, maybe it *was* a miracle; I don't know what I would have done without that five hundred bucks until Dad came home.

The house, an old Victorian with a wraparound porch, sits a short way down the beach from the island's ferry slip. Only the second floor is lit, dimly. Ruth asks about Mom, says Dad is sleeping. A lamp glows low on the battered old card table next to his hospital bed. There, his beat-up digital clock radio reads 5:15. We've tried unsuccessfully to get him a fancier radio so he can listen to CDs or pick up the BBC on shortwave or get the local news from Chicago to hear about his grandson, a rising star in city politics there. But all the newfangled radios have too many dials, too many options for an old blind guy who just wants to push a button from time to time, hold the radio next to his ear, take his mind off whatever it's on. I've asked him what he thinks about, confined to his bed twenty-four hours of every day. Usually he hesitates before he answers, then says, Oh, nothing much, crazy stuff—dreams, you know?

Now his breathing is deep and regular, not labored exactly but a little too fast and hungry to seem restful, as if he's in a hurry to get somewhere. I can't say it's any different from what I've been seeing lately but I remember what the hospice nurse said on the phone. I sit down, stay with him for a while.

The big bag hanging from the railing of his hospital bed is nearly full, blood-red, flecks of clot percolating through the tube that drains urine from his bladder. A good sign, sort of: He's still making urine. I put my fingers lightly on his wrist to feel his pulse. It's a bit rapid but still strong, and he doesn't stir at all when I touch him. His fingernails need trimming again, like his hair and his beard. I do this for him every few weeks. He says the others don't shave him right, and it's something I will remember until I die myself, first trimming his beard with the ancient electric hair-cutter he once used himself to cut his boys' hair in the bathroom—four trips to the barber shop every month was more than Dad wanted to spend—and then lathering his snow-white stubble with that newfangled shaving gel he likes so much and then carefully, oh so carefully, angling the razor under his nose and just beneath his lips and down his neck where his carotid arteries bound with life, my face close to his, concentrating, leaning over him, Dad sightless and silent but grateful for the closeness, you can tell, and then finally that big smile you can see right through the warm damp towel that I drape over his face when we're done, such a simple thing, but for him such a sensual pleasure, like chocolate. He never asks to be shaved, it isn't his way. But he never refuses me either. I just tell him he's starting to look like Howard Hughes again, and he laughs at the memory of the eccentric billionaire's photos during his final wacko recluse days and Dad says, Okay, okay, I don't want them carrying me out of here in a straitjacket.

He would know about straitjackets. He never talked about it, almost a full year in the VA hospital, first for detox and his liver, then for his head. Dad never talked about his brother Fred either but Fred would have known about straitjackets, too. A brilliant guy with a Columbia law degree who spoke six languages, including Russian and Japanese, Fred could never relax after returning from the war, where he had served as an interpreter at the Japanese surrender.

He died in a state mental hospital at age thirty-four, no treatment then for manic depression. (Back then, no one even knew what it was.) Our family disease didn't kill Dad's sister, too, not directly anyway, but Dad had learned enough from her—she was in and out of Payne Whitney, Cornell's famous inpatient psychiatry service, for decades—to know what to watch for in his own kids. This had come in handy more than once. Even so, some in our family blamed Dad (and his genes) for their troubles, ignoring the fact that Mom's side carried the gene, too. I was closer to Dad than the others but none of us, including me, ever really got to know him. Occasionally, in his later years, Dad would reminisce about his youth and say wistfully, You know, it's strange, I never really got to know my own father, and I and my siblings would just roll our eyes.

Next to his bed now, I look at the old photo of Dad's father. The strong chin, like Dad's, and the kind, wary eyes. Dad had pronounced his own father dead at home, signed the death certificate himself, as he knew I would do for him one day. Other than the photo, all Dad had kept as mementoes were a gold watch and a worn piece of parchment that Grandpa folded into his wallet. Handwritten in a fine tight cursive script, it read:

> A wise old owl sat on an oak.
> The more he saw the less he spoke.
> The less he spoke the more he heard.
> I want to be like that wise old bird.

Sitting here now, watching Dad breathe, fast and deep, I recall that Grandpa died when I was eight. His heart attack happened shortly after his son Fred died in the mental hospital. It was a few months after that when Dad wound up in the hospital himself.

My cell phone buzzes on my belt. It's a nurse at the hospital in Greenport. Hold, please, she says, while I get the doctor. A cardiologist comes to the phone, introduces himself. He's not one of the ones I've met before. When I hang up, I wish I could wake Dad, talk it through with him. Despite everything, he knows Mom better than anyone.

His breathing still looks strong, so I take another long look, tell Ruth where I'm going, and head back to the ferry slip along the beach. It's dark now. Out on the bay, its running lights aglow on the water, a ferryboat glides silently toward me, more than halfway here. I'll be with Mom in fifteen minutes.

An hour later, I've seen the new heart tracings and discussed them with the cardiologist. He seems to understand my position, why I say what I say. But, as I walk back to Mom's room, I hear him asking the nurse about my power-of-attorney document.

I sit by Mom's bedside for a while, hold her hand. Then I kiss her good-bye.

Am I going home now? she asks.

Not yet, Mom, not yet. Soon. You'll be going soon.

Outside, in the empty hospital parking lot, I look out over the harbor and across the bay. Just barely, I can see the house from here, the lights still lit on the second floor. What would Dad say? I don't know. But I think he would say it's not a bad way to go, your heart just winding down, slower and slower, sleepy and sleepier, and then it's done and you're home free. Compared to what Dad's been dealing with, not such a bad way to go.

He'll be glad for her, I think.

Several weeks after the events described here, I found myself sitting in a restaurant in lower Manhattan having lunch with Nobel Prize winner Daniel Kahneman. I had come with Dr. Lisa Rosenbaum, a cardiology fellow at Cornell, who arranged the meeting. The daughter and granddaughter of distinguished physicians, Lisa writes articles in the *New England Journal of Medicine* and the *New York Times* about how it *feels* to be a doctor, the dilemmas doctors face when trying to do the "right thing" for their patients. (When she was a kid, Lisa's grandfather wrote a book that became a hit Hollywood movie, *The Doctor*, starring William Hurt, the story of a successful, arrogant surgeon who, transformed by his own diagnosis of cancer, begins to see life and doctoring through different eyes.) After training at world-class hospitals in San Francisco, Boston, and New York, Lisa wants to learn more about what makes doctors tick, why we do what we do, how our feelings help, hurt, and get hurt by our work with patients. After we'd met at Cornell and talked about mutual interests, Lisa, who runs marathons and thinks big, said: Why don't we talk to the guy who knows more about this stuff than anyone on the planet?

We rode downtown together in a cab. Lisa said I looked tired, asked how I'd been. I told her about my parents, what I'd done, and why. She offered her condolences, then whistled when I told her that this had all happened in the midst of a busy time on-service in the hospital. I told her about Mr. Warner, described his last few days, our uncertainties, what his autopsy showed. *Wow*, Lisa said. I found myself saying that I wished I could do it over again, that in the old days it might have gone down differently. Lisa's grandfather had told her about the old days. *Have you had any experience with house calls, Dr. Reilly? My grandfather says it was the best thing he did.* I didn't tell her about Fowler House or Fred.

When we arrived at the restaurant, Dr. Kahneman was sitting with his wife, Dr. Anne Treisman, at a balcony table. Dr. Treisman is one of the most distinguished academic psychologists in the world, a member of both the U.S. National Academy of Sciences and the Royal Society of London. A professor of psychology at Princeton (like her husband), Dr. Treisman's polite British reserve didn't hide her sparkling intelligence or wry sense of humor, and it was obvious immediately that her more famous spouse revered her. After brief chitchat and a look at the menu, Kahneman looked at Lisa and asked gently, So, how can we help you?

Lisa expressed our admiration for Kahneman's research and told him that we wanted to learn more about the psychology of medical decision-making. If we can understand better how doctors and patients think and feel when confronted with hard decisions, it can only make us better doctors, don't you think?

Maybe so, Kahneman said, but I must admit I don't know much about medicine.

His wife seemed amused by his remark and I thought I knew why. I'd read an interview in the *Times* a few years ago in which Kahneman said he really didn't know much about economics. At the time, he had just been awarded the Nobel Prize—in Economics. So

I figured that if this guy doesn't know even one-tenth as much about medicine as he doesn't know about economics, Lisa and I might still learn something.

Since the 1970s, Kahneman and his late colleague, Amos Tversky, had done groundbreaking research demonstrating that most human beings don't think like quants. This may seem obvious until you realize that leading philosophers and economists had assumed for centuries that human beings behave as "rational agents." But Kahnemanandtversky—the names of the two psychologists are linked inseparably—proved that the rational agent model doesn't describe most people. It's not that people are *irrational*, unresponsive to reason, but that human rationality is limited—constrained in various ways by emotion, bias, logical inconsistencies, tricks of memory. The implications of this research have been profound, important whenever people make decisions, whether buying a car or considering treatment for cancer.

In medicine, for example, Kahneman and Tversky had helped us understand why patients are more likely to agree to risky surgery when told that the operation gives them a 90 percent chance of survival than when told it carries a 10 percent chance of death. (These two outcomes are identical but patients "see" the decision differently, depending on how it is "framed.") Their research explained why most people, when faced with a small risk—for example, a 1 percent chance of a heart attack—either ignore the risk completely or "weight" it excessively, exaggerating its importance. They showed that first impressions (like my own about Mr. Principo) and vivid memories (like Mr. Principo's about his first wife) influence doctors' and patients' decisions more than a purely "rational agent" would allow. They showed how hindsight distorts our view of the past. Why we mistake random chance for causality. How and why we jump to conclusions, or "close" our thinking prematurely. Most important, they discovered that these and many other "mind tricks" are universal, essential features of what makes us human.

While we waited for lunch, at Lisa's urging I told Kahneman and his wife about Mr. Warner.

Kahneman listened quietly. When I was done, he asked, What is the usual treatment in a case like this?

I told him that Mr. Warner had met none of the generally accepted criteria for surgery. We had treated him according to the consensus standard of care.

Why, then, Kahneman asked, does this case bother you? Even now, all these weeks later?

I told him I wished I had done more. I wished I had *acted* on my sense that Mr. Warner was in trouble, that he probably wouldn't make it. I didn't know this for sure, but . . .

Kahneman waited.

. . . I just wish I had *done* more.

Kahneman nodded and pinched his nose where his eyeglasses sat. (Later, Lisa would say he looked tired, too. We didn't know it but, at the time, Kahneman was deep into the writing of his future bestseller—the instant classic *Thinking, Fast and Slow*—and was feeling fatigued and frustrated by his slow progress.) He turned deferentially to his wife.

Sounds like asymmetric regret, he said.

Yes, Dr. Treisman said confidently, it does.

Lisa and I glanced at each other, then back at them.

What's *that*? we asked.

The intensity of regret, Kahneman answered, varies under different conditions. Psychologists have long believed that regret is asymmetric in the sense that people feel more regret about an outcome linked to an action than one linked to an inaction. If this were true, for example, doctors would regret a patient's dying after surgery more than they regret a patient dying without surgery. But regret, Kahneman explained, is more complex than just the difference between commission and omission. Regret, it seems, is also about comparing one's decision to a "default" decision—the decision that is the accepted norm in that situation. Thus, action will cause greater regret when the norm is inaction. But if action (like performing surgery) is the norm in a given case, then inaction (not performing surgery) will cause greater regret.

Oh, we said.

I didn't talk about Fred and Martha. (What was the "norm" in their case?) And I don't remember much else about the rest of our lunch. But afterward I felt admiration for these two distinguished folks who had shared their time and expertise with people they didn't even know. And I felt a little better about Mr. Warner. Most likely I would have felt even more regret had we done the surgery (which, not the accepted norm in his case, almost certainly would have failed). When Kahneman's great book was published, he explained it this way:

> Intense regret is what you experience when you can most easily imagine yourself doing something other than what you did. . . .
>
> The asymmetry in the risk of regret favors conventional and risk-averse choices. . . . Imagine a physician with a gravely ill patient. One treatment fits the normal standard of care; another is unusual. The physician has some reason to believe that the unconventional treatment improves the patient's chances, but the evidence is inconclusive. The physician who prescribes the unusual treatment faces a substantial risk of regret, blame, and perhaps litigation. In hindsight, it will be easier to imagine the normal choice. . . .
>
> True, a good outcome will contribute to the reputation of the physician who dared but the potential benefit is smaller than the potential cost.

Not bad, I thought, for a guy who doesn't know much about medicine.

Even so, after our meeting, decisions I had made for Mr. Warner and my mother gnawed at me. In Mom's case, the clinical facts (and Kahneman's discourse on regret) seemed to leave little room for counterfactual thinking. Unequivocally, the standard of care for Mom's heart problem was *action*: She needed a pacemaker. Surely, this would be the least regrettable decision. But two considerations had suggested otherwise. One: Mom, when mentally competent to decide, had refused any "heroic" life-sustaining treatments. Fair enough, but a pacemaker? It's such a simple, everyday thing today. What does "heroic" mean, anyway? Two: The pacemaker would treat

Mom's heart but not her brain. Save her heart but lose her brain? As in Mr. Warner's case, can one justify such a decision? Could you? Do you know a person like Mom? Someone you love? A person with severe dementia, after it has progressed—as dementia *always* does—to a stage even worse than Mom's? Such a person is more alone than any widow, any orphan, any prisoner on death row will ever be; in some ways, no longer a person at all, really. Do you have a loved one like Mom? Have you sat with her, stayed with her, tried to put yourself in her place? For this—*knowing you were saving her for this*—would you save her heart? Would you?

The science of medicine cannot answer such questions. Neither can the science of psychology. Would Mom be better off dead? It's a question for philosophers or God, not for scientists or one doctor—no matter how well the doctor knows his patient.

Science didn't have the answers in Mr. Warner's case, either. In the end, this was the source of my regret about him: We were flying blind. There was no widely accepted, evidence-based standard of care for Mr. Warner's problem. (The science is lacking.) But if regret is largely about comparing one's decision to the "accepted norm," whence comes my regret about Mr. Warner? In his case, no such norm existed. The answer to this question—and perhaps much more—lay in Kahneman's comments about the "asymmetric" regret of action versus inaction.

The hard reality is that doctors lack an accepted norm—an evidence-based, "right" thing to do—for patients we see every day, not just in rare cases like Mr. Warner. But decisions must be made and, when we make them, most doctors in the United States lean toward action, not inaction. In other words, the "culture" of U.S. medicine is interventionist: When in doubt, doctors' default mode tends to be "don't just stand there, do something"—get the CT scan, give the chemotherapy, perform CPR—even when the patient is ninety years old with dementia or incurable cancer. It was this "cultural imperative" to intervene that drove my regret about Mr. Warner: If only I had . . . done more.

But, precisely *because* doctors often lack an accepted norm for our tough decisions, our interventionist "culture" is an incubator of regret. As Kahneman noted, when there is no conventional solution to an urgent problem, action ("do something") is more likely to cause regret than inaction ("stand there"). Why, then, do doctors embrace this interventionist culture? Surely, it fosters regret; doctors don't talk about it but it's there—and it festers, affecting all doctors in (personal and professional) ways that most of us don't understand. Why do we let this happen? Is the medical profession's interventionist culture really better for patients? If so, is regret the price all doctors must pay to help them? Certainly, patients suffer harms as well as benefits from modern medicine's wondrous interventions. And, certainly, doctors must continue their efforts to reduce these harms. But what about the other casualties of medicine's "friendly fire"? What about the doctors?

We have a lot to learn about such things. I suspect this is part of what Kahneman meant when he disclaimed knowing much about medicine. In that sense, I don't know much about medicine either. The reality is that we have barely begun to understand how doctors and patients can best "share" decisions, especially in the many cases in which the relevant clinical science is weak and the "standard of care" is unproven. No doubt more and better clinical research will help; one day we will *know* what to do for patients like Mr. Warner.

But while we wait for greater knowledge, we must aspire to greater wisdom. This won't come from a test tube or petri dish. Medical wisdom will grow only with help from giants *outside* the biomedical sciences, giants like Kahneman, because the mysteries of medicine extend far beyond the purview of biology. And so do their solutions.

Dad went first.

After I left the hospital, Mom staring blankly out her window at the harbor lights, I drove west out of Greenport, thinking. Soon I found myself on an old country road that ended in a small, empty parking lot on a beach, the big bay shimmering in the moonlight. The place looked familiar. As I parked my car, its headlights shone on an old stone wall where a brass engraving read: Founders Landing 1640. I had been here once before, with my wife, the place where her Pilgrim ancestors had disembarked so long ago. I got out of my car, looked across the water toward Shelter Island, a thin dark line on the horizon. I thought for a while about what I'd done. I was still thinking about it when, a short while later, I crossed on the ferry and went back to the house. Dad was asleep, the single lamp lit low at his bedside. He seemed fitful. He groaned. I went to him, watched him breathe, took his pulse.

He turned his head toward me and opened his eyes, unseeing.

That you, Bren?

Yes, Dad.

How's Mom?

His speech was clear and sharp.

She's fine, Dad. She's gonna be fine.

Oh . . . good. That's good.

He closed his eyes and turned away. His breathing seemed to slow. Then he spoke again.

Thanks, Bren. Thanks . . .

I was tired. I took a shower. Before I did, I looked in on him again, his breathing regular and deep, just like before. Ten minutes later, my skin steamy warm, I looked into his room again. It seemed the same, the light low, Dad peacefully asleep. I stood there watching, waiting for him to breathe. Sometimes it's like that near the end; our breathing stops, then starts again. More than once in my career I've thought people dead who weren't. Dad was.

He had been more than a father to me. He had been my friend. Next to my wife and my kids, he was the one I loved the most. I sat down in the chair next to his bed. I missed him already. But I was glad for him. Finally, it was done. I stayed for a while, just looking. I thought more about Mom, what I had done. Then, back to the hospital, to tell Mom about Dad.

Those next few days, there was a lot to do. I discovered that they had purchased only one gravesite, not two, registered in Dad's name. It's a pretty spot under a big shade tree where the sun rises over the island graveyard. Luckily, another gravesite—the two of them side by side together under that same tree—was still available. As I made the swap and wrote the check, I couldn't help wondering about all the other times Mom and Dad had gone their separate ways. Mom had always said she wanted to go to the family mausoleum in the city. She liked the idea of having her name and dates engraved on that fine red marble, together with the mother she never knew and those other names from long ago. That wasn't Dad's style. He didn't like the ostentation, the marble, those stone angels preening astride the vault. When the chance had come a few years ago to buy a solo shady sunrise spot here on the island, Dad had said, Good enough for me. As Mom faded, she began to waver about her mausoleum, then forgot it altogether. When the time came, I made the call to keep them together.

It doesn't look like a graveyard—it looks like a wide sun-drenched lawn with shade trees—until you walk out on the grass yourself and come upon the headstones, all of them humble and small, laid flat to the earth, bouquets of flowers and tiny American flags here and there. No mausoleums. Shelter Island had been Mom's dream, not Dad's, but he had learned to love it, too. Like so much of their life together, its ending would be a compromise.

I don't say so in the little church when it's my turn to come up on the altar and speak about Dad.

It's a strange day, even the weather. Overnight, the temperature has risen thirty degrees. As the few of us take our seats, warm sun streams through the chapel windows. This balmy surprise, so un-expected in the first week of February, reminds me of something, somewhere, but I can't place it. I look at the date printed on the Mass card. Today is the day for Mr. Warner's Morbidity and Mortality Conference at Cornell. Now, as I rise to speak about Dad, Tina is rising to speak about Mr. Warner. She understood, of course, when I told her why I can't be there to help—to defend her, if necessary, when the questions fly. She'll do fine without me.

Here, in the chapel, there won't be any questions. The pews are mostly empty. A few old folks, accompanied by caregivers and walk-ers and wheelchairs, have come to pay their respects and wonder when their turn will come. At the lectern, on the altar, I wonder aloud what a son can say in just a few minutes about a good man who lived a full life for more than ninety years. Dad had never been one to talk about himself, so I tell them briefly about his life—the war, his medical work, his family. I tell them I wonder what it means that his heart and Mom's, together for almost seventy-five years, decided to stop on the very same day. I tell them that science doesn't understand such things. Then I tell them what Mom had said that night, the night I went back to the hospital to tell her Dad was gone.

Her eyes were closed, her heart monitor bleeping soft and slow. She recognized me, said something about my height, thanked me for coming. She didn't remember that I'd been with her just two hours before. I told her I had terrible news. She didn't understand at first. Then her eyes grew wide and she turned away to look out the bayside window into the night.

He had a lot of pain? she asked.

No, Mom. He just went to sleep. He asked for you. He wanted to be sure you were all right. Then he fell asleep. It was very peaceful.

Oh . . . good. That's . . . good.

Then she was quiet. She looked out the window. For a few minutes, we just sat there, in silence. Then she turned to me.

How's Dad doing, Bren?

So I told her again.

He had a lot of pain, didn't he? Mom asked.

I told her about my visit the week before when I'd had to help him in his bed, turn him on his side despite his painful, cancerous hip. I told Mom it had hurt me just to watch him. Mom nodded, as if she understood. Then I told her what Dad had said, in that wisecracking voice of his, as he struggled to compose himself and catch his breath. Sensing, somehow, my own distress at his pain, Dad said, Well, Bren, I guess I'm not as young as I thought I was!

Mom laughed, her eyes flashing. Then she shook her head.

He never complained. He was a good patient, wasn't he, Bren?

And then she began to remember. As she spoke, a dreamy look came into her eyes. He was tall, athletic, handsome. Mom said he made her heart go pitter-pat. She remembered how they would sneak into the night clubs and ballrooms where the great forties bands were playing—Benny Goodman, Tommy Dorsey, people like that. They couldn't afford the cover charge but they would dance every dance until the maître d' caught them and kicked them out and then they just left and went on to the next place and did the same thing. Just the two of us, Mom said, doing the town, dancing the night away.

We had a lot of fun, she said.

I told her that a few weeks ago Dad had asked me how I felt about becoming a grandfather for the first time. I told him that Janice and I had been speaking recently to friends about the different names they chose for their grandkids to call them, not just Nana or Grandpa but Mimi and G-dad and names like that. I told Dad that one of our friends had decided that her grandchildren should call her "Gorgeous" and now, whenever she visits them, these cute little two- and three-year-olds come running up to her, yelling "Hiya, Gorgeous!" Dad had laughed and laughed, a big loud belly laugh that shook the bed. He was dying but, even then, he could laugh like that.

Dad loved to laugh, Mom said.

There was a pause, then dead silence but for the slow bleep of Mom's heart monitor. She was far away again.

So . . . I said.

Mom turned, surprised to see me.

Oh, hi, Bren! Thanks for coming, dear.

Glad to, Mom.

How's Dad doing, Bren?

Today, I don't tell the folks in the church about this last part. I remind them how gracefully Dad had handled his blindness, how much he had missed his art, the sunsets on the water, his books. He never said a word about it. Many people who met him for the first time didn't even know he was blind. When I would ask him privately, from time to time, about his vision, try to get him to talk about it, all he would say was: You know, Bren, there's a lot of really good stuff on the radio these days.

Finally, in the church, I am reading from the *Four Quartets*, the part Dad loved, the part about how we die with the dying and are born with the dead, the part about the rose and the yew-tree. Then, I am looking down from the altar and speaking directly to Mom. She's sitting in the front pew.

Mom . . .

Her voice rings out, loud and clear in the little church.

Yes?

Dad's in a good place now, Mom. He has no pain. He laughs a lot. His vision is 20/20. He's sitting on a big porch looking out over the water. The view is to die for.

Mom laughs.

We had a lot of fun, Mom says to no one in particular.

And that was that.

As it had happened, when I went back to the hospital the night Dad died, I'm not really sure what made the difference, why I undid what I had done. Maybe it was what Mom had said about Dad and Benny Goodman and dancing the night away. Maybe I just wasn't able to let go, not both of them, not the very same day. But, looking back now, I think it was that look on Mom's face when she gazed out at the bay from her hospital bed. The window was closed but, for just a few fleeting seconds, her chin rose and her eyelids fluttered and she sighed with pleasure, as if she could actually feel the sea breeze blowing gently through her hair. Was she remembering? Hallucinating? Does it matter?

She doesn't know she has a pacemaker. Her past is largely lost, her future unthinkable. But yesterday, after Dad's wake, she looked out her bedroom window and smiled as she watched the gulls play on the water. Sometimes, in the present, Mom's still here.

This will change, I know. But I keep that to myself. The others will find out soon enough.

Just yesterday, at Dad's wake, my brother asked Mom if she wanted to kiss Dad good-bye. (Willie's in show business, what can I say?) All but a few of the visitors had left. The casket was open—a hideous custom, in my opinion, but I had been overruled by others—and there lay Dad, horizontal on a satin pillow, unnaturally blushed, waiting for the damned casket to finally get shut.

At first, Mom didn't understand. She was exhausted, her face a blank. So Willie asked her again and led her gently to the casket, directing the final scene.

Mom took a long look at Dad. Then she stepped back, and turned away.

No, she said, shaking her head with great conviction.

Willie persisted.

Why, Mom? Are you sure?

Yes, William, I'm sure.

Her voice was strong, her tone assured. She knew exactly what she was saying. This was the Mom I knew.

But why, Mom? Willie asked.

Why? Look at the poor man!

What do you mean, Mom?

Well! I don't want to wake him up!

EPILOGUE

We live forwards; we understand backwards.

—William James (1890)

September 2012

The foghorn blows long and loud as the northbound ferry pulls out of its slip. The island, lush green in the early fall, drifts away, left behind in the mist. Mom's doing fine, as these things go—less mobile and more frail but still aware, at least some of the time, that she's in her own home. That fact, as best I can tell, is what matters to her most. Mom's new caregiver, Mavis, is a godsend but it isn't easy to find substitutes when she needs a break. So, we'll see. One day at a time.

When it was all happening, I didn't connect the dots. Looking back, how could I? There was a lot going on: Mom and Dad, Warner and Principo, Tina and Ashley and Dan. Maybe I would have made the connections eventually, even if I hadn't seen the piece in the *Times*, the one about the new search in the Pacific. They're looking for Amelia Earhart again. A big expedition to Nikumaroro, fancier equipment than ever before. New evidence, the *Times* reported, something about an old shoe found on a beach. Her plane went down before I was born, back when Mom and Dad were sneaking into dance clubs, and yet we're still searching for her today. It made me wonder why we care about connecting dots. So I dug out the old letters, the pictures of Martha's family, my memories of that hill and their house, the birch-dappled meadow in summertime. I even dreamed about it again, once. I Googled Fred, something I hadn't done since Chicago. That's when I noticed the date, the one that started me connecting the dots myself.

A coincidence? Certainly. What else could it be? Still, it got my attention. Was it really the same date? That sudden thaw, so unexpected in early February, both times? Dad's funeral and Fred's death, *exactly* twenty-five years apart? Could that be?

It got my attention.

So now, on the ferry, I settle in for the ride. This isn't the eight-minute crossing from Shelter Island. It's the ninety-minute trip to Connecticut. I'm heading north, to Vermont.

It's been decades since I moved away but I've heard that my world is changing there, too. The primary care crisis hasn't hit God's country as hard as other places, but it's coming. Then, inevitable as winter, the fragmentation and depersonalization of care will follow, the new reality of medicine commoditized. They will be shaking their heads at the folly of it, the weavers and stonemasons and dairy farmers, good neighbors all. But the medical commons is national now, not local. We're all connected, all of us grazing in the same pasture, whether you live in my Manhattan or the one in Kansas.

Fred would have had some ideas about this.

I telephoned ahead. Margaret still lives in Norwich with her husband, Steve. She was surprised, of course. It's been a long time. But she seemed glad to hear from me. I told her I'd like to see her, show her a story I've been writing.

It's about your mom and dad, I said.

Margaret laughed.

Mom always said you would do that someday.

Yeah, well, we'll see. It's not done yet.

The ferry's foghorn blasts again, longer and louder this time. Something up ahead, invisible in the haze. These pilots know the Sound like the back of their hand but, still, they show respect. The currents, the showboaters, the storms, you can't be too careful. The new ferries are faster and safer than the old ones—real progress, certainly—but they're bigger, too, more passengers on board. Best to slow down, sound the horn, take no chances.

On the starboard side, Plum Island looms into view. It's a spooky, flat place, barren except for the animal disease research laboratory operated by the U.S. Department of Homeland Security. "Anthrax Island," Hannibal Lecter called it in *The Silence of the Lambs*. Personally, I'm glad it's here but some of the local folks think otherwise. A few years ago, the feds almost sold it to some tycoon so he could make the island his own private refuge, like Gardiner's Island and Fisher's Island nearby, beachy enclaves of the rich and famous. Those folks say they're all for homeland security, just not in their backyard. It's a tricky business, this thing about protecting the national commons. The part about medicine is just that, just one part of it.

The fog begins to lift off the water. Now I can see the coastline up ahead, the place where the big river from the north country flows down into the Sound. From there, it's a straight shot up the Connecticut to that high meadow of my dreams. If you had the time and the inclination, you could paddle a birch canoe from Fred and Martha's house in Vermont directly to my hospital on the East River. It's all connected.

While you're up here, Margaret had said on the phone, maybe you'd like to look around a little. We could use a doctor like you. (My wife nodded when I told her this; Janice has been saying the same thing for years.)

In the moment, on the phone, I said something polite, noncommittal. After all, Margaret may feel different after she reads my story. But, hey, you never know. I'm beginning to think some things are meant to be.

NOTES

Prologue

4 *the legacy of Libby Zion, who died at this hospital:* The unexpected, tragic death in 1984 of this eighteen-year old woman less than twenty-four hours after her admission to New York Hospital (now New York Presbyterian Weill Cornell Medical Center) catapulted concerns about hospital safety and residents' long work hours onto the national stage. (See, for example, Asch and Parker, *New England Journal of Medicine* 1988;318:771.) The Bell Commission subsequently recommended sweeping changes in New York State that eventually transformed national policies about these issues. See also note for page 30 and page 62.

Chapter 1: Lost and Found

9 *mortality rates go up on the weekend:* Studies in the United States and other countries have shown that in-hospital mortality is higher among patients admitted from the emergency department on weekends than among those admitted on weekdays (see, for example, Bell and Redelmeier, *New England Journal of Medicine* 2001;345:663; Aylin and colleagues, *Quality and Safety in Health Care* 2009;doi:10.1136/qshc.2008.028639.) This "weekend effect" has been documented as a general phenomenon and also among patients with specific medical diagnoses, such as heart attack (see Kostis and colleagues, *New England Journal of Medicine* 2007;356:1099) or pulmonary embolism (see Aujesky and colleagues, *Circulation* 2009;119:962). The absolute increase in hospital mortality rates on weekends is small; for example, the increase ranged from 0.2 percent to 2.3 percent in the four studies cited above. Nevertheless, this difference is real—careful statistical analyses show that the probability is less than one in one thousand that these study findings occurred by chance alone—and, when applied to the millions of patients at risk, it translates into thousands of excess deaths per year in the United States. This is not a simple problem to understand or solve (see Halm and Chassin, *New England Journal of Medicine* 2001;345:692; Redelmeier and Bell, *New England Journal of Medicine* 2007;356:1164). But, literally a matter of life and death, this is one of countless reasons why "health services research" (which studies such phenomena) requires much more attention and public funding.

9 *This is doctor-talk:* Doctors tend to lean toward optimism when discussing their patients' prospects. There are many reasons for this, not least the fact that doctors deal daily with the

emotional burden of sick or dying patients; thinking positively not only can raise patients' spirits, it can raise doctors' spirits, too. In some cases, this optimism reflects the fact that medical prognostication is not an exact science. In one study, for example, cancer specialists overestimated their patients' remaining days of life by 500 percent! (See Christakis and Lamont, *British Medical Journal* 2000;320:469.) But, in other cases, doctors' optimism is a deliberate strategy, a well-intentioned effort to offer patients hope. For example, as many as one-third of cancer specialists *purposely* overestimate life expectancy when discussing prognosis with their patients. (See Lamont and Christakis, *Annals of Internal Medicine* 2001;134:1096.) Achieving the right balance here is difficult, as Peter Ubel has explained: "The truth we communicate to patients should help them prepare for the worst while allowing them to hope for the best" (see *Annals of Internal Medicine* 2001;134:1142).

10 *one of them fainted dead away:* The student was unhurt. Nevertheless, this incident illustrates how the transition from the classroom to the "real world" of medicine can be traumatic for medical students even when, as at Cornell, every effort is made to prepare them. Much has been written about the emotional turmoil experienced in anatomy class when students first "meet" the corpse whose body they will dissect over the course of several months. But, for many students, the anatomy lab is a piece of cake compared to their first encounter with a real, live sick patient. Our student's experience gave our team of young doctors an opportunity to learn about syncope (the medical term for fainting), a common problem that will appear more than once in subsequent chapters of this book. But it also gave us a chance to talk about physicians' emotional reactions to their clinical experiences, an issue that receives insufficient attention in medical education.

10 *recovering from antibiotic-induced colitis: Clostridium difficile* colitis is a classic example of a "disease of medical progress," one that occurs as an unintended consequence of the treatment of another disease. Usually caused by antibiotic therapy, "*C. diff.*" is most regrettable when the offending antibiotic is prescribed unnecessarily for a condition well known not to require antibiotics, such as the common cold (as in our patient's case). Sometimes fatal, the current epidemic of *C. diff.* is one of many reasons why patients' uneducated demand for antibiotics—and physicians' willingness to accede to those demands—has become a major public health problem today.

11 *and we have no one to talk to about what to do:* Patients have the right to make final decisions about their own medical care. This has been recognized as the legal standard in the United States since 1914 when Justice Benjamin Cardozo, then serving on the New York State Court of Appeals, recognized the right of competent adult patients to refuse or consent to medical treatments in *Schloendorff v. The Society of New York Hospital* (now called New York Presbyterian Hospital, where I work). However, in some cases, an adult patient is not "competent" to make these decisions, in which case the patient is said to lack decision-making capacity. The determination of capacity can be complex (see Sessums and colleagues, *Journal of the American Medical Association* 2011;306:420). For example, establishing whether patients with serious psychiatric illness have "capacity" can be especially troubling. In general, decision-making capacity requires that the patient appreciate her medical situation; understand the risks, benefits, and consequences of proposed treatment (and alternative treatments); and can make and communicate a choice that is stable over time, consistent with her own personal goals and values, and that does not result from delusions or hallucinations. Ms. Jackson was considered

to lack capacity because she was consistently and flagrantly delusional. In such cases, then, it is crucial to identify an appropriate "surrogate" decision-maker to decide in the patient's best interests. (See also Chapter 4.) Sadly, one of the many tragedies that befall psychiatrically incapacitated, homeless people like Ms. Jackson is that their relationships with family and friends may be broken irrevocably; utterly alone, they have no one to speak for them. In such cases, only the attending physician can decide what to do, usually in consultation with other physicians (or a hospital's ethics committee) who can help the attending physician "reduce hidden bias, identify unwarranted assumptions and unconvincing arguments, and suggest new alternatives." (See Lo, *Resolving Ethical Dilemmas* [Baltimore: Williams and Wilkins, 1995], p. 120.) This difficult responsibility is not one that attending physicians savor (notwithstanding old jokes about doctors who like to "play God").

12 *elderly people with HIV are rare:* The accuracy of this statement depends on the definition of "elderly" and how one frames the data. Fewer than one in every one thousand people in the United States above age seventy have HIV infection today. In this sense, Mr. Warner is a rarity. On the other hand, 10 to 15 percent of all HIV infections in the United States today afflict people older than age fifty. (In New York State alone, tens of thousands of people above age fifty are HIV-infected.) Thus, HIV-positive elderly patients like Mr. Warner will not be rare, by any definition, in the coming decades.

13 *It's like working in an auto repair shop:* Some people may find this simile inapt, even insulting to physicians. It is neither. Any medical doctor who has listened carefully to *Car Talk*, the hilarious public radio show about car repair, will appreciate the similarity between doctors' diagnosis of human ailments and Tom and Ray ("Click" and "Clack") Magliozzi's diagnosis of automobile malfunction. In fact, I suspect that some medical students would become better doctors faster if their premedical education included not only biology and chemistry but also machine repair. Related ideas and implications have been explored brilliantly by Matthew Crawford in his popular book *Shop Class as Soul Craft*, (New York: Penguin Press, 2009). Crawford, who holds a Ph.D. in philosophy from the University of Chicago, earns his living as a motorcycle repairman.

14 *when Gladwell wrote in* Blink: More precisely, Gladwell wrote in *Blink* about three physicians involved in this research: myself; Dr. Arthur Evans, who directed our research team in Chicago (and who now is the chief of Hospital Medicine at Cornell); and Dr. Lee Goldman, whose original research in Boston was the basis for the work done by Evans, myself, and our Chicago team. (Dr. Goldman is now the dean of Columbia's medical school, which, like Cornell's medical school, is the academic partner of New York Presbyterian Hospital.)

16 *the history (what the patient tells you) is 90 percent of diagnosis:* This statement, an oft-repeated "pearl" of clinical medicine, probably exaggerates the impact of the patient's history on doctors' diagnostic accuracy—but not by much. The few studies that have addressed this question suggest that the patient's history—a description of the quality, location, and timing of symptoms; the tempo of the illness; related medical complaints; past medical care; and other "historical" data about the patient—is the pivotal clue to the patient's diagnosis (as opposed to the patient's physical examination, laboratory tests, or radiologic tests) in 60 to 80 percent of all cases. (See, for example, Peterson and colleagues, *Western Journal of Medicine* 1992;156:163.) This explains why experienced clinicians will often say that they can make

an accurate diagnosis *over the telephone* at least three times out of four. It also explains why savvy patients often wish to talk to their physician by telephone or email before taking the time to come to the doctor's office. (Health care reform should provide reimbursement for doctors to provide these "remote" consultations, a cost-efficient use of both their time and their patients' time.) Unfortunately, some doctors take shortcuts on history-taking and rely more on tests, a strategy that may generate more income and save time (in the short term) but also may lead to serious mistakes.

16 *can learn only so much from the patient's physical examination:* Even in the modern era of CT and MRI scans, expert physical examination can make a critical difference to patients' care in about 10 to 20 percent of patients with new or previously undiagnosed medical conditions. (See, for example, Reilly, *Lancet* 2003;362:110.) In one sense, such estimates are spurious because physical examination was never intended to be performed *in isolation from* the other essential parts of the diagnostic process, especially the patient's history (see above). Even so, this issue is noteworthy for two reasons. First, if doctors' skills in physical examination decline, they will rely even more heavily on technological diagnosis, which is always more expensive, sometimes less accurate, and occasionally harmful when compared to physical examination. Second, many patients today, especially sick or elderly ones like Mr. Warner, are unable to communicate a cogent history. As a result, the medical diagnostician must "become a veterinarian" (rely on physical examination and tests alone) more often than we like.

16 *the racket in the corridor:* New York Presbyterian Hospital (NYPH), like many other acute care hospitals, has made a concerted effort to reduce "noise pollution" in order to improve patients' experience in hospital. For example, every afternoon between 2:00 p.m. and 4:00 p.m. is "quiet time" at NYPH: Lights are dimmed, voices are lowered, and unnecessary intrusions into patients' rooms are minimized. The latter effort is especially important; studies have shown that hospital staff (of various types) enter each patient's room, on average, three to four times *per hour* over a twenty-four-hour period (a total of seventy to ninety times per day)! At a time when sleep deprivation among doctors and nurses is an important medical care issue (see note, p. 62), sleep deprivation *among patients* deserves attention, too. One study found that elderly patients described a "good" (versus "poor" or "fair") night's sleep on only 25 percent of their total nights in hospital. (See Lee and colleagues, *The Open Sleep Journal* 2008;1:29.) This is not a trivial problem when one considers that sleep deprivation (and sleeping medication) contributes importantly to patients' developing delirium in hospital. (See also Chapter 7.) No doubt sleep deprivation also contributes to patients' posthospitalization fatigue; many patients report that they require a long time to recover fully from even a brief hospitalization.

17 *reasons why this practice has fallen out of favor today:* Currently, the only components of the annual physical examination (the "routine checkup") proved to provide cost-effective benefit to patients are measurement of blood pressure and body weight (BMI) and screening tests for hearing and visual loss, none of which require examination by a physician. (Pap smears make the cost-effective list but only for young, sexually active women who have a cervix; and, even for these patients, Pap smear is not recommended every year.) This does not mean that preventive health care is cost-ineffective. To the contrary, many preventive services, ranging from advice about seatbelts to flu shots, are indisputably worthwhile. (See, for example, Chacko and Anderson, *American Journal of Medicine* 2007;120:581.) Rather, it is

the doctor's annual "laying on of hands" whose cost-effectiveness is unproven. But measures of cost-effectiveness may not be the only ways to judge the value of this traditional "healing ritual," as the author Abraham Verghese has described the physical examination (see *Annals of Internal Medicine* 2011;155:550). *Annals* editor Christine Laine agrees: "If careful study documents that patients who get annual physical examinations feel better, behave healthier, undergo more appropriate screening, and trust their physicians more . . . skeptics would need to reconsider the value of this yearly ritual" (see *Annals of Internal Medicine* 2004;136:701).

18 *Systemic Inflammatory Response Syndrome:* The presence of two or more of the following clinical findings define the syndrome of SIRS: 1) an abnormally high (or abnormally low) body temperature; 2) rapid heart rate; 3) rapid breathing; and 4) abnormally high (or abnormally low) white blood cell (WBC) count. Many different diseases can cause SIRS; most (but not all) of them are infections. The key to saving a patient with SIRS is to identify the syndrome early and then identify and treat the specific disease causing it. (When infection is the cause, it is essential to identify the specific type and location of the infection.) The "SIRS criteria" are helpful to doctors because many patients with serious infections do not meet *all four* criteria (unlike Mr. Warner). Elderly patients, for example, may not develop a fever even when suffering from a life-threatening infection. Thus, knowledge and use of the SIRS criteria can alert doctors to the presence of serious infection even when the patient's clinical presentation is atypical (as it often is in elderly patients).

20 *The normal response in this Babinski reflex:* Infants are the exception to this rule. Before the human brain is fully developed, infants will demonstrate an "abnormal" (upgoing) Babinski response. This response typically disappears one or two years after birth. Like many tests, however, the Babinski reflex can be difficult to interpret. (For example, this reflex must be elicited without actually tickling the patient's foot; when tickled, a normal patient's toe will respond in a manner that appears abnormal.) This is one example of the many "tests" performed by doctors during the physical examination, whose results are valid and reliable only insofar as the examiner's method and interpretation are rigorous. Many people, including some doctors, don't understand physical examination for what it really is: a series of tests.

21 *because the study of expertise in any field requires:* See Ericsson and colleagues, *The Cambridge Handbook of Expertise and Expert Performance* (Cambridge: Cambridge University Press, 2006).

21 *two different ways of human thinking complement each other:* These ideas are explored in great detail in two fine books: Evans and colleagues, *In Two Minds: Dual Processes and Beyond* (Oxford University Press, 2009); and Kahneman, *Thinking, Fast and Slow* (New York: Farrar, Strauss and Giroux, 2011). (See also Chapter 10.)

23 *I do a more sensitive test:* In medicine, the term "sensitive" has a special meaning when applied to diagnostic tests, including tests done during the physical examination (see McGee, *Evidence-Based Physical Diagnosis* [Philadelphia: W.B. Saunders, 2001]). A test's sensitivity is defined as the percentage of all patients with a particular disease in whom the diagnostic test is positive (i.e., abnormal). Thus, it refers to the frequency with which a test detects an abnormality when, in fact, an abnormality exists. By this definition, then, "pronator drift" on the neurological examination is a more sensitive indicator of (mild) unilateral motor weakness than other tests of strength. See also note, p. 27, about diagnostic test "specificity," the flip side of test sensitivity.

24 *these drugs don't help nearly as many people as they could:* Despite clear evidence that "thrombo-lytic" drugs improve outcomes for acute stroke patients (see Wechsler, *New England Journal of Medicine* 2011;364:2138), fewer than 10 percent of eligible patients receive them, both in the United States (where only 1 to 7 percent receive "clot-busters") and elsewhere (about 3 percent of stroke patients in Canada and Europe receive them). There are many reasons for this failed opportunity to help stroke patients (see Wardlaw and colleagues, *British Medical Journal* 2009;339:1251), most prominently the fact that patients fail to seek attention as soon as stroke symptoms begin. For this reason, public health campaigns have labeled strokes as "brain attacks" to alert patients that a stroke, like a heart attack, is a dire emergency for which life-saving treatment is available (if provided in a timely manner). Many large hospitals have created on-site "stroke teams" of doctors and nurses to respond immediately to these emergencies, but they remain greatly underutilized.

24 *Most patients having a stroke don't have a fever and heart murmurs:* This is a classic example of a "pattern" of symptoms and signs (see text pp. 20–22) readily recognized by clinicians as a powerful diagnostic clue. Ask one hundred experienced internists what comes to mind when presented a patient with fever, heart murmurs, and a stroke, and every one will give the same answer: bacterial endocarditis. Thus, suspecting this diagnosis is obvious when all parts of the "pattern" are apparent. The difficulty in Mr. Warner's case involves recognizing the subtle signs on his neurological examination that suggest that he has, in fact, had a stroke. When these subtle signs are missed (as they were initially in Mr. Warner's case), the diagnosis of endocarditis is not so obvious, because its recognizable diagnostic "pattern" is incomplete.

26 *what was scribbled in his chart:* At the time these events occurred, New York Presbyterian Hospital (NYPH) had successfully adopted an electronic medical record (EMR) system throughout the hospital, *with the exception of its emergency department.* (Special challenges exist for EDs when "going electronic.") Today, unlike the great majority of U.S. hospitals, NYPH is fully electronic, including the ED. (See Jha and colleagues, *New England Journal of Medicine* 2009;360:1628.)

27 *an abnormal but nonspecific finding:* The "specificity" of tests in medicine (see also note, p. 193) refers to the frequency with which a test is negative (i.e., normal) when the disease in question is *not* present. Thus a nonspecific test is one that is frequently positive (i.e., abnormal) even in patients who do not have the disease in question. For example, urine specimens are tested for the presence of white blood cells in order to diagnose bladder or kidney infections; this test is nonspecific because white blood cells can be found in the urine of many patients who do *not* have such infections. (See also Chapter 6 about interpreting diagnostic tests.)

27 *abnormalities have been attributed erroneously to "old age":* Some test abnormalities are more frequently observed in elderly patients than in young patients. For example, eighty-year-old people, *as a group*, have slightly lower red blood cell counts, slightly reduced kidney function, and slightly less brain tissue volume (as seen on CT scans) than forty-year-old people, *as a group*. But each individual eighty-year-old person is unique. Thus, many individual eighty-year-olds will have red blood cell counts, kidney function, and brain CT scans indistinguish-able from that of the average forty-year-old. Therefore, doctors should never assume that abnormalities in these (or any other) tests are *caused* by old age. Indeed, this is rule number 1 for geriatricians, experts in aging who do what all elderly patients want and deserve: "Treat

me, not my age." (This is also the apt title of the wonderful book published recently by Dr. Mark Lachs, the co-chief of geriatrics at Cornell and New York Presbyterian Hospital.)

29 *hospitals no longer are reimbursed for every day:* See also Chapter 3 about hospital reimbursement.

29 *In 2000, the Institute of Medicine reported that medical errors:* See *To Err is Human: Building a Safer Health System* (Washington, D.C.: National Academy Press, 2000). See also Chapter 2.

30 *Most doctors don't do hand-offs:* A recent study from the University of Chicago illustrates this phenomenon (see Chang and colleagues, *Pediatrics* 2010;125:491). Pediatric interns (first-year residents) who were completing a thirty-hour shift on-duty "handed off" their hospital patients to interns scheduled to care for those patients on the next thirty-hour shift. Hand-offs occurred at a dedicated time and place, included the interns' clinical supervisors, and involved a relatively small number of patients (an average of only four patients per intern). Despite these favorable conditions, the single piece of information considered "most important" by the off-going intern was *not* communicated successfully to the on-coming intern *in 60 percent of all patients* handed off. (In these cases, the off-going intern believed that this information *had* been communicated successfully, and all participants in these hand-off sessions rated highly the overall exchange of information.) Thus, even when a great effort is made to do hand-offs well in a very fine hospital, effective communication of critical patient information is far from perfect. This is one of many ways in which medical care in the United States has become increasingly fragmented and "chaotic"; it has important implications for physicians as well as their patients. (See, for example, Detsky and Berwick, *Journal of the American Medical Association* 2013;309:987.)

30 *Tina, by law, must leave the hospital:* National accreditation agencies for postgraduate medical training programs set rigorous standards that limit on-duty hours for interns and residents (see Blanchard and colleagues, *New England Journal of Medicine* 2009;360:2242). These standards have continued to evolve—and have become even more restrictive—after the events described in this book. See also note, p. 62.

33 *aortic stenosis and mitral regurgitation:* The former refers to a stenotic (narrowed) aortic valve, the latter a regurgitant (leaking) mitral valve. Usually, but not always, these heart valve abnormalities can be diagnosed (and differentiated) on physical examination, using a stethoscope. As in other aspects of physical examination, the more experienced the examiner, the more accurate the diagnosis.

35 *The elevator arrives, empty:* Patient confidentiality is closely guarded in hospitals. My team would not have discussed Mr. Warner's case on the elevator had any other passengers been present.

Chapter 2: Caught in the Middle

38 *Would strongly consider palliative care:* Many doctors are not trained to relieve patients' symptoms as well as they are trained to treat disease. As a result, many patients today suffer unnecessarily because their doctors don't focus enough on how to make them *feel* better. (See

Eric Cassell's classic work *The Nature of Suffering and the Goals of Medicine* [Oxford University Press, 2004, (2nd ed.)].) Palliative care is a relatively new phenomenon in American medicine, an offshoot of the hospice movement begun in Great Britain in the 1970s. Originally intended for patients with terminal cancer, palliative care (which focuses on relieving symptoms such as pain, shortness of breath, and anxiety) can help patients who suffer from any type of serious illness. Unfortunately, many doctors and patients have resisted its ministrations because they equate palliative care with "giving up"—and dying. However, palliative care should complement, not replace, efforts to treat the patient's underlying disease, as illustrated by a recent study of patients with advanced, incurable lung cancer. Patients who received palliative care in addition to cancer treatment (chemotherapy and radiation treatments) not only felt better (experienced less depression and a higher "quality of life") *but also lived longer* than patients who received cancer treatments alone (see Temel and colleagues, *New England Journal of Medicine* 2010;363:733). The impact of palliative care on longevity is not well understood; nevertheless, in patients with serious disabling illnesses, there is no reason *not* to consider palliative care.

38 *Ordinarily, I prefer the bedside:* The past several decades have witnessed a profound transition from a culture of medicine in which doctors made treatment decisions without much input from the patient to one in which doctors require the patient's informed consent for treatment. In the coming decades, it is likely that a subsequent transition will occur, this time from a culture of informed consent to one of "informed choice" in which patients literally "share" decision-making with their doctors. One way teaching hospitals can facilitate this transition is for attending physicians and physicians-in-training to discuss their decision-making about a patient, when possible, *in the presence of the patient*. The medieval notion that most patients would be upset by hearing their own case discussed by their doctors was debunked more than thirty years ago when doctors at Duke University reported that 95 percent of patients reported being pleased by a "bedside" style of clinical decision-making (see Linfors and Neelon, *New England Journal of Medicine* 1980;303:1230). Nevertheless, in most U.S. teaching hospitals today, this practice remains the exception, not the rule; typically, physicians will discuss the case outside the patient's room, in the hospital corridor or in a conference room. This practice not only isolates the patient from the decision-making process, it also decreases the amount of "face time" doctors spend with their hospitalized patients.

38 *this rare type of pancreatic cancer sometimes has a better prognosis:* The most common type of pancreatic cancer, which arises in the glandular cells of this digestive organ, is one of the deadliest cancers of all. Unless it is discovered and treated before it causes symptoms—as in the lucky case of Supreme Court Justice Ruth Bader Ginsburg, whose pancreatic cancer was discovered serendipitously during a routine check-up for another kind of cancer—it is often rapidly fatal. In contrast, Mr. Atkins's less common type, which arises in the islet cells of the pancreas, tends to have a better prognosis, sometimes causing the patient relatively little trouble over the course of many years. Unfortunately for Mr. Atkins, his islet-cell cancer was highly malignant and spread widely despite best treatment. "Cancer" is an umbrella term for hundreds of different diseases that arise in different cell types as a result of thousands of unique genetic and environmental influences. Regrettably, President Nixon's "War on Cancer," begun in 1971, gave credence to the notion that cancer is a single disease whose ravages will end when scientists find "the cure." In fact, each different type of cancer is a unique

disease that requires its own treatment. (See Siddhartha Mukherjee's masterful "biography of cancer," *The Emperor of All Maladies* [New York: Scribner, 2010].)

40 *myxedema, the life-threatening thyroid deficiency:* Underactivity of the thyroid gland (called hypothyroidism) is life-threatening only when it remains undiagnosed and untreated for many months or years. In such cases, it can cause coma ("myxedema coma") or fatal heart disease. But in most cases it is easily diagnosed and treated without need for hospitalization.

41 *Medical care in the United States is a buyer's market:* This is true only in the very narrow sense described here. In all other respects, medical care in the United States is a *seller's* market, its prices exorbitant and unconstrained by typical free market economic forces. See, for example, Brill, "Bitter Pill," *Time*, 2/26/2013.

41 *Medical care is far more expensive in the United States:* Per capita expenditures for health care in the United States are higher than those in any other country in the world. Unfortunately, this does not result in the highest quality. For example, the World Health Organization in 2000 ranked the United States number 1 in cost, number 37 in overall performance, and number 72 in overall health among 191 nations whose health care systems were compared.

42 *about one-third of all medical care in the United States is unnecessary:* This is a complex issue, but the most telling evidence derives from Dartmouth researchers' findings that Medicare enrollees in high-spending regions of the United States receive 30 percent more care than those in low-spending regions *but do not have better health outcomes or satisfaction with care* (see Fisher and colleagues, *Annals of Internal Medicine* 2003;138:273; *Annals of Internal Medicine* 2003;138:288). Not surprisingly, many observers disagree with the Dartmouth researchers' methods (see Bach, *New England Journal of Medicine* 2010;362:569) and conclusions (see Romley and colleagues, *Annals of Internal Medicine* 2011;154:160). Much of this disagreement implicitly revolves around the definition of "unnecessary" and the "value" of health care (see Skinner and colleagues, *New England Journal of Medicine* 2010;362:569). See also Chapter 5 about the Dartmouth research efforts.

42 *U.S. hospitals now spend enormous sums to upgrade their "hotel" accommodations:* This is a relatively new phenomenon in U.S. medicine, largely driven by new business models that encourage hospitals to market themselves directly to patients. Although all U.S. hospitals receive similar financial reimbursements for patients with a given diagnosis, luxurious hospital amenities attract a *larger number* of patients, thus improving the hospital's bottom line. (See Goldman, *New England Journal of Medicine* 2010;363:2185; Grote, *The McKinsey Quarterly* 2007.) This is an important issue for many reasons, including the fact that patients' reported "satisfaction" with their hospital care may affect hospitals' reimbursement for the services they provide, independent of more objective measures of the quality of clinical care patients receive. Patient-reported satisfaction often correlates with, but is not a surrogate for, outcome measures of quality care. (See Manary and colleagues, *New England Journal of Medicine* 2013;368:201.) For example, in one large national study, higher patient satisfaction was associated with higher costs of care and *increased* mortality rates (see Fenton and colleagues, *Archives of Internal Medicine* 2012;172:405).

43 *Then performing annual mammograms:* There is no question that screening mammography saves lives when performed regularly on women between ages fifty and sixty-nine. This mor-

tality benefit is less than many people assume, but it is real. (See Welch, *New England Journal of Medicine* 2010;363:1276; Welch and Frankel, *Archives of Internal Medicine* 2011;171:2043.) Among fifty-year-old women, the ten-year risk of death from breast cancer is about 4 per 1,000 women who undergo annual screening and about 4.4 per 1,000 women who don't have annual mammograms. (This means that the number of such women who will *not* die from breast cancer increases from 995.6 to 996 per 1,000 women as a result of annual mammography screening.) Even so, when applied to millions of such women, this small difference translates into thousands of lives saved. In younger women (under age fifty), however, there is no conclusive evidence that screening mammography saves lives. This does *not* mean that no young woman's life has been saved by such screening; it means that screening *all* such women has not been shown to be cost-effective. (See Warner, *New England Journal of Medicine* 2011;365:1025.) For this reason, the U.S. Preventive Services Task Force does not recommend annual breast cancer screening in younger women (unless there is a high genetic risk of cancer). This recommendation remains controversial for many reasons. (See, for example, Groopman, *The New York Review of Books*, February 11, 2010.)

43 *offering these men a PSA test:* There is no evidence that PSA (prostate specific antigen) testing or any other screening procedures for prostate cancer in older men (above age seventy) saves lives. (See Hoffman, *New England Journal of Medicine* 2011;365:2013.) In fact, the U.S. Preventive Services Task Force has concluded that, even in younger men (aged fifty to sixty-nine), "there is moderate or high certainty that [PSA testing] has no net benefit or that the harms outweigh the benefits" (see McNaughton-Collins and Barry, *New England Journal of Medicine* 2011;365:1951). This is controversial largely because a European trial, arguably the best to date, found a small mortality benefit of screening in men aged fifty to sixty-nine: This study found that among ten thousand such men screened, there were seven fewer deaths due to prostate cancer over a period of nine years when compared with men not screened (see Schroder and colleagues, *New England Journal of Medicine* 2009;360:1320). For this reason, many authorities recommend that each individual man, after learning the pros and cons of prostate cancer screening, make his own informed decision in this matter.

43 *at least the antibiotics make the patient feel better:* Various treatment trials for acute bronchitis ("chest cold") have concluded that antibiotics do not help patients with this common, self-limited illness in any significant way (see Evans and colleagues, *Lancet* 2002;359:1648; Little and colleagues, *Lancet Infectious Diseases* 2013;13:123).

43 *But try telling these folks that the mammogram:* This does not imply that screening mammography in young women or prostate cancer screening in elderly men is "wrong" or should never be done. Such decisions must be individualized. However, based on current evidence, such testing cannot be recommended as a general rule and must be considered a cost-*ineffective* use of medical resources that can also cause very real *harm* to patients.

44 *what Daniel Callahan calls "regnant social expectations":* See Callahan, *Setting Limits: Medical Goals in an Aging Society* (New York: Simon & Schuster, 1987). See also Chapter 9.

44 *reflects a local "culture" of medical practice that tacitly condones:* See Chapter 5 about John Wennberg's decades-long efforts to understand this phenomenon.

45 *I check his IV; it's running slowly:* Intravenous (IV) tubes are connected to plastic bottles or bags containing salt or sugar solutions that infuse through the tubing into the patient's vein. Drugs or blood products (transfusions) can be administered together with these solutions by "piggy-backing" a bottle of drug or blood product into the same IV tubing, thereby sparing the patient an additional needle puncture for every such treatment. Whenever a patient develops a serious new problem in the hospital—for example, if the patient drops his blood pressure or becomes short of breath or confused—one of the first things an experienced doctor will do is to check which drugs and solutions the patient is receiving through his IV, because, not infrequently, such new and unanticipated problems result from complications (allergic reactions or other side effects) of our treatment rather than from the patient's disease. This is a rule of thumb I impart to all physicians-in-training: If a patient develops a problem in hospital that he didn't have before he came to the hospital, it is likely that "we" caused it. Such "iatrogenic" complications—literally, from the Greek meaning "caused by a physician"—are often unavoidable, but recognizing them quickly (and stopping the offending treatment) often limits the harm.

46 *Get me an amp of Narcan:* Narcan is the trade name for naloxone, a drug used to reverse the harmful effects of opiate drugs (such as morphine or heroin). A "fingerstick" refers to rapid blood glucose (sugar) testing performed by pricking the patient's finger and measuring the blood glucose level in a drop of blood. In any patient found unresponsive but alive, opiate overdose (reversible with naloxone) and hypoglycemia (reversible with glucose) must always be excluded urgently, given their life-threatening effects and easy reversibility.

47 *let's hold the Narcan:* Tightly constricted (small) pupils are typically present in a patient who is comatose from an opiate overdose. In addition, Narcan (naloxone) can cause uncomfortable side effects in a patient like Mr. Atkins who has been using opiate drugs for a long time. Both of these considerations support Chris's decision temporarily to withhold Narcan in this case.

47 *somewhere in my brain an idea is aborning:* It is commonly believed that the practice of medicine is largely a matter of "technical rationality," a professional process whereby problems are solved through the selection of means best suited to established ends. This notion sounds right from a patient's perspective. For example, if you break your leg or have a heart attack, you expect your doctors to know the "right" thing to do to solve your problem, based on their knowledge of the various possible treatments and which one will work best for you. This notion also rings true for many medical subspecialists whose job largely *is* a matter of technical rationality: These specialists solve well-defined problems that come to their attention precisely because the problem *is* well-defined and known to require their special expertise (e.g., an orthopedist for your broken leg or a cardiologist for your heart attack). However, this emphasis on problem-*solving* ignores what all patients need their doctors to do first: problem-*setting,* the process by which, as Donald Schon says, professionals "make sense of an uncertain situation that initially makes no sense" (see Schon, *The Reflective Practitioner: How Professionals Think in Action* [New York: Basic Books, 1983]). This process can be humbling, as it was for me in Mr. Atkins's case, especially because I had been humbled by this very same problem before (see Reilly, *Annals of Internal Medicine* 2001;135:467). This may be one reason why many doctors choose to become subspecialists rather than generalists: The "problem domain" of the subspecialist is narrower and more manageable than that of the generalist, who must "make sense of" an intimidating breadth of clinical problems.

49 *The combination of his sick liver and not eating:* Normally, sugars are stored in the liver in the form of glycogen to help maintain blood glucose levels when patients fast (or metabolize glucose rapidly). Patients with severe liver disease lose this ability to store glucose and are especially vulnerable to hypoglycemia after prolonged fasting. Cancer in the liver rarely causes this problem unless the cancer has replaced most of the normal liver tissue (as, unfortunately, Mr. Atkins's cancer had done).

50 *he can't have a liver transplant:* Patients with cancer confined *only* to the liver may be candidates for liver transplantation. Almost always, these patients have a cancer that began in the cells of the liver ("primary" liver cancer) and has not spread outside the liver. *Very* rarely, patients whose cancer began outside the liver (for example, in the breast or intestine) may be eligible for a liver transplant if the metastatic cancer ("secondary" liver cancer) is confined to the liver *and* there is no evidence of the original cancer (for example, in the breast or intestine) after treatment. Ironically, this can occur in Mr. Atkins's type of cancer where the prognosis may be sufficiently good (see note, p. 38) to consider liver transplantation when the residual cancer, after treatment, is detectable only in the liver. (This was not true in Mr. Atkins's case.) The late Steve Jobs, the founder and CEO of Apple, had the same type of pancreatic cancer as Mr. Atkins and did receive a liver transplant. Given the long waiting list for liver transplants, Jobs's receipt of a new liver raised many eyebrows about wealthy patients "gaming the system" and "jumping the queue," especially because it is so rare for patients with metastatic cancer of any type to be considered transplant candidates. (See Grady and Meier, *New York Times*, 6/23/2009.)

52 *today number in the tens of thousands:* At the time of this writing, hospitalists comprise the fastest-growing medical specialty in the United States, approximately thirty thousand strong. It is unknown whether this trend will continue, and especially whether these physicians will make a lifelong career of hospital medicine. (Many hospitalists today are fresh out of residency training, "treading water" in their career path, pending future decisions about further subspecialization.) If hospital medicine continues to grow as its own specialty—and I believe it will—its main challenge will be to improve "transitions" of care between hospitalists and the physicians who care for the patients before and after they leave the hospital. See also Chapters 3 and 8 about discontinuity and transitions of care.

53 *hospitalists are more cost-effective:* This statement has been well-documented in the limited context of an acute, episodic hospitalization. In general, hospitalists discharge patients from the hospital in fewer days than nonhospitalists. (In hospital vernacular, hospitalists reduce patients'"length of stay.") This is "cost-effective" from the perspective of the hospital, which receives the same reimbursement from insurers whether a patient with a given diagnosis stays for two days or ten. (See also Chapters 3 and 8.) More study is needed to learn whether these length-of-stay reductions for acute hospitalizations are cost-effective from a more global perspective, i.e., when the cost and inefficiency of transitions of care are included in the analysis.

54 *published results of the SUPPORT trial:* See The Support Principal Investigators, *Journal of the American Medical Association* 1995;274:1591; Knaus and colleagues, *Annals of Internal Medicine* 1995;122:191.

54 *calls human beings "the temporarily immortal":* See Lynn, Chapter 8 in *To Improve Health and Health Care 1997: The Robert Wood Johnson Foundation Anthology* (Jossey-Bass, 1997).

55 *for a long time most doctors believed:* Many studies have shown that this is not true for the majority of hospitalized patients. (See, for example, Reilly and colleagues, *Archives of Internal Medicine* 1994;154:2299.)

56 *There's a formal hospital process to get to the bottom of such things:* In most U.S. hospitals today, "patient safety" events—preventable incidents that cause (actual or potential) harm to patients—initiate a careful review by a team of hospital staff charged with investigating these events and, whenever possible, preventing their recurrence. For example, a patient found to have a dangerously low blood sugar in hospital would initiate a review to determine not only whether proper procedures had been followed in this case (to prevent, or to diagnose and treat, the low blood sugar in a timely and effective manner) but also to ensure that *hospital-wide* policies adequately address this "safety" issue for all patients. In some cases, rigorous "root cause analyses" are performed to dissect possibly flawed "systems issues" raised by the incident in question (see Vincent, *New England Journal of Medicine* 2003;348:1051).

57 *They're not accustomed to their attending physician admitting:* See also Chapter 7.

57 *In one year recently, 98,609 hospitalized patients:* See Brennan and colleagues, *New England Journal of Medicine* 1991;324:370; Leape and colleagues, *New England Journal of Medicine* 1991;324:377.

57 *About one-third of these health care "crashes":* See Leape and colleagues, *Quality Review Bulletin* 1993;8:144.

57 *an average of 1.7 errors* per day per patient: See Gopher and colleagues, Human Factors Society presentation, October 18, 1989; Denver, Colorado.

57 *as Lucien Leape pointed out in his classic analysis:* See Leape, *Journal of the American Medical Association* 1994;272:1851.

58 *Anesthesiologists, for example, have reduced deaths:* See Saidman and Smith (eds.), *Monitoring in Anesthesia* (Butterworth, 1993). Some experts have questioned whether anesthetic deaths have declined to the extent enumerated here but all agree that great progress has been made (see Gabel, *Journal of the American Medical Association* 2002;288:2404).

58 *"perfect" doctors don't want to see their mistakes:* See Wu, *British Medical Journal* 2000;320:726; Hilfiker, *New England Journal of Medicine* 1984;310:118.

58 *many of us freak out:* See Wu, *Journal of the American Medical Association* 1991;265:2089; Wu, *British Medical Journal* 2000;320:726; Scott and colleagues, *Quality and Safety in Health Care* 2009;18:325.

60 *we may need to include a "stop order":* This strategy is used frequently today in many electronic medical records systems, but it can cause unintended harms as well as benefits. Too many such "stop orders," especially if trivial or redundant, seriously impede health care professionals' work flow and efficiency.

61 *a smart system can protect patients from one doctor's:* See Reason, *British Medical Journal* 2000;320:768; Reason, *Human Error* (Cambridge University Press, 1990).

61 *In the current vernacular of patient safety efforts:* See Leape, *Journal of the American Medical Association* 1994;272:1851.

61 *I "closed" the problem prematurely:* See Kassirer and colleagues, *Learning Clinical Reasoning* (Philadelphia: Lippincott Williams and Wilkins, 2010 [2nd ed.]).

62 *well-known "cognitive dispositions" and biases:* See Kahneman and colleagues (eds.), *Judgment Under Uncertainty: Heuristics and Biases* (Cambridge University Press, 1982); Kahneman, *Thinking, Fast and Slow* (Farrar Strauss and Giroux, 2011).

62 *Regulations allow exceptions to this rule:* This is a complex, evolving issue. Residents' work hours have been strictly regulated for the past decade, primarily due to concerns about residents' sleep deprivation contributing to serious medical errors, especially when caring for critically ill patients (see Landrigan and colleagues, *New England Journal of Medicine* 2004;351:1838). These work hours regulations have been controversial, for two principal reasons. First, residents have long been a cheap source of labor in U.S. teaching hospitals; replacing their hours with other workers will add an estimated 1.1 to 2.5 *billion* dollars annually to U.S. health care costs. Second, many physicians-in-training *want* to work longer hours because they believe that, by "being there" more often, they will learn more, serve their patients better, and, ultimately, become better prepared for careers as autonomous physicians (see Drolet and colleagues, *New England Journal of Medicine* 2012;e35). Strictly speaking, current regulations allow residents, on their own initiative, to remain in hospital beyond the maximum limit of work hours in exceptional situations. However, these exceptions are difficult to monitor and easily abused. For these and many other reasons, it is likely that the work hours issue will remain contentious for many years to come.

Chapter 3: A Safe Bet

64 *as soon as we can find you a bed upstairs:* In some cases, waiting for a bed in the ED is an inconvenience only, but unfortunately, there are many other "waits that matter," as discussed poignantly by John Maa, a surgeon, in the case of his own mother (see Maa, *New England Journal of Medicine* 2011;364:2279). See also note, p. 325. Many observers believe that such waiting has resulted in "an increasingly interventionist ED practice style," not always a good thing. (See, for example, Pitts, *New England Journal of Medicine* 2012;367:2465. See also Chapter 10.)

65 *More than 120 million Americans:* See Tang and colleagues, *Journal of the American Medical Association* 2010;304;664.

66 *I'm on-service in the hospital this month:* Because my job at Cornell involves considerable academic and administrative work, I am no longer what I call a "real doctor," one who practices clinical medicine full-time. Instead, I am a part-time clinician who spends month-long "rotations" as a hospitalist, supervising teams of residents and students. I am ambivalent about this because, in my opinion, full-time clinicians (like my former self) are better doctors than

part-time clinicians (like my current self). Many influential people in academic medicine disagree with me about this. They believe that so-called "triple threat" doctors—who, because they also teach and do research, spend only part of their time taking care of patients—are just as good (or better) at clinical medicine than those who practice it full-time. In rare cases, this may be true. (Exceptional people do exceptional things.) But, in general, it's not true, based on my interaction with thousands of full-time and part-time clinicians over the past forty years. Practicing clinical medicine expertly is a hard thing to do; it requires *never-ending* improvement of one's knowledge and skills. Think about it: If your brain needs fixing, do you want a "real" neurosurgeon who operates every day or a researcher who operates only twice a month? Teaching hospitals accommodate part-time clinicians like me more forgivingly because the residents we "supervise" are very talented young people who make our lives easier (and often compensate for their teachers' weaknesses) as we try to make their education better. But this is a slippery slope. In some cases, residents in teaching hospitals seem to "supervise" their attending physician more than the other way around.

66 *syncope—the medical term for transient loss:* Derived from the Greek word meaning to "cut short"—as when musical meters are interrupted by "syncopation"—syncope in medicine means "transient loss of consciousness with loss of postural tone." (In some cultures, the slang expression for syncope is "falling out," an apt description, because a person who faints not only "passes out" but also *falls down*.) This precise definition is important, because syncope results from a temporary decrease of blood flow to the entire brain, a phenomenon that may be caused by many different disorders, some (a minority) of which are life-threatening. See also Chapters 5 and 6. In contrast, people who appear to "pass out" yet don't fall—or those who fall but don't pass out—usually suffer from very different disorders than those that cause "true" syncope. For this reason, a detailed description of the fainting episode by an eyewitness is the most important step in deciding whether a patient has experienced syncope.

67 *the cardiac arrest team is working frantically:* In most hospitals (and in all large teaching hospitals), designated individuals compose the cardiac arrest team (or "code team") that responds immediately to calls for assistance from anywhere in the hospital when a patient suffers (actual or impending) cardiac arrest. By definition, these events are unexpected life-threatening emergencies that typically require expertise in cardiopulmonary resuscitation (CPR), including endotracheal intubation (inserting a breathing tube into the patient's windpipe) and advanced cardiac life support (including such procedures as insertion of a temporary pacemaker into the heart or draining fluid from the pericardial sac with a large needle). Thus, the code team usually consists of at least one medical doctor (e.g., an internist), an anesthesiologist, and a nurse who, on-call in the hospital 24/7, drop everything they are doing and run to the "code" when it is announced on the hospital's overhead public address system (and on special pagers carried by each member of the code team). In hospitals with large, well-staffed emergency departments like New York Presbyterian, codes that occur in the ED may be handled primarily by ED staff, but even then, the hospital's code team typically responds to offer assistance. Strong scientific evidence supports the deployment and cost of code teams in hospital. Although cardiac arrests that occur outside the hospital have a very poor prognosis, as many as 40 percent of patients who suffer in-hospital cardiac arrests may survive, at least temporarily, thanks to the quick response and expertise of hospitals' code teams. See also Chapter 8.

68 *twice the rate of U.S. population growth, despite the fact:* See Tang and colleagues, *Journal of the American Medical Association* 2010;304;664.

68 *more than 3 out of 4 walk in:* See National Hospital Ambulatory Medical Care Survey: 2008 Emergency Department Summary Tables.

68 *reported a sixfold increase:* See Shortliffe and colleagues, *New England Journal of Medicine* 1958;258:20.

69 *EDs today account for 11 percent of all:* See Kellerman and Martinez, *New England Journal of Medicine* 2011;364:24; Pitts and colleagues, *Health Affairs* (Millwood, 2010;29:1620.

69 *One of every six patients today is uninsured:* See National Hospital Ambulatory Medical Care Survey: 2008 Emergency Department Summary Tables.

70 *there are 25 percent fewer hospital beds:* See Baker and colleagues, *National Institute for Health Care Management Research Brief,* November 2008; U.S. Census Bureau, Statistical Abstract of the United States: 2011.

70 *In New York State, for example, only two-thirds:* See Statewide (New York State) Planning and Research Cooperative System (SPARCS) database 2006 report, Table 6.

71 *as many as 70 percent of all patients discharged:* See Wong and colleagues, *Annals of Pharmacotherapy* 2008;42:1373.

71 *can result in patients' being* readmitted *to the hospital unnecessarily:* About one of every five Medicare patients discharged from the hospital "bounces back" into the hospital within the ensuing thirty days. Many of these readmissions are "necessary" but some are not.

71 *simply refuse to leave:* This is a difficult problem that requires careful attention. (See, for example, Moran and colleagues, *The Primary Care Companion to the Journal of Clinical Psychiatry* 2010; Vol. 12, No. 6.) In New York State, patients who refuse discharge are permitted a twenty-four-hour extension of their hospital stay for review of their case by their physicians and social workers.

72 *A CT scan of his chest was negative:* In Mr. Tosca's case, performance of this imaging test of the lungs made good clinical sense. However, the use of diagnostic radiology services—and their attendant radiation risks—has increased dramatically over the past fifteen years (see Smith-Bindman and colleagues, *Journal of the American Medical Association* 2012;307:2400). Remarkably, there are few data that quantify the actual benefits and harms to patients of this increased use of radiological technology. See Smith-Bindman, *New England Journal of Medicine* 2010; 363:1 and *Archives of Internal Medicine* 2009;169:2078. This is an especially important issue as these diagnostic technologies are used ever more frequently, even among patients whose probability of disease is very low (see, for example, Litt and colleagues, *New England Journal of Medicine* 2012;366:1393; Prevedello and colleagues, *American Journal of Medicine* 2012;125:356; Adams and colleagues, *American Journal of Medicine* 2013;126:36).

72 *a repeat electrocardiogram and two sets of troponins:* Elevated blood levels of a protein called troponin are found in virtually every patient with acute myocardial infarction when the blood tests are performed within eight to twelve hours after the onset of symptoms. In many cases, elevated troponin levels appear in the blood even before eight to twelve hours have elapsed. For this reason, standard procedure in all emergency departments for patients with a possible heart attack calls for these blood tests every four hours up to twelve hours after the patient's arrival. (This is why such patients typically spend at least twelve hours in the ED, awaiting the results of a full sequence of troponin tests.) Interpreting troponin tests, however, is not always easy. Some patients who are not having a heart attack will have abnormal troponin tests. Conversely, some patients whose troponin tests are normal are still in great danger because they are on the brink of having a heart attack that hasn't happened yet. See also Chapter 6 regarding "false-positive" and "false-negative" diagnostic tests.

72 *a diagnosis of acute coronary syndrome:* This term refers to a spectrum of clinical presentations that indicate the possibility of an impending acute myocardial infarction.

73 *whether he'll need a cath:* This term is shorthand for "cardiac catheterization," the procedure whereby a cardiologist inserts a catheter into the patient's heart and injects dye into the coronary arteries (coronary angiography). This allows the cardiologist to visualize with X-rays any blockage or narrowing in the coronary arteries that may require treatment. Coronary angiography, the "gold standard" test to diagnose coronary artery disease, is not performed in *every* patient with *possible* coronary disease because, rarely, the test itself can cause serious complications, including stroke (or even myocardial infarction, the outcome it is intended to treat or prevent). Often, then, when the diagnosis is in doubt, other "noninvasive" (essentially risk-free) tests are done first. When these tests, generically called "stress tests," are normal, the need for cardiac catheterization can usually (but not always) be avoided.

73 *It is my heart, yes?:* See also note, p. 38.

74 *This practice is countercultural:* See also Reilly, *Lancet* 2007; 370:705.

75 *No dynamic ECG changes:* This refers to changes in the patient's electrocardiogram at different points in time, for example, when the patient is experiencing chest pain and after the pain has subsided. See also note, p. 89.

77 *What doesn't make sense is what we think:* This is an example of reflection-in-action, the process whereby one's own thinking undergoes intense scrutiny in real time, sometimes resulting in a changed decision. (See Schon, *The Reflective Practitioner: How Professionals Think in Action* [New York: Basic Books, 1983] and note, p. 47). This in-the-moment "meta-cognition" is essential to the expert practice (and teaching) of all professions, including medicine. Some critics argue that sharing this process with the client can undermine the professional-client relationship by exposing the uncertainty and fallibility inherent to all professional decision-making. In my view, to the contrary, involving the patient in this process is likely to improve patient satisfaction, because, whatever the outcome of the decision, the patient will have participated in its determination. See also Barry and Edgman-Levitan, *New England Journal of Medicine* 2012;366:780; Kon, *Journal of the American Medical Association* 2010;304:903; Quill and Holloway, *New England Journal of Medicine* 2012;366:1653; Bardes, *New England Journal of Medicine* 2012;366:782.

77 *Heart pains typically happen during physical exertion:* This does not mean that symptoms of coronary artery disease occur *only* during physical exertion. When partial blockages in coronary arteries impede blood flow to heart muscle, any situation resulting in an increased rate or force of heart muscle activity may cause symptoms. (For example, severe emotional stress can precipitate these symptoms in the absence of any physical activity.) In addition, patients with very severe coronary disease may develop symptoms at rest when the blockages in their arteries (and their exertional symptoms) have progressed to the point where little or no provocation is needed. Rarely, spasm of a coronary artery may cause symptoms at rest even when there are no fixed blockages in the artery (see also subsequent notes, pp. 78 and 94).

78 *I was worried that he'd ruptured a plaque:* A "plaque" is a cholesterol deposit in the wall of an artery. When the artery in question is a coronary (heart) artery, such plaques represent coronary artery disease, the usual underlying cause of acute myocardial infarction ("heart attack"). Not long ago, it was widely assumed that most heart attacks occur when coronary arteries become blocked as the end result of a gradual and progressive narrowing of the artery by such plaques. In fact, it is now known that these plaques can "rupture" unpredictably and cause sudden blockage of a coronary artery even in patients who have not had previous progressive narrowing of the artery. This explains why some patients develop an acute (sometimes fatal) heart attack with no prior warning symptoms. Theoretically, this disease mechanism could explain Mr. Tosca's symptoms, hence Tina's concern.

78 *very low risk:* Here, Tina is quoting evidence from the best study to date on this subject: Goldman and colleagues, *New England Journal of Medicine* 1996;334:1498. This is the same research that interested Malcolm Gladwell in *Blink* (see also note, p. 14).

79 *reduced mortality from coronary heart disease by more than half:* See, for example, Meyer, *Journal Watch Cardiology* 2012 (February 29); Bandosz and colleagues, *British Medical Journal* 2012;344:d8136; Hunink and colleagues, *Journal of the American Medical Association* 1997;277:535.

80 *between 1 and 4 percent of all patients:* See, for example, Pope and colleagues, *New England Journal of Medicine* 2000;342:1163; McCarthy and colleagues, *Annals of Emergency Medicine* 1993;22:579; Goldman and Kirtane, *Annals of Internal Medicine* 2003;139:987.

80 *single most costly cause:* See, for example, Rusnak and colleagues, *Annals of Emergency Medicine* 1989;18:1029.

81 *consider a 1-in-200 chance so remote that it's not even worth their thinking about:* This kind of thinking is not restricted to medical decisions. For example, authoritative ("power-law") decision-making models suggest that there is about a 1-in-200 chance that a terrorist attack will kill one million people or more in a NATO country at some time in the next decade (see Silver, *The Signal and the Noise* [New York: Penguin Press, 2012]). Despite this risk, there has been no mass exodus from NATO countries.

82 *Many of us do this in an irrational way:* For example, the difference between probabilities of 0 percent and 1 percent is the same as the difference between probabilities of 50 percent and 51 percent; by simple arithmetic, the difference in both cases is 1 percent. But for many people

these differences don't feel the same at all. For them, the difference between a probability of 0 percent (absolute certainty) and a probability of 1 percent (very slight uncertainty) feels much bigger than it really is. See Kahneman and Tversky, *Econometrica* 1979;47,2:263; Tversky and Kahneman, *Journal of Risk and Uncertainty* 1992;5:297.

82 *when emotion complicates the calculus:* See Kahneman, *Thinking, Fast and Slow* (New York: Farrar Strauss and Giroux, 2011).

82 *words like tachyarrythmia, hypertrophic cardiomyopathy, or pheochromocytoma:* Each of these conditions can cause symptoms like Mr. Tosca's. *Tachyarrythmias* are pathologically rapid heart rhythms—there are many different types—that may occur with or without underlying heart disease. *Hypertrophic cardiomyopathy* is a disorder of heart muscle that can cause symptoms similar to coronary artery disease even when the coronary arteries themselves are normal. *Pheochromocytoma* is a rare tumor of the adrenal gland that can cause unpredictable episodes similar to Mr. Tosca's.

82 *we talk about cocaine:* Illicit use of cocaine is a well-known cause of chest pain and palpitations—cocaine causes spasm of the coronary arteries—whether the user has underlying heart disease or not. For this reason, patients in many EDs are tested for cocaine use when they present with these symptoms.

83 *Our job is to* know, *isn't it?:* How we know what we know and whether we ever know anything with certainty are questions for philosophers and cognitive neuroscientists, not medical doctors. Nevertheless, an important phenomenon in modern medicine is doctors' overconfidence in their own knowledge and judgment (see, for example, Friedman and colleagues, *Journal of General Internal Medicine* 2005;20:334; Johnson and Fowler, *Nature* 2011;477:317; Croskerry and Norman, *American Journal of Medicine* 2008;121[5A]:S24). *Certainty* in medical diagnosis is actually the exception, not the rule, because most patients never undergo a "gold standard" diagnostic test, i.e., a test that is considered *definitive proof* of the disease or disorder in question. Why not? Because most such tests are "invasive" tests—they require invasion of the patient's body with cameras, biopsies, catheters, or surgical procedures—which, in general, are more cumbersome, more expensive, and potentially more harmful than less invasive (but less definitive) tests such as blood analyses or CT scans. See also Chapter 6 about diagnostic testing.

84 *to see if they show any signs of cardiac ischemia:* The electrocardiogram (ECG), invented about one hundred years ago, records on a strip of paper the waveforms created by the electrical activity of the heart. These waveforms depict the timing and circuitry of electrical currents as they spread through the heart, and their various components, named P, Q, R, S, and T waves. Distortions in these waveforms, e.g., abnormal Q waves or deviations of T waves, indicate abnormalities of the structure and function of the heart. Even today, the ECG is the single most important predictor of the patient's diagnosis and prognosis when a heart attack is suspected.

85 *the single most common cause of palpitations:* The best prospective study to date about the causes of palpitations found that various cardiac disorders were responsible in 43 percent of patients, various psychiatric disorders in 31 percent, and miscellaneous causes such as drugs or thyroid

problems in 10 percent; in the remaining 16 percent, the cause could not be determined. (See Weber and Kapoor, *American Journal of Medicine* 1996;100:138.) However, panic disorders (with or without other coexisting psychiatric disorders) were the single most common cause, accounting for 27 percent of all study patients.

86 *No physical cause can be found to explain patients' physical symptoms:* See Barsky and Borus, *Journal of the American Medical Association* 1995;274:1981; Kroenke and colleagues, *Archives of Internal Medicine* 1990;150:1685.

86 *Medical students, for example:* My own "medical student disease" was amyotrophic lateral sclerosis (sometimes known as Lou Gehrig's disease), a devastating neurological disorder characterized by muscle fasciculations—visible twitches in calf or biceps or eyelid muscles, which I, like millions of other healthy people, sometimes experience.

87 *How the brain achieves these mysterious "disconnections":* Although we don't understand the biology of these disorders, Barsky and Borus have described eloquently their phenomenology: "Distressing symptoms are omnipresent in daily life. They result from benign dysfunctions and self-limited ailments. . . . Under the influence of medical scrutiny . . . a process of symptom amplification that alters the perception of these endemic symptoms can be set in motion. . . . A self validating and self-perpetuating cycle of symptom amplification and disease conviction ensues: The suspicion of disease heightens bodily awareness, symptom perception, and distress, and these, in turn, reinforce the belief that the sufferer is sick." See Barsky and Borus, *Annals of Internal Medicine* 1999;130:910; Barsky, *New England Journal of Medicine* 1988;318:414.

87 *panic attacks, defined as:* See *DSM-IV* (2000), American Psychiatric Association.

88 *Patients with panic attacks, for example:* See Barsky and colleagues, *Psychosomatics* 1999;40:50; Barsky and colleagues, *Archives of Internal Medicine* 1995;155:1782; Barsky and colleagues, *Archives of General Psychiatry* 2005;62:903.

88 *the more hypochondriacal (and angry) they become:* Hypochondriasis and panic disorder are considered two different "psychosomatic" syndromes, but they overlap in about 25 percent of patients (see Barsky and colleagues, *Archives of General Psychiatry* 1994;51:918).

88 *the "hidden reasons" that patients visit medical doctors:* See Barsky, *Annals of Internal Medicine* 1981;94:492.

89 *The doctor has recognized some clue:* Malcolm Gladwell's *Blink* (New York: Little Brown, 2005) provides interesting insights about these subconscious processes, but academic psychologists like Daniel Kahneman tend to believe that these processes are not "mysterious" at all (see Kahneman, *Thinking, Fast and Slow* [New York: Farrar Straus and Giroux, 2011]). See also Goldman, *The Yale Journal of Biology and Medicine* 1990;63:47; Polanyi, *The Tacit Dimension* (University of Chicago, 1966); D'Amasio, *Descartes' Error* (New York: G.P. Putnam, 1994); D'Amasio, *The Feeling of What Happens* (Boston: Houghton Mifflin Harcourt, 1999); D'Amasio, *Looking for Spinoza* (Boston: Houghton Mifflin Harcourt, 2003).

90 *I don't tell them about Fred and Martha:* See Chapters 5 through 7.

91 *pretty gutsy to send him home:* Diabetes, now a national (indeed global) epidemic, greatly increases the risk of vascular disease (such as heart attack and stroke) in addition to causing "diabetic complications" such as blindness and kidney failure. This is the reason Mr. Tosca's diabetes is so pertinent to his presentation in the ED with symptoms of a possible heart attack: The risk of heart attack increases two- to sevenfold in diabetics compared to nondiabetics.

Chapter 4: What's the Plan?

94 *the reason for his groin pain:* Pain in the hip joint typically is localized to the groin (the frontal crease between the genitals and the upper thigh).

94 *which means we can't cure the cancer:* At the time of this writing, bladder cancer that has metastasized to bone is incurable (except in extraordinarily rare cases).

94 *the "minor" kind that means he is on the brink:* Heart attacks (myocardial infarctions) are never "minor" but some cause less permanent heart damage than others. In general, however, "minor" heart attacks often augur "major" ones; for this reason, heart attack patients receive the same careful evaluation, regardless of whether the initial test results suggest major or minor heart damage.

95 *the hospital's social workers perk up:* This does not mean that the social workers wanted Mr. Mukaj to receive anything less than the best care. But uninsured patients create enormous financial burdens for hospitals, and the social workers (who are employed by the hospital) do all they can to help the hospital as well as the patient. Theirs is a very challenging, underappreciated role in U.S. medicine today.

95 *nor any of the doctors here will be reimbursed:* Hospitals in New York State (and other states) receive some reimbursement for "charitable" care of uninsured patients. (Physicians do not.) Medicaid provides the lion's share of these hospital reimbursements through its Disproportionate Share Hospital (DSH) Payments program, which gives financial assistance to hospitals that serve a large number of low-income patients. In 2009, for example, New York State received $1.6 billion from the federal Medicaid program for distribution to hospitals that met criteria for DSH payments (see *National Health Policy Forum*; June 15, 2009; George Washington University). Because these federal payments flow through state governments, state politics and budget problems may have a substantial impact on hospitals' reimbursement (see, for example, Hartocollis, *New York Times*, February 22, 2010).

99 *a feeding tube inserted into her stomach:* This can be done on a temporary basis by inserting the tube through the patient's nose down into the stomach, or, more permanently, by inserting the tube through a small incision in the patient's abdomen directly into the stomach.

100 *90 percent of Hodgkin's patients are cured:* There is still some debate about the best way to cure patients with Hodgkin's Disease, largely due to controversy about the *harms* of curative chemotherapy (see Connors, *New England Journal of Medicine* 2011;365:264).

High-dose chemotherapy for patients with advanced disease has an impressive cure rate but at a cost: a 3 percent rate of treatment-related death, a 2 to 3 percent rate of secondary leukemia, infertility in men and premature menopause in women, and high rates of hospitalization. Less toxic chemotherapy followed by bone marrow transplant is a common alternative today.

101 *it's the "permanent" kind of catheter:* Central vein catheters can be inserted and removed easily when intended for short-term use in hospital. However, patients with cancer (and some other diseases) often require these catheters for longer periods of time (months) and for use in both inpatient and outpatient settings. In these cases, more durable devices are inserted into the vein, typically by means of a minor surgical procedure. A similar procedure is needed to remove the catheter.

102 *what I knew about rebuttals to Pascal:* See Connor, *Pascal's Wager: The Man Who Played Dice with God* (New York: HarperCollins, 2006). Ironically, doctors sometimes adopt Pascal's wager to "hang crepe," exaggerating the patient's probability of dying in order to create a "no-lose" situation—for the doctor! (See Siegler, *New England Journal of Medicine* 1975; 293:853.)

103 *try to open his coronary arteries:* In general, cardiologists treat coronary artery disease by dilating narrowed arteries with a catheter-guided balloon (a procedure called angioplasty) and then "stenting" the dilated artery with a wire mesh device that maintains patency of (and blood flow through) the artery. Thus are coronary arteries "opened."

103 *surgically remove his entire bladder:* Removal of the urinary bladder requires rerouting the two ureters (ducts that carry urine from the kidneys to the bladder) either to external drainage bags or to a surgically reconstructed "new bladder," typically fashioned from a piece of the patient's intestine.

103 *suffered from postherpetic neuralgia:* A minority of patients who develop shingles (herpes zoster), a reactivation of the chicken pox (varicella zoster) virus, are afflicted subsequently by chronic nerve pain in the area of the body affected by the shingles skin rash (which, unlike the pain, disappears). In some patients, including my father, the shingles develops at the site of a recent surgical incision. Ironically, in my father's case, the surgical incision that preceded his shingles was unnecessary, the result of a "false-positive" PET scan that incorrectly led to an (unnecessary) operation for suspected lung cancer. (See also Chapter 6 about the pitfalls of diagnostic testing.) In many patients with a history of chicken pox, shingles (and postherpetic neuralgia) can be prevented by the new varicella zoster vaccine. My father did not receive the vaccine; I wish he had.

105 *a not-so-closely-guarded secret: Some fates are worse than death:* Among adults, this issue seems most relevant to patients with chronic severe pain, dementia, coma (see Patrick and colleagues, *Medical Decision Making* 1994;14:9) or major strokes (see Kelly and Holloway, *Neurology* 2010;75:682), but see also Pearlman and colleagues, *Journal of Clinical Ethics* 1993;4:33. One difficulty in understanding this issue is that healthy individuals typically "rate" disabled health states (like stroke) lower than patients who actually suffer from the disability in question. This systematic bias is important because the issue here is patients' perceptions of future health states when making informed decisions about their own future care. In one study of

patients *at risk for* future stroke, 45 percent reported feeling that a stroke that produced major functional impairment (in ambulation, speech, etc.) would be a fate worse than death (see Samsa and colleagues, *American Heart Journal* 1998;136:703). This does not mean that these patients would rate their disability as worse than death if they actually suffered a major stroke.

105 *"Do everything" really means:* See Quill and colleagues, *Annals of Internal Medicine* 2009;151:345.

105 *about three of every four such patients focus on quality:* See Quill and colleagues, *Journal of Palliative Care* 2006;9:382.

106 *for some of us, remaining physically active:* Ibid.

106 *many of us change our minds:* See, for example, Fried and colleagues, *Archives of Internal Medicine* 2006;166:890 and *Journal of the American Geriatrics Society* 2007;55:1007; Ubel and colleagues, *Health Psychology* 2005;24:557.

107 *Patients who want everything:* See Quill and colleagues, *Annals of Internal Medicine* 2009;151:345, Quill and Holloway, *Journal of the American Medical Association* 2011;306:1483.

109 *"leaves of absence":* Strictly speaking, leaves of absence from acute care (nonpsychiatric) hospitals can be arranged in extraordinary situations but are rarely done today.

112 *Papers to sign and witness:* Because cardiopulmonary resuscitation (CPR) is the de facto "default" option for all patients in U.S. hospitals, documentation is required for patients (or their surrogate) to "opt out" and consent to a do-not-resuscitate (DNR) order. The attending physician and a second party (witness) must sign papers that document the patient's wishes to forgo resuscitation (and/or other life support measures) and place them in the patient's hospital chart. This longstanding practice of performing resuscitation measures unless explicitly refused, even in imminently dying patients, deserves careful reconsideration (see, for example, Blinderman and colleagues, *Journal of the American Medical Association* 2012;307:917). See also Chapter 8.

113 *Median survival statistics?:* See Chapter 8 and Stephen Jay Gould's experience.

113 *clinical prognostication is far from an exact science:* Nicholas Christakis has discussed this issue brilliantly in *Death Foretold: Prophecy and Prognosis in Medical Care* (University of Chicago, 1999). Christakis and Elizabeth Lamont have studied this problem in greatest detail in patients with cancer (see Lamont and Christakis, *Journal of the American Medical Association* 2003;290:98 and *Annals of Internal Medicine* 2001;134:1096; Christakis and Lamont, *British Medical Journal* 2000;320:469). Cancer patients who overestimate their survival chances—with or without doctors' help—often suffer as a result. (See Weeks and colleagues, *Journal of the American Medical Association* 1998;279:1709; Smith and Swisher, *Journal of the American Medical Association* 1998;279:1746.)

113 *This surrogate responsibility is a big deal:* In general, surrogates base their decisions on three different standards, in order of preference: 1) the patient's known wishes; 2) "substituted

judgment" (what the surrogate thinks the patient would want); and 3) "best interests" (what the surrogate believes is in the patient's best interest). Each of these standards can be problematic to apply and all of them underestimate the complexity of this process (see Berger and colleagues, *Annals of Internal Medicine* 2008;149:48). Nevertheless, decision-making for patients who lack surrogates is even more problematic (see, for example, White and colleagues, *Annals of Internal Medicine* 2007;147:34).

113 *After the patient's death, surrogate decision-makers often feel guilty, regretful, depressed:* In one systematic review of this subject, at least one-third of surrogates experienced a "negative emotional burden" as a result of making end-of-life treatment decisions for others. These negative effects were often substantial and long-lasting (see Wendler and Rid, *Annals of Internal Medicine* 2011;154:336).

114 *the Federal Patient Self-Determination Act:* See Greco and colleagues, *Archives of Internal Medicine* 1991;115:639.

114 *The law's purpose is* not *to save money:* See Lewinsky (*New England Journal of Medicine* 1996;335:741), who argues eloquently that advance care planning "should not become a subtle or subconscious mechanism whereby physicians shift their role from that of caregivers to that of propagandists for limited medical treatment." That said, advance directives do tend to reduce aggressive care (and medical costs) at the end of life, increase hospice care, and improve quality of life for terminally ill patients and their caregivers (see, for example, Wright and colleagues, *Journal of the American Medical Association* 2008;300:1665; Deterling and colleagues, *British Medical Journal* 2010;340:1345; Nicholas and colleagues, *Journal of the American Medical Association* 2011;306:1447).

115 *Most Americans haven't done them either:* Completion rates for advance directives or health care proxy designations vary in different settings and patient populations but no more than one-quarter of people in the United States have done either (see Lo and Steinbrook, *Archives of Internal Medicine* 2004;164:1501; Perkins, *Annals of Internal Medicine* 2007;147:51; Gillick, *New England Journal of Medicine* 2010;362:1239). Remarkably, outpatients with metastatic cancer (see Temel, *Journal of General Internal Medicine* 2009;25:150) and seriously ill inpatients cared for by hospitalists (see Anderson and colleagues, *Journal of General Internal Medicine* 2009;26:359) seem to discuss and document these issues no more frequently than others. Some experts believe that U.S. society may be "retreating" from advance care planning, an ominous trend. (See Tinetti, *Journal of the American Medical Association* 2012;307:915.)

115 more than two-thirds *had become incapacitated:* See Silveira and colleagues, *New England Journal of Medicine* 2010;362:1211. Surprisingly, among those patients who needed to have a decision made, *most had completed* an advance directive, far more than expected (see preceding note). This encouraging recent finding has raised hopes that the Physicians Orders for Life Sustaining Treatment (POLST) program (see Hickman and colleagues, *Hastings Center Report* 2005;35:Spec No:S26) will gain wider public support. Notably, its success "depends on the strength of the underlying patient-doctor communication and on the establishment of a statewide system for communicating and honoring those orders" (see Gillick, *New England Journal of Medicine* 2010;362:1239).

115 *at or above the twelfth-grade reading level:* See Institute of Medicine, *Health Literacy: A Prescription to End Confusion* (National Academy Press, 2004). The mean reading level of U.S. adults today is eighth grade; among the elderly, the mean is fifth grade.

115 *Each state has a different law:* See Castillo and colleagues, *Annals of Internal Medicine* 2011;154:121, for an excellent summary of the "unintended consequences of advance directive law on clinical care."

116 *Verbal directives, even from duly appointed surrogates:* In some states, innovative programs have begun to address this issue (see Feder and colleagues, *Annals of Internal Medicine* 2006;144:634).

116 *simply don't know what the patient would want:* See, for example, Shalowitz and colleagues, *Archives of Internal Medicine* 2006;166:493 for a review of the "accuracy" of surrogate decision-makers.

116 *doctors don't always honor advance directives:* See Hardin and Yusufaly, *Archives of Internal Medicine* 2004:164:1531.

116 *some impressive local successes in their use:* See for example, Silveira and colleagues, *New England Journal of Medicine* 2010;362:1211 (see note, p. 115).

116 *this new approach focuses on preparing the patient's chosen surrogate:* See Sudore and Fried, *Annals of Internal Medicine* 2010;153:256; White and Arnold, *Journal of the American Medical Association* 2011;306:1485. This new approach involves: 1) choosing an appropriate surrogate; 2) clarifying and articulating the patient's values over time; and 3) establishing leeway in surrogate decision-making.

117 *these same insurers refuse to reimburse doctors for spending time:* This is an evolving issue. Health care reform in the United States, instigated by President Obama's Affordable Care Act, may reverse the current status quo.

118 *to involve the hospital's Ethics Committee:* All U.S. hospitals are required by accreditation agencies to empower a formal mechanism for adjudication of ethical issues that may arise in the care of hospitalized patients. Extraordinarily helpful in some cases, these mechanisms vary widely from hospital to hospital in their timeliness, quality, and effectiveness. No panacea, hospital Ethics Committees have both positive and negative attributes. See Lo, *Resolving Ethical Dilemmas: A Guide for Clinicians* (Philadelphia: Lippincott, Williams and Wilkins, 2009 [2nd ed.]).

121 *Despite her visible grief:* There has been much controversy recently about how to "classify" grief, especially its relationship to clinical depression (and its need for medical treatment). There is much overlap between these conditions—and they frequently coexist—but, as Friedman has concluded, "grief resolves naturally on its own. . . . The medical profession should normalize, not medicalize, grief" (see Friedman, *New England Journal of Medicine* 2012;366:1855). That said, grief is neither simple nor fleeting. (See Rousseau, *Archives of Internal Medicine* 2012;172:360.)

121 *first personal experience with being sued for medical malpractice:* Much has been written about the perverse incentives and deleterious effects of malpractice litigation on U.S. medical care and physicians in all specialties (see Jena and colleagues, *New England Journal of Medicine* 2011;365:629). "Defensive medicine" certainly is a real phenomenon, but its cost, causes, and solutions remain highly controversial. One compelling, if contrarian, view can be found in Tom Baker's *The Medical Malpractice Myth* (University of Chicago, 2005). See also Atul Gawande's "The Malpractice Mess" (*The New Yorker*, November 14, 2005).

122 *what initially looked like septic shock turned out to be:* When first evaluated, patients with severe dehydration may have low blood pressure, impaired mental status, and signs of kidney dysfunction easily mistaken for septic shock, a much more serious problem.

122 *lifelong sickle cell disease is no picnic:* Sickle cell anemia is a genetic disorder that predominantly affects patients of African and Mediterranean descent. In many patients it is a devastating, debilitating disease punctuated by frequent, sometimes life-threatening complications. Bone and joint disorders are especially common, including infections and avascular necrosis (bone destruction caused by inadequate blood supply).

123 *but there's nothing I can do about it:* This is one of many reasons why a universal electronic medical record—whereby a patient's medical information can be made accessible to health care providers in any location—is so important. Without easy access to patients' medical records, doctors at one site often repeat unnecessarily tests and procedures already performed at other sites. Unfortunately, patients who "game" the system—most prominently, patients with substance abuse disorders—capitalize on this information gap to get what they want. There is no way, for example, to "alert" all emergency departments in New York City to "get wise" to Ms. Tate and other drug-seeking patients.

123 *Marfan syndrome, a plastic aorta and:* Marfan syndrome is a heritable disorder of connective tissue that predisposes patients to many disabling and life-threatening complications, most notably "dissection" of the aorta and serious joint abnormalities.

124 *make sure his morphine pump was doing its job:* Morphine "PCA" pumps—PCA refers to "patient-controlled analgesia"—are devices attached to intravenous infusions that can be programmed to deliver designated amounts of morphine (or other analgesics) to the patient with the simple push of a button. This allows the patient to control when and how much morphine is delivered (within limits programmed into the device) without the need for frequent nursing visits and injections. The issue here is not whether the pump itself is working, but rather whether the doses of morphine programmed into the device are meeting the patient's needs.

126 *False negative, Chris shrugs:* See also Chapter 6 about "false-negative" and "false-positive" diagnostic tests. A savvy senior resident like Chris has learned that false-negative test results are hurdles all doctors face.

127 *This "fee-for-service" reimbursement system:* See, for example, Wilensky, *New England Journal of Medicine* 2009;360:653. However, this is a complex issue; it is not at all clear whether there is a better way (see, for example, Vladeck, *New England Journal of Medicine* 2010;362:1955; Atul Gawande, "Piecework," [*The New Yorker*, April 4, 2005]). What does seem clear is that the

high *price* of medical services in the United States is the principal reason national health care costs are higher in the United States than in other countries (see Anderson and colleagues, *Health Affairs* 2003;22:89).

128 *The other half pays for medical malpractice premiums:* Operational expenses for outpatient medical practices have grown enormously during the past few decades, largely due to the need for more office personnel to perform nonclinical work: scheduling, billing, pre-certification, dispute resolution with insurers, compliance with payer-dictated "quality assurance" requirements. It is not uncommon for a solo physician practitioner to employ a half-dozen or more office staff. In general, practice expenses consume between 40 percent and 60 percent of all revenues collected for the clinical care provided in most outpatient practices. Thus, these "administrative" expenses represent a significant financial burden for the U.S. health care system (see Woolhandler and colleagues, *New England Journal of Medicine* 2003;349:768).

128 *radiologists, ophthalmologists, or dermatologists:* Among medical educators, this widespread phenomenon has achieved its own popular acronym, typically invoked with what-can-I-say resignation. Many medical students today, especially those with the largest educational debts, are said to be heading down the "ROAD," i.e., toward lucrative (and lifestyle-friendly) careers in radiology, ophthalmology, anesthesiology or dermatology.

128 *whose health care systems perform better:* See note, p. 41, and Starfield, *Journal of the American Medical Association* 2000;284:483. Editors of a recent report from the Institute of Medicine have summarized the problem thus: "The United States spends more on health care than does any other country, but its health outcomes are generally worse than those of other wealthy nations. . . . U.S. males and females in almost all age groups— up to age 75— have shorter life expectancies than their counterparts in 16 other wealthy, developed nations. . . . The scope of the U.S. health disadvantage is pervasive and involves more than life expectancy: the United States ranks at or near the bottom in both prevalence and mortality for multiple diseases, risk factors, and injuries. . . . Now the question is what U.S. society is prepared to do about it." (See Woolf and Aron, *Journal of the American Medical Association* 2013;309:771.)

Chapter 5: An End

138 *she has no hemiparesis or headache or anything else:* Patients who suffer a stroke causing unilateral facial weakness often (but not always) also have unilateral weakness of their arm and leg (hemiparesis). The "pattern" of weakness and other signs depends on which part of the brain is damaged by the stroke.

138 *make sure she wouldn't need more Benadryl:* Benadryl (trade name for diphenhydramine) is an antihistamine typically used to treat allergies. But Babs's problem was not an "allergy" to Compazine, the antinausea drug she had taken earlier in the day, but a "dystonic" effect, which Benadryl can also counteract.

140 *their new blood test for HIV:* The first HIV blood test became available for clinical use in the spring of 1985.

140 *Back then, HIV was rare in small-town America:* Abraham Verghese's fine book about this phenomenon (*My Own Country: A Doctor's Story* [Vintage, 1995]) depicted the "arrival" of AIDS in rural communities in 1985.

145 *helping old folks die at home wasn't part of the medical curriculum:* Unfortunately, this essential skill set for physicians isn't part of the curriculum in most medical schools today either.

148 *Is grief a disease?:* See note, p. 121.

148 *"The Boundaries of Medicine":* See Seldin, *Transactions of the American Association of Physicians* 1981;94:75. For a different view, see Perkoff, *Journal of Chronic Diseases* 1985;383:271; Haggarty, *Pharos* 1972;35:106.

149 *not to make people happy. Medicine's task:* Seldin's argument, in part, was a response to the World Health Organization's definition of health as "a state of complete physical, mental and social well-being and not merely the absence of disease or infirmity." See *World Health Organization: Basic Documents*, 26th ed. (Geneva: World Health Organization, 1976).

149 *George Engel, a legendary professor:* See Engel, *Science* 1977;196:129.

150 *what matters to patients is how they feel, the impact of their "ill-ness":* See also Eric Cassell, *The Nature of Suffering and the Goals of Medicine*, 2nd ed. (Oxford, 2004).

151 *a few brief periods in the 1970s:* Ensuring adequate numbers of primary care physicians in the United States has been a roller-coaster ride for decades, brief surges in interest followed by prolonged periods of disillusionment and decline. Whether primary care will survive in its traditional form is unknown. (See, for example, Bodenheimer, *New England Journal of Medicine* 2006;355:861; Sandy and Schroeder, *Annals of Internal Medicine* 2003;138:262.) Some doctors of my generation still consider primary care "the best job in medicine" (see Woo, *New England Journal of Medicine* 2006;355:864). Others wonder how it can be resurrected as a sustainable foundation of U.S. medical care in the twenty-first century (see Showstack and colleagues, *Annals of Internal Medicine* 2003;138:268).

151 *recently the college trustees had recognized the female sex:* Dartmouth's trustees voted to matriculate women undergraduates in 1972. My own clinical experiences with this change began in 1977. Decades later, many women students at Dartmouth in those early days of coeducation recalled a wonderful undergraduate experience (see Rosenbaum, *New York Times*, October 9, 2009), but others saw it differently (see Merton, *Esquire*, June 19, 1979).

152 *female analogs of Dartmouth men:* Dartmouth's student body has become much more diverse, both ethnically and socioeconomically, in the years since the events described here.

154 *when quantum mechanics and Thomas Kuhn:* Kuhn's *The Structure of Scientific Revolutions* upended many prevailing dogmas about the "certainties" of scientific discovery and progress.

158 *a phrase in my textbook's Introduction:* See Reilly, *Practical Strategies in Outpatient Medicine*, 1st ed. (Philadelphia: W.B. Saunders, 1984).

160 *one of the largest multispecialty practices in the United States:* At the time, there were relatively few such groups in the United States—at Mayo in Minnesota and Kaiser Permanente in California, for example. Today, there are many more, but Dartmouth's remains one of the largest.

161 *"small area analysis," a term he had invented:* Wennberg's original work in this field was done in collaboration with Dr. Alan Gitelson of Johns Hopkins University (see Wennberg and Gitelson, *Science* 1973;182:1102).

162 *trained in sociology as well as medicine:* See Wennberg, *Tracking Medicine: A Researcher's Quest to Understand Health Care* (Oxford: 2010)

162 *differences in physicians' use of hospital services in Boston versus New Haven:* See Wennberg and colleagues, *Lancet* 1987;1:1185.

162 *"Medical Commons: Who Is Responsible?":* See Hiatt, *New England Journal of Medicine* 1975;293:235. The inspiration for Hiatt's seminal article was an article written five years earlier by Garrett Hardin, a biologist, entitled "The Tragedy of the Commons" (see Hardin, *Science* 1968;162:1243).

164 *these novelties included computed tomography:* See Griner, *Annals of Internal Medicine* 1972;77:501.

164 *"prehospital rescue units":* See Liberthson and colleagues, *New England Journal of Medicine* 1974;291:317.

164 *health care spending had grown more than 2,000 percent:* These figures (see www.usgovernmentspending.com: *Government Spending Chart in United States 1960–2010*) are not adjusted for inflation. (Neither is the growth in population.)

164 *more intensive care units than hospitals:* See, for example, Zilberberg, *Seminars in Respiratory and Critical Care Medicine* 2010;31:13.

164 *CT scans will cause fifteen thousand:* See Brenner and Hall, *New England Journal of Medicine* 2007;357:2277. See also Brenner, *Radiation Research* 2010;174:809.

165 *who is tracking their effectiveness and cost?:* Currently, Medicare reimbursement for out-of-hospital emergency care is tied to subsequent transport to an emergency department. This policy, which is not always in the patient's (or health care system's) best interest, deserves reappraisal. (See, for example, Munjal and Carr, *Journal of the American Medical Association* 2013;309:667.) See also Chapter 8 regarding cost-effectiveness of emergency personnel treatment for out-of-hospital cardiac arrest.

165 *and around the world:* See, for example, McPherson and colleagues, *New England Journal of Medicine* 1982;307:1310.

165 Dartmouth Atlas of Health Care: See Wennberg and Cooper, eds. (American Hospital Publishing, 1998). Not everyone agrees with the analysis and methodology of Wennberg and his colleagues (see, for example, Bach, *New England Journal of Medicine* 2010;362:569) or their

conclusion that greater use of services may not correlate with better outcomes for patients (see, for example, Romley and colleagues, *Annals of Internal Medicine* 2011;154:160). But no one doubts the importance of the questions Wennberg and his colleagues have raised by their careful research (see especially Fisher and colleagues, *Annals of Internal Medicine* 2003;138:273 and 2003;138:288). In 2008, the prestigious Institute of Medicine, noting that Wennberg had "shown conclusively that more care is not always best and that patient outcomes are often better with more conservative treatment," awarded him its highest prize "for his impact on the evolution of health care delivery in the United States."

165 *Countless sick patients are discharged:* See Jencks and colleagues, *New England Journal of Medicine* 2009;360:1418.

165 *could just pick up a telephone, "any time, day or night":* It is no coincidence that researchers recently have confirmed Hiatt's commonsense notion that a "telephone-care management strategy" can help patients while also reducing their medical care costs and hospitalization rates. One of Jack Wennberg's many contributions to health care is the work of his son, David Wennberg, the lead author of one such important research effort (see Wennberg and colleagues, *New England Journal of Medicine* 2010;363:1245.

Chapter 6: The Postman Rings Twice

175 *in the Section of General Internal Medicine:* Academic departments of medicine are divided into sections or divisions, according to the subspecialty of internal medicine. The section, or division, of General Internal Medicine includes physicians who specialize in internal medicine but not any of its subspecialties (which include allergy/immunology, cardiology, endocrinology, gastroenterology, geriatrics, hematology, infectious diseases, nephrology, oncology, pulmonary/critical care, and rheumatology; some would also include dermatology and neurology in this list).

176 *to see patients who didn't really need their services:* See note, p. 47.

177 *and handled sundry other unscheduled tasks:* In the modern era, these "other" tasks of primary care physicians are so time-consuming that many "full-time" physicians can be scheduled for only twenty-four scheduled visit-hours per week, or only 60 percent of my scheduled visit-hours in the 1980s (See Baron, *New England Journal of Medicine* 2010;362:1632). Most of these "other" tasks are not reimbursable, an important impediment to the fiscal sustainability of primary care practice.

178 *My "hospitalist" experiment:* The hospitalist model had been operational in a number of U.S. hospitals before 1985 but it became popular, and acquired its name, after an influential journal article was published in 1996 by researchers at the University of California, San Francisco (see Wachter and Goldman, *New England Journal of Medicine* 1996;335:514).

179 *add "value" to the patient's care?:* The concept of "value" in health care has a specialized meaning. Here, value refers to a dividend: the quality of care (measured as the outcome of patient care) *divided by* its cost. Thus, for example, value increases if (objectively measurable) quality of care increases with no increase in its cost; if quality increases proportionately more than

the increase in its cost; if quality remains the same but its cost decreases; or, theoretically, if quality decreases but its cost decreases proportionately more. Decreases in "value" refer to the converse of these dynamics in the ratio of quality to cost.

180 *the chief medical resident, with occasional comments:* Academic departments of medicine are led by a chair, typically a distinguished educator and/or researcher. The chief resident is a postgraduate physician who, after completing residency (and, in some institutions like Cornell, subspecialty fellowship) training, spends an additional year overseeing the clinical and educational experience of the department's residents and medical students.

181 *this kind of internal bleeding was a well-known complication:* See also Chapter 8.

182 *The aneurysm was small, only four centimeters in diameter:* The normal adult aortic diameter is three centimeters. Aortic aneurysms, then, range in size from four centimeters to more than ten centimeters. In general, the larger the aneurysm, the more likely it is to rupture. See, for example, Lederle and colleagues, *New England Journal of Medicine* 2002;287:2968.

182 *There was no way to tell for sure:* Depositions of calcium within the wall of the adult aorta are frequently localized and discontinuous, i.e., not perfectly circumferential. Thus, the "break" visualized in this patient's line of calcification does not necessarily mean that the aneurysm has ruptured.

183 *only about one patient in ten survived:* This statistic refers to patients with *ruptured* abdominal aortic aneurysms, not all patients with aortic aneurysms. Most patients who undergo repair of unruptured aortic aneurysms have an excellent prognosis (see, for example, Greenhalgh and Powell, *New England Journal of Medicine* 2008;358:494).

183 *emphysema, severe pulmonary hypertension, and right ventricular overload:* When emphysema (one form of chronic obstructive pulmonary disease, or COPD) is severe and longstanding, it causes increased pressure in the lung circulation (pulmonary hypertension) and in the right ventricular chamber of the heart (right ventricular overload). These circulatory complications greatly worsen the patient's prognosis.

184 *he could "probably" be weaned off the machine again:* Patients with respiratory failure who require mechanical ventilation sometimes require "weaning" from the ventilator, i.e., mechanical ventilatory assistance must be gradually reduced over a period of time to allow the patient to resume breathing on his own. Some patients with very severe lung disease cannot be weaned from the ventilator and thus become "ventilator-dependent," sometimes permanently.

184 *Osler told family and friends:* See Bliss, *William Osler: A Life in Medicine* (Oxford: Oxford University Press, 1999).

185 *A high autopsy rate strengthened a hospital's reputation:* See Locks and colleagues, eds., *The Oxford Illustrated Companion to Medicine* (Oxford, 2001); Bliss, *William Osler: A Life in Medicine* (Oxford, 1999); Ludmerer, *A Time to Heal: American Medical Education from the Turn of the Century to the Era of Managed Care* (Oxford, 1999).

185 *Since 1761:* This was the publication date for Giovanni Battista Morgagni's classic treatise *On the Sites and Causes of Disease*, which included detailed drawings of more than seven hundred autopsies that the author had performed at the University of Padua.

185 *about 50 percent of all patients who died in U.S. hospitals:* See, for example, Roberts, *New England Journal of Medicine* 1978;299:332.

185 *Osler's own autopsy revealed no surprises:* Osler's autopsy was unusual because his brain was transported back to the United States from England, where he died, by his longtime collaborator, Dr. Thomas McCrae. McCrae was the brother of Dr. John McCrae, the author of the famous World War I poem "In Flanders Fields." Osler's own son, Revere (the great-great-grandson of Paul Revere), died in the same World War I battlefield area where John McCrae served as a military surgeon during World War I. See Bliss, *William Osler: A Life in Medicine* (Oxford, 1999) and Bliss, *Harvey Cushing: A Life in Surgery* (Oxford:2005).

185 *In 1983, researchers at Brigham and Women's Hospital:* See Goldman and colleagues, *New England Journal of Medicine* 1983;308:1000.

186 *regulatory agencies eliminated minimum mandatory autopsy:* Medicare stopped paying directly for autopsies in 1986, but the Joint Commission on Accreditation of Healthcare Organizations eliminated its requirement for a minimum autopsy rate in 1970 (see Shojania and Burton, *New England Journal of Medicine* 2008;358:873).

187 *the autopsy rate in U.S. hospitals is less than 5 percent:* See Burton and Nemetz, *Medscape General Medicine* 2000; 2000:E8 and Nemetz and colleagues, *MedGenMed* 2006;8:80. This decline in autopsy rate is most evident among elderly patients (see Ahronheim and colleagues, *Journal of the American Medical Association* 1983;250:1182).

187 *a new generation of researchers:* See Shojania and colleagues, *Journal of the American Medical Association* 2003;289:2849.

187 *would range from a low of 8.4 percent:* This wide statistical range reflects the uncertainty created by the fact that the actual autopsy rate today is less than 5 percent, not 100 percent.

187 *the Institute of Medicine's sobering estimate:* See Institute of Medicine, *To Err Is Human: Building a Safer Health System* (National Academy Press, 2000).

187 *at least one-third of all death certificates are incorrect:* This estimate derives primarily from studies in Great Britain (see Roulson and colleagues, *Histopathology* 2005;47:551), but similar concerns apply in the United States (see Lundberg, *Journal of the American Medical Association* 1998;280:1273).

187 *keep medical educators honest, showing medical students:* George Lundberg, longtime editor of the *Journal of the American Medical Association*, has been one of the most vocal advocates of this idea but to little avail. In support of his position, Lundberg quoted one Fred Raber who in 1947 said: "Doctoring must be very easy to do because the doctors always bury their mistakes" (see Lundberg, *Journal of the American Medical Association* 1983;1199).

187 *Autopsies . . . identify new or emerging diseases.:* See Lundberg, *Journal of the American Medical Association* 1998;280:1273 and Xiao and colleagues, *American Journal of Medical Sciences* 2009;337:41. It has been estimated that between 1950 and 1996 at least eighty-seven disorders were newly discovered or clarified through autopsy investigations (see Hill and Anderson, *Archives of Pathology and Laboratory Medicine* 1996;120:702). These include such relatively uncommon disorders as Legionnaire's disease, toxic shock syndrome, and sudden infant death syndrome, but also such common ones as myocardial infarction (heart attack). See also Dobbs, *New York Times*, April 24, 2005; Horowitz and Naritoku, *Human Pathology* 2007;38:688.

187 *How else can one study cells deep in the brain:* New imaging techniques, such as "functional magnetic resonance imaging (fMRI)," have helped in this regard. For the same reasons, "virtual autopsy" using postmortem computed tomography (CT) scanning has been proposed as an alternative to the traditional medical autopsy (see Wichmann and colleagues, *Annals of Internal Medicine* 2012;156:123), but many questions remain about the utility of this proposal (see Burton and Mossa-Basha, *Annals of Internal Medicine* 2012;156:158).

188 *responsible for the decline of nonforensic autopsies:* See Nemetz and colleagues, *Mayo Clinic Proceedings* 1989;64:1055 and 1065. Forensic autopsies, i.e., those performed in criminal investigations, are different from medical autopsies. See also Shojania and Burton, *New England Journal of Medicine* 2008;358:873.

188 *Finally, many doctors are conflicted:* See Bove and Iery, *Archives of Pathology and Laboratory Medicine* 2002;126:1023; Burton and colleagues, *American Journal of Medicine* 2004;117:255.

189 *like a mushroom on a stalk:* Most atrial myxomas are pedunculated, i.e., attached by a stalk to the interior surface of the heart chamber.

190 *the usual incidental findings, unsurprising in an eighty-year-old man:* These findings, including the small area of prostate cancer, are "incidental" in the sense that they have no clinical relevance to the patient's clinical care. For example, up to 80 percent of men in this age group will have prostate cancer, which, in most cases, will require no treatment. (See also Welch and colleagues, *Overdiagnosed: Making People Sick in the Pursuit of Health* (Beacon, 2011).

190 *this myxoma was in the right atrium, the rarest kind of all:* About 90 percent of all myxomas are found in the left atrium, the heart chamber that receives oxygenated blood from the lungs before it is pumped into the arterial circulation. In contrast, the right atrium receives unoxygenated blood from the venous circulation before it is pumped into the lungs.

191 *Fred's blue color, called cyanosis:* Unoxygenated blood is blue, not red, in color. Because Fred's myxoma transiently obstructed all blood flow into his lungs, his circulating blood (and thus his lips and skin) turned blue.

191 *we had eyewitnesses to prove it:* See also note, p. 66. Eyewitness accounts are often the most important information doctors use when evaluating patients with syncope (see, for example, Kapoor, *New England Journal of Medicine* 2000;343:1856; Strickberger and colleagues, *Circulation* 2006;113:316).

192 *the only one we haven't excluded:* This is true only if we consider the possibility that the echocardiogram, the test typically used to diagnose myxoma, might be "falsely negative" in Fred's case. See also note, p. 193.

192 *the M-mode and 2-D ultrasound examinations:* Cardiac ultrasound testing (echocardiography) has evolved over the past several decades. The old-fashioned two-dimensional images available in the 1980s have evolved to three-dimensional, "color flow Doppler" imaging whose sensitivity and specificity for most cardiac abnormalities, including atrial myxoma, is superior to the older ultrasound imaging modalities (see Feigenbaum, *Echocardiography* [Williams and Wilkins, 2009]).

192 *would the cardiologist have agreed to perform* two *of these procedures:* To investigate the left atrium, the site of most atrial myxomas, the cardiologist inserts a catheter into a large *artery* (typically in the groin) and then threads the catheter backward (against the flow of blood) into the left side of the heart. To investigate the right atrium, however, the cardiologist inserts a catheter into a large *vein* (also typically in the groin) and then threads the catheter forward (in the direction of venous blood flow) into the right side of the heart. These two procedures, called left heart catheterization and right heart catheterization, are performed on the same patient only in unusual circumstances.

192 *Even exhaustive diagnostic testing does not reveal the cause:* See, for example, Kapoor, *New England Journal of Medicine* 2000;343:1856.

193 *I would remember this story if I ever heard one like it again:* As of this writing, I have not personally cared for another patient with a (diagnosed) right atrial myxoma.

193 *This was a well-known limitation of cardiac ultrasound technology:* See also note, p. 192. Modern cardiac ultrasound technology does not have the same limitations.

193 all *tests in medicine have a "false-negative rate":* This statement is a slight oversimplification. For many medical tests, it is possible to minimize, or even eliminate, false-negative results but only at a cost: Almost always, reducing the false-negative rate of a test also increases its "false-positive" rate. This trade-off of a test's sensitivity (true-positive rate) and specificity (true-negative rate) is inherent in all medical testing. See also Griner and colleagues, *Annals of Internal Medicine* 1981;94(Part 2):559–87; Sox, *Annals of Internal Medicine* 1986;104:60; Ransohoff and Feinstein, *New England Journal of Medicine* 1978;299:926.

195 *the false-negative rate of a screening mammogram is about 25 percent:* See, for example, Poplack and colleagues, *Radiology* 2000;217:832 where, among 53,803 women screened in New Hampshire, the false-negative rate was 27.6 percent. Mammograms are graded on a "BI-RADS" scale of 1 to 5, with grades 4 or 5 considered "suspicious" or "highly suspicious," respectively (see Lieberman and Menell, *Radiology Clinics of North America* 2002;40:409; Eberl and colleagues, *Journal of the American Board of Family Medicine* 2006;19:161). Fewer than 1 percent of women whose screening mammogram result is "BI-RADS 1, 2, or 3" have breast cancer, but no mammogram result can predict the absence of breast cancer with 100 percent certainty.

195 diagnostic *tests, which are done to evaluate:* Diagnostic mammograms are more sensitive but less specific than screening mammograms. About 20 percent of diagnostic mammograms, i.e., mammograms performed to evaluate a known abnormality (such as a palpable breast lump), are false negative and about 10 percent are false positive (see Poplack reference in previous note, p. 195).

196 *the cause of FUO is never found in a significant minority of patients:* In the modern era, FUO is subclassified according to various clinical contexts, e.g., FUO in hospitalized patients versus outpatients, or FUO in immune-compromised patients versus patients with normal immune status. The frequency of negative workups, i.e., cases in which the cause is not identified, varies in these different contexts.

200 *how probable the diagnosis needs to be:* See Sox and colleagues, *Medical Decision Making* (Boston: Butterworth-Heineman, 1988).

200 *the ultrasound detects a myxoma that, in fact, isn't there:* Various technical "red herrings" (e.g., turbulent blood flow or blood clots) can cause an ultrasonographer to suspect an intracardiac tumor like a myxoma when, in fact, no such tumor is present.

201 *during the Nazi blitzkrieg of London:* See, for example, Green and Swets, *Signal Detection Theory and Psychophysics* (New York: Wiley and Sons, 1966).

206 *I was careful not to prescribe other drugs that could interact:* Various drugs can raise or lower the serum level of digitalis drugs, thereby potentially increasing the toxicity or reducing the effectiveness of digitalis.

206 *His letter quoted extensively from the writings of John King:* See King, *Transactions of the American Clinical and Climatological Association* 1949;61:65. More than a decade earlier, Alvah Gordon had reviewed previous literature on the "mental complications of heart disease" and its treatment (see Gordon, *Transactions of the American Clinical and Climatological Association* 1937;53:53) and concluded, quoting MacBeth: "Throw physic to the dogs! I'll none of it!" Nevertheless, in the modern era, efforts to remind physicians about the side effects of digitalis tend not to mention neuropsychiatric symptoms (see, for example, Yang and colleagues, *American Journal of Medicine* 2012;125:337).

Chapter 7: Lost Marbles

216 *her breathing had nothing to do with her inability to walk or lie down:* Patients with severe heart disease have trouble walking or lying supine because doing these things makes them feel short of breath. Despite her known heart disease, then, this fact means that Martha's current problem has a different cause.

219 *what they really wanted to know: So, what's wrong:* Physicians-in-training learn best when expected to analyze a patient's problem "from scratch," i.e., unprejudiced by other physicians' previous opinions. Time pressure and trainees' burdensome workloads make this ideal learning environment uncommon in U.S. hospitals today. The impact of this reality on trainees' diagnostic skills and their maturation as effective clinicians has been poorly studied.

220 *I had seen a patient with polymyositis:* Polymyositis is an inflammatory muscle disease of unknown cause that typically presents as subacute weakness of large muscle groups, most prominently the shoulders and thighs. In unusual cases, it can progress rapidly, involve small as well as large muscles, and impair swallowing and breathing.

221 *patients with factitious illness—people who purposely made themselves sick:* Factitious illness refers to the intentional production or feigning of physical (not psychological) symptoms or disease caused by a patient's need to assume the "sick role" (without other external incentives, such as economic gain), which behavior does not occur exclusively during the course of any other major psychiatric disorder, such as schizophrenia (see Eisendrath, *Western Journal of Medicine* 1994;160:177). Unlike patients with somatization disorders (see Chapter 3), conversion reactions, or hypochondriasis (see Chapter 5), patients with factitious illness produce their symptoms or disease *consciously*. They are fully cognizant of their actions; it is the motivation for their actions that is subconscious. Many patients with factitious illness have had training or jobs in health care fields (see Krahn and colleagues, *American Journal of Psychiatry* 2003;160:1163). Effective management of these patients is poorly understood (see Eastwood and Bisson, *Psychotherapy and Psychosomatics* 2008;77:209), largely because the disorder is uncommon (see Sutherland and Rodin, *Psychosomatics* 1990;31:392) and most patients decline psychiatric care and follow-up.

222 *Staphylococcus aureus, a bad bug:* See also Chapters 1, 4, and 9.

222 *she might have had a harmless "transient bacteremia":* It is not unusual to grow bacteria from cultures of patients' blood that cause no illness and require no treatment. (Such blood culture "contaminants" are daily events in all hospitals.) *Staphylococcus* bacteria are among the most commonly isolated contaminant organisms but, because *Staph* also commonly causes life-threatening disease, distinguishing benign contaminants from a serious condition can be difficult in patients with Staphylococcal bacteremia.

225 *She wasn't a malingerer:* See note, p. 221.

220 *Alice's Munchausen psychopathology:* Strictly speaking, I don't know that Alice has Munchausen's syndrome, which refers to patients who *make a career* of manufacturing diseases (see Asher, *Lancet* 1951;1:339), a sociopathic phenomenon. This group probably constitutes only a small minority (perhaps 10 percent) of all patients with factitious illness, who, like Alice, typically are lost to follow-up.

226 *rating Martha's surgical risk from general anesthesia:* There are many different "prediction rules" used to estimate patients' risk (and hence suitability) for surgical procedures that require general anesthesia. Anesthesiologists tend to use rules developed by anesthesiologists, but they often defer to cardiologists (who use different rules), because most (but not all) risks pertain to the heart.

229 *at least 20 percent of the 12.5 million people aged sixty-five years or older:* See Inouye, *New England Journal of Medicine* 2006;354:1157. Prevalence of delirium varies with the type of patients and the settings studied (see Wong and colleagues, *Journal of the American Medical Association* 2010;304:779).

229 *This problem adds billions of dollars to annual Medicare costs:* See, for example, *CMS (Centers for Medicare and Medicaid Services) Statistics* 2004, U.S. Department of Health and Human Services. One study found that delirium increased the one-year health care costs of affected patients between $16,303 and $64,421 per patient, which, if extrapolated to the entire United States, amounts to incremental health care costs of $38 billion to $152 billion annually.

230 *the in-hospital* mortality *rate for patients with delirium:* See Inouye, *New England Journal of Medicine* 2006;354:1157. The harmful effects of delirium extend beyond the patient's hospitalization (see, for example, Witlox and colleagues, *Journal of the American Medical Association* 2010;304:443). Longer-term consequences of delirium include shortened life span, increased risk of institutionalization, and increased subsequent diagnoses of dementia.

230 *Z. J. Lipowski called delirium the "Cinderella" of American medicine:* See Lipowski, *Journal of Nervous and Mental Diseases* 1967;145:227.

230 *But other cases that Lipowski described:* Ibid.

231 *prevalence of delirium among very elderly people:* See Folstein and colleagues, *International Psychogeriatrics* 1991;3:169; Rahkonen and colleagues, *International Psychogeriatrics* 2001;13:37; Inouye, *New England Journal of Medicine* 2006;354:1157.

231 *The most common predisposing conditions are elderly age:* See Inouye, *New England Journal of Medicine* 2006;354:1157; O'Mahony and colleagues, *Annals of Internal Medicine* 2011;154:746; Marcantonio, *Journal of the American Medical Association* 2012;308:73.

231 *classic medical experiments about the effects of fever:* See Ebaugh and colleagues, *American Journal of Psychiatry* 1936;23:191.

231 *The most common precipitating factors are drugs, infections:* This is such a reliable list that some doctors use a mnemonic "DIMS Neurologically" to remember the five common precipitating causes of delirium, a syndrome in which patients literally "dim" neurologically. "DIMSN" lists, in order of prevalence, these precipitating (and largely reversible) factors: Drugs, Infections, Metabolic disturbances (e.g., low blood sugar), Sleep deprivation or Surgery. Neurological disorders (e.g., stroke) are the *least* common precipitating cause.

231 *in the Yale Delirium Prevention Trial:* See Inouye and colleagues, *New England Journal of Medicine* 1999;340:669.

231 *Similar preventive studies have reduced delirium:* See, for example, Marcantonio and colleagues, *Journal of the American Geriatrics Society* 2001;49:516.

232 *Although one-third of delirium cases in hospital may be preventable:* See Inouye and colleagues, *New England Journal of Medicine* 1999;340:669.

232 *hospital staff often assume that the patient has* dementia: This is not surprising, given the frequency with which dementia patients are hospitalized (see, for example, Phelan and colleagues, *Journal of the American Medical Association* 2012;307:165) and the sometimes subtle

differences between delirium and dementia (see Lipowski, *American Journal of Psychiatry* 1980;137:674 and *New England Journal of Medicine* 1989;320:578; Mahler and colleagues, *Western Journal of Medicine* 1987;146:705; Rahkonen and colleagues, *Journal of Neurology, Neurosurgery and Psychiatry* 2000;69:519). Improved prevention and treatment of delirium is especially important in patients with dementia, some of whom will suffer *permanent* adverse outcomes due to delirium in hospital (see Fong and colleagues, *Annals of Internal Medicine* 2012;156:848).

232 *his hands had been restrained (painlessly) with soft straps:* One of many reasons to prevent delirium in hospital is to avoid the need for physical restraints, which, like all medical interventions, may cause harm as well as benefit. Considerable judgment may be needed to decide whether "soft" (less harmful) restraints are sufficient to protect the patient.

234 *Neither of us knew that this particular antibiotic could cause delirium:* In my father's case, this actually happened with two different, commonly prescribed antibiotics: erythromycin and levofloxacin. Rare side effects of drugs often are not discovered until "postmarketing" surveillance is done in a systematic way. See, for example, *eHealthMe: Real world drug outcomes,* specifically, www.ehealthme.com/ds/erythromycin/delirium and www.ehealthme.com/ds/levaquin/delirium.

235 *In those days, surgery for this condition required a team:* This is sometimes still true today, but most large academic medical centers have "spine surgeons," typically orthopedists or neurosurgeons with special training and expertise in this area.

237 *many patients—especially elderly patients:* Varying degrees of spinal stenosis will be found in 6 to 23 percent of asymptomatic adults. Those percentages are even higher in elderly patients (see Kalichman and colleagues, *The Spine Journal* 2009;9:545). For this reason, imaging procedures alone cannot determine the need for treatment of this condition (see Suri and colleagues, *Journal of the American Medical Association* 2010;304:2628).

238 *Clearly, there are major risks:* Even today, this kind of surgery (which is performed in more than thirty thousand Medicare patients annually) is associated with 5 to 6 percent risk of life-threatening complications (see Deyo and colleagues, *Journal of the American Medical Association* 2010;303:1259).

238 *Insurers had begun talking about publishing "report cards" of surgeons' success:* Such report cards have been used most prominently for cardiac surgeons, most notably for the most common type of heart surgery (coronary artery bypass procedures). Although some observers consider this attempt at transparency "a watershed event in health care accountability" (see Ferris and Torchiana, *New England Journal of Medicine* 2010;363:1593), others are concerned that it may discourage treatment of more difficult, severely ill patients, a problem that has been documented in several parts of the United States (see Dranove and colleagues, *Journal of Political Economy* 2003;111:555).

239 *His infection, called subacute bacterial endocarditis:* This is essentially the same disease as Mr. Warner's (see Chapter 1 and Part III), but its tempo is more indolent, hence the term "subacute" rather than "acute."

244 *He took time off, wrote a book:* See Hilfiker, *Healing the Wounds: A Physician Looks at His Work* (New York: Pantheon, 1985).

244 *the (nonreligious) "Samaritan" role of doctors:* David Hilfiker's second book provides insight into this role. See Hilfiker, *Not All of Us Are Saints: A Doctor's Journey with the Poor* (New York: Ballantine, 1996).

244 *This new culture has even changed our vocabulary:* See, for example, Hartzband and Groopman, *New England Journal of Medicine* 2011;365:1372.

244 *Guilt is about self-disappointment:* See Gaylin, *Feelings: Our Vital Signs* (New York: Harper and Row, 1979).

245 *many doctors, like Hilfiker, have become:* See Wu, *British Medical Journal* 2000;320:726.

245 *Fewer than 10 percent of all U.S. medical school graduates:* See, for example, Bodenheimer, *Health Affairs* (Millwood) 2010;29:799 and *New England Journal of Medicine* 2006;355:861; Rieselbach and colleagues, *Annals of Internal Medicine* 2010;152:118 Rabinowitz and colleagues, *Journal of the American Medical Association* 2001;286:1041.

246 *If we didn't do harm, we couldn't do good:* The origin of the ambiguous caveat "First, do no harm" is discussed in Smith, *Journal of Clinical Pharmacology* 2005;45:371. Its deeper meaning has been reviewed in Jonsen, *Annals of Internal Medicine* 1978;88:827; Lasagna, *Science* 1967;158:246; Shelton, *Journal of the American Medical Association* 2000;284:2687; Lenert and colleagues, *Clinical Pharmacology and Therapeutics* 1993;53:285.

246 *more African-American women got mammograms:* See Weber and Reilly, *Archives of Internal Medicine* 1997;157:2345.

249 *his eulogist had written:* Accessed in *Memorial Tributes: National Academy of Engineering.*

249 *an international authority on "evidence-based medicine":* See Sackett, Richardson, and colleagues, *Evidence-Based Medicine: How to Practice and Teach EBM* (London: Churchill Livingstone, 1997).

253 *Mark's efforts are making digitalis obsolete:* "Radiofrequency catheter ablation" of atrial fibrillation is not for everyone, but, increasingly, it is replacing drug therapy as the treatment of choice for many patients. (See Stevenson and Albert, *New England Journal of Medicine* 2012;367:1648; Nielsen and colleagues, *New England Journal of Medicine* 2012;367:1587).

Chapter 8: Never Say Never

258 *When I examined Mom myself:* This is the test done to detect "orthostatic hypotension," the medical term for an abnormal drop in blood pressure associated with assuming an upright (standing) position. Many different disorders can cause this problem, whose typical symptom is fainting (or light-headedness) precipitated by standing up, but among the most common causes are dehydration and prolonged bed rest.

260 *Considered by many the "father of open-heart surgery":* This unofficial honorific has been be-
stowed on several cardiac surgeons of the era—Michael DeBakey, Denton Cooley, and Frank
Austen, among others—but Lillehei was one.

262 *Ms. Dubois was a "full code":* Lacking a written do-not-resuscitate order, all hospitalized patients are considered a "full code," i.e., expected to receive full resuscitation ("code") efforts
by hospital personnel, including cardiopulmonary resuscitation and mechanical ventilation.
See also notes, pp. 67, 112, and 269.

263 *We have no reason to believe that our own treatment:* Some will consider this wishful thinking on
our part. Maybe so. But the point here is that there are two plausible hypotheses about the
role of the blood clot in Ms. Dubois's death, and there is no direct evidence to support one
hypothesis over the other. However, one hypothesis is far more likely—Dan's contention that
the clot played no causative role—because the alternative hypothesis "almost never" happens.

264 *After we clean the clot out of it:* This was done for sanitary, not exculpatory, reasons. Ms. Dubois's
son was thoroughly informed about what we had found at autopsy.

264 *two case reports from Belgium and Texas published years ago:* See Young and colleagues, *Texas Heart
Institute Journal* 2001;28:53; Denis and Hoffer, *Acta Anaesthesiologica Belgica* 2006;57:153.

265 *just ten days after his dilemma had seemed impossible:* See Chapter 4.

267 *pharmaceutical companies and medical device manufacturers promote:* In recent years, several
companies have been fined heavily in criminal prosecutions by the U.S. federal government.
Whether these substantial penalties ($3 billion in a recent judgment against the British drug
maker GlaxoSmithKline) will reduce this kind of "creep" remains uncertain (see Thomas
and Schmidt, *New York Times,* July 3, 2012). Experts at the Mayo Clinic recently reviewed
common questions about off-label drug use (see Wittich and colleagues, *Mayo Clinic Proceedings* 2012;87:982). Legal issues abound as well. (See Boumil, *New England Journal of
Medicine* 2013;368:103; Kesselheim and colleagues, *Journal of the American Medical Association*
2013;309:445.)

267 *a new CPR technique called closed-chest cardiac massage:* See Kouwenhoven and colleagues,
Journal of the American Medical Association 1960;173:94.

267 *who had also developed the external cardiac defibrillator:* See Kouwenhoven and colleagues,
Surgery 1957;42:550.

267 *the National Academy of Sciences issued its own report:* See Ad Hoc Committee on Cardiopulmonary Resuscitation, *Journal of the American Medical Association* 1966;198:138.

267 *U.S. communities funded "mobile intensive care units":* See Pantridge and Geddes, *Lancet* 1967;II:
271; Grace and Chadbourn, *Diseases of the Chest* 1969;55:452.

268 *higher than the success rate for patients who suffer cardiac arrest in hospital today:* Success, defined as "meaningful recovery" and discharge from hospital, varies in different settings and

different patient populations (see, for example, Bedell and colleagues, *New England Journal of Medicine* 1983;309:569; Taffet and colleagues, *Journal of the American Medical Association* 1988;260:2069; Nichol and colleagues, *Journal of the American Medical Association* 2008;300:1423; Aufderheide and colleagues, *New England Journal of Medicine* 2011;365:798). It is unclear whether these survival rates are improving (see, for example, Ehlenbach and colleagues, *New England Journal of Medicine* 2009;361:22; Girotra and colleagues, *Circulation* 2011;124:A509; Girotra and colleagues, *New England Journal of Medicine* 2012;367:1912). Nevertheless, important research continues to test new methods of resuscitation (see, for example, Holzer, *New England Journal of Medicine* 2010;363:1256; Hagihara and colleagues, *Journal of the American Medical Association* 2012;307:1161) and determinants of its success (see Sasson and colleagues, *New England Journal of Medicine* 2012;367:1607).

268 *studies involving* only *elderly patients:* See Kim and colleagues, *Archives of Internal Medicine* 2000;160:3439; Murphy and colleagues, *Annals of Internal Medicine* 1989;111:199; Ehlenbach and colleagues, *New England Journal of Medicine* 2009;361:22. The good news here is that most of (the relatively few) elderly patients who survive CPR are still alive one year later. The bad news is that a majority of these survivors are discharged from hospital with either "moderate-to-severe" neurological disability or in a coma or vegetative state. (See Chan and colleagues, *New England Journal of Medicine* 2013;368:1019.) In other words, "successful" CPR in such patients is not only uncommon, it is also not uncomplicated.

268 *the first study of out-of-hospital CPR:* See Pantridge and Geddes, *Lancet* 1967;II: 271.

268 *Recent studies have shown that survival rates after out-of-hospital CPR:* See, for example, Becker and colleagues, *Annals of Emergency Medicine* 1991;20:355; Longstreth and colleagues, *Journal of the American Medical Association* 1990;264:2109; Kim and colleagues, *Archives of Internal Medicine* 2000;160:3439.

269 *(fictional) cardiac arrests portrayed on* ER: See Diem and colleagues, *New England Journal of Medicine* 1996;334:1578.

269 *"CPR can lead to prolonged suffering, severe neurologic damage":* See, for example, Edgren and colleagues, *Lancet* 1994;343:1055; de Vos and colleagues, *Archives of Internal Medicine* 1999;159:249. However, as noted recently, "There is currently a paucity of data on long-term outcomes of patients who survive an in-hospital cardiac arrest and are discharged home" (see Chan and Nallamothu, *Journal of the American Medical Association* 2012;307:1917). Recent data about out-of-hospital cardiac arrests, however, are troubling. A Japanese study of almost 650,000 patients found that 4.7 percent survived at least one month, but more than one-half of these survivors were vegetative or had severe cerebral disability (see Hasegawa and colleagues, *Journal of the American Medical Association* 2013;309:257).

269 *One geriatrician, who cared for elderly patients in a long-term care facility:* See Murphy, *Journal of the American Medical Association* 1988;260:2098. The author had estimated a 3 percent chance of survival in these patients, based on strong empirical evidence (see Murphy and colleagues, *Annals of Internal Medicine* 1989;111:199). In some long-term care facilities today, CPR is performed only for patients who "opt out" of an institution-wide default policy *not* to perform CPR. (See Kane and colleagues, *Journal of the American Medical Association* 2012;307:917.)

269 *doctors and patients are susceptible to the notion that:* See, for example, Grimes, *Journal of the American Medical Association* 1993;269:3033 on "Technology Follies: The uncritical acceptance of medical innovation."

270 *in 1965, a surgical team replaced the infected heart valve:* See Wallace and colleagues, *Circulation* 1965;31:450. Four years earlier, a surgical team had successfully cured a fungal infection of a patient's tricuspid (right-sided) heart valve (see Kay and colleagues, *New England Journal of Medicine* 1961;264:907).

270 *Ten years later, 239 endocarditis patients worldwide:* See Parrott and colleagues, *Annals of Surgery* 1976;183:289.

270 *These (highly selected) patients are offered such risky surgery because:* As described in Mr. Warner's case, this is a complex decision affected by many variables. See, for example, Kiefer and colleagues, *Journal of the American Medical Association* 2011;306:2239; Schick and colleagues, *UptoDate* (accessed 11/28/2011). These and many other authorities note that much remains uncertain about the advisability (and timing) of surgery for endocarditis patients, especially those with bleeding strokes (see, for example, Schick and colleagues [above] and Ruttmann and colleagues, *Stroke* 2006;37:2094).

270 *new chemotherapy treatments can extend this median survival:* As with all types of cancer, this is an ever-evolving area of study—new treatment regimens are introduced frequently—but see, for example, Hussain and colleagues, *Journal of Clinical Oncology* 2001;19:2527; von der Maase and colleagues, *Journal of Clinical Oncology* 2005;23:4602. In general, many patients offered chemotherapy for advanced cancer do not understand that the treatment is rarely curative (see, for example, Weeks and colleagues, *New England Journal of Medicine* 2012:367:1616).

271 *Frail, elderly patients . . . are typically excluded from research studies:* Prognosis is often affected by patients' "comorbidities," i.e., coexisting diseases. For example, patients with cancer who also have heart disease or AIDS will have worse prognoses than patients whose only disease is cancer. The Charlson comorbidity index is commonly used to measure comorbidity (see Charlson and colleagues, *Journal of Chronic Diseases* 1987;40:373). Estimates of the risks as well as the benefits of any treatment for elderly patients should always include an assessment of competing risks related to comorbidities (see, for example, Welch and colleagues, *Annals of Internal Medicine* 1996;124:577; Casarett, *Annals of Internal Medicine* 2006;145:700). However, especially in older cancer patients, comorbidity does not necessarily correlate with "functional status," a measure of patients' ability to work, perform daily activities, and care for personal needs (see Extermann and colleagues, *Journal of Clinical Oncology* 1998;16:1582). Assessment of cancer patients' functional status should include input from both the patient and the oncologist (see Blagden and colleagues, *British Journal of Cancer* 2003;89:1022).

271 *Statistical analyses of large groups:* This has long been the basis for physicians' complaints about "evidence-based medicine": incongruence between the overall effects of a treatment in a study *population* and deciding the best treatment for an *individual* patient. Thus, understanding better how the benefits and harms of a treatment vary across different *subsets* of a study population—sometimes called the "heterogeneity of treatment effect"—deserves greater attention from researchers (see, for example, Kent and colleagues, *Trials* 2010;11:85).

271 *"The Median Is Not the Message"*: See Gould, *Discover* magazine, June 1985.

274 *new, handheld portable echo machine*: Point-of-care ultrasonography refers to ultrasound testing performed and interpreted by the clinician at the patient's bedside, not by a trained radiologist (or cardiologist). This practice, which has increased greatly in recent years, can be clinically useful and cost-effective, but it is poorly regulated and incompletely understood. (See note, p. 267, about technology creep.) More research is needed because "indiscriminate use of ultrasonography could lead to further unnecessary testing, unnecessary interventions in the case of false-positive findings, or inadequate investigation of false-negative findings" (see Moore and Copel, *New England Journal of Medicine* 2011;364:749).

274 *intravenous infusions of Vitamin K and blood plasma*: Warfarin inhibits Vitamin K–dependent clotting factors. These infusions provide the deficient clotting factors immediately and also begin to reverse the antagonism of Vitamin K.

274 *this time with a Russian interpreter, not his daughter*: Whenever possible, a trained language interpreter, not a family member, should be recruited to aid in communicating with a patient whose language is foreign to the physician. (See, for example, Regenstein and colleagues, *Journal of the American Medical Association* 2013;309:145.)

275 *sometimes a sign of heart or lung problems*: Because the large veins of the neck drain directly into the right side of the heart (and thence into the lungs), careful visual inspection of these veins—a dying art in modern times—can raise the physician's "bedside suspicion" of various cardiopulmonary disorders.

275 *bleeding into his retroperitoneum*: See also Chapter 6.

276 *After undergoing heart surgery, many elderly patients seem different*: This complex problem has been best studied in patients who undergo coronary artery bypass surgery, the procedure Mr. Barensky underwent (see Selnes and colleagues, *New England Journal of Medicine* 2012;366:250). It is not at all clear how many of these postoperative changes, e.g., subjective memory problems and anxiety, are caused by the surgical procedure itself (see, for example, Djikstra and colleagues, *Neuropsychology Reviews* 2002;12:1). It is now known that many recently hospitalized patients experience a transient period of susceptibility to various adverse events, sometimes called the "post-hospital syndrome," even if their hospitalization did not involve a surgical procedure. (See Krumholz, *New England Journal of Medicine* 2013;368:100.)

276 *classic somatic symptoms of psychological distress*: See also Chapter 3 and note, p. 87.

279 *spend more time interacting with the damn computer than with the patients*: Whether in the hospital or in outpatient settings, this issue is ubiquitous, frustrating to many physicians and patients alike.

280 *Hickam's Dictum, not Occam's razor*: See also Chapter 1.

282 *it comes and goes*: Patients with pericardial tamponade, Mr. Barensky's problem, manifest a phenomenon called "pulsus paradoxus" whereby their blood pressure declines abnormally

during the inspirational phase of their breathing cycle. An important diagnostic clue, this "paradox" can cause confusion during blood pressure measurement.

283 *He pulls a laryngoscope out of his metal case:* A laryngoscope is a handheld, lighted instrument that is inserted into the patient's mouth and used to visualize the patient's trachea (windpipe) before inserting a breathing tube.

285 *Hemopericardium, most likely:* Pericardial fluid collections can be caused by different types of fluid. Hemopericardium refers to a collection of blood in the pericardium.

285 *it's not like I've never seen a false-negative echocardiogram before:* See also Chapter 6 and note, p. 193.

286 *among elderly patients, warfarin is the most common cause of medication-related emergency hospitalizations:* Such serious drug-related events are not rare, numbering approximately one hundred thousand annually in the United States (see Budnitz and colleagues, *New England Journal of Medicine* 2011;365:2002). They also represent just the tip of the iceberg, given the prevalence of all serious adverse drug events in the United States (see Bates and colleagues, *Journal of the American Medical Association* 1995;274:29).

287 *transitions of care between the hospital and home:* See Coleman, *Journal of the American Geriatrics Society* 2003;51:549; Coleman and Berenson, *Annals of Internal Medicine* 2004;140:533. Among many other issues, helping patients (and families) find the right "level" of posthospital care deserves much more attention (see Kane, *Journal of the American Medical Association* 2011;305:284). Many interventions have shown promise in improving patient "handovers" from hospital to primary care, but it has been difficult to generate firm conclusions about what works best (see Hesselink and colleagues, *Annals of Internal Medicine* 2012;157:417; Bray-Hall, *Annals of Internal Medicine* 2012;157:448). Transitions of care near the end of life deserve special attention. (See Teno and colleagues, *Journal of the American Medical Association* 2013;309:470.)

288 *the lack of a universal electronic medical record:* To address this problem, the Health Information Technology for Economic and Clinical Health (HITECH) Act was enacted; its implementation faces many challenges (see Blumenthal, *New England Journal of Medicine* 2010;362:382; 2011;365:2323; 2011;365:2426). A history of the "evolving medical record" in the United States since the early 1800s provides an interesting perspective about this critically important issue (see Siegler, *Annals of Internal Medicine* 2010;153:671).

288 *the administrative morass created by our smorgasbord of different health insurers:* See Woolhandler and colleagues, *New England Journal of Medicine* 2003;349:768. These authors compare the administrative costs in the United States with costs in Canada, whose national health insurance system is less expensive. Predictably, not all experts agree with these authors' questions or answers (see, for example, Aaron, *New England Journal of Medicine* 2003;349:801). But even in the absence of a single-payer system in the United States, many opportunities exist to reduce administrative costs (see, for example, Cutler and colleagues, *New England Journal of Medicine* 2012;367:1875).

288 *hospitals have had no incentive to dismantle their revolving door:* This will change soon. The Centers for Medicare and Medicaid Services have begun to track hospital readmission rates

and plan to reduce reimbursement to hospitals with high (risk-standardized) readmission rates. This is a step in the right direction but many experts point to the challenges involved (see, for example, Jha and colleagues, *New England Journal of Medicine* 2009;361:2637; Epstein, *New England Journal of Medicine* 2009;360:1457; Epstein and colleagues, *New England Journal of Medicine* 2011;365:2287; Kansagara and colleagues, *Journal of the American Medical Association* 2011;306:1688; Vaduganathan and colleagues, *Journal of the American Medical Association* 2013;309:345; McCarthy and colleagues, *Journal of the American Medical Association* 2013;309:351).

288 *a lucrative "line of business":* See Mor and colleagues, *Health Affairs* 2010;29(1):57.

289 *in 25 percent of U.S. hospitals today, one-quarter of all admissions are thirty-day readmissions:* See Jencks and colleagues, *New England Journal of Medicine* 2009;360:1418. In general, readmissions are less frequent in pediatric hospitals (see Berry and colleagues, *Journal of the American Medical Association* 2013; 309:372).

289 *"post-acute care" patients today account for more than 70 percent of all new patient admissions:* See Mor and colleagues, *Health Affairs* 2007;26:1762.

289 *This revolving door is speeding up, not slowing down:* See Mor and colleagues, *Health Affairs* 2010;29(1):57.

289 *patients with congestive heart failure in Bend, Oregon:* See Jha and colleagues, *New England Journal of Medicine* 2009;361:2637; Dharmarajan and colleagues, *Journal of the American Medical Association* 2013;309:355.

289 *Patients in Utah who are discharged from hospitals:* See Mor and colleagues, *Health Affairs* 2010;29(1):57.

289 *Various interventions designed specifically to address:* Multifaceted interventions in Philadelphia (see Naylor and colleagues, *Journal of the American Medical Association* 1999;281:613) and Denver (see Coleman and colleagues, *Archives of Internal Medicine* 2006;166:1822), for example, reduced rehospitalization rates and decreased costs for chronically ill elderly patients. However, increasing access to primary care (an important effort) may be insufficient to solve this problem (see Weinberger and colleagues, *New England Journal of Medicine* 1996;334:1441; Vashi and colleagues, *Journal of the American Medical Association* 2013;309:364; Dharmarajan and colleagues, *Journal of the American Medical Association* 2013;309:355; Brock and colleagues, *Journal of the American Medical Association* 2013;309:381).

289 *the National Pilot Program on Payment Bundling:* This new effort presents many opportunities and challenges, as discussed by Mechanic, *New England Journal of Medicine* 2011;365:777; Cutler and Ghosh, *New England Journal of Medicine* 2012;366:1075. Bundled care in the Netherlands, for example, has had both positive and negative consequences (see, for example, Struijs and Baan, *New England Journal of Medicine* 2011; 364:990). It may also have unintended consequences in the United States (see, for example, Weeks and colleagues, *Annals of Internal Medicine* 2013;158:62).

290 *Bundling will not be easy to do well:* See, for example, Hackbarth and colleagues, *New England Journal of Medicine* 2008;359:3; Hussey and colleagues, *Health Affairs* 2011;30:2116; Sood and colleagues, *Health Affairs* 2011;30:1708; Mechanic and Tompkins, *New England Journal of Medicine* 2012;367:1873.

292 *it's best to clear the infection before trying to repair:* Like so many other issues about this disease, there is no definitive scientific evidence to support this practice (see, for example, Kiefer and colleagues, *Journal of the American Medical Association* 2011;306:2239). Even if such studies could be performed, it is unlikely that they would include many patients like Mr. Warner, who was unusual in many respects, with a high risk of mortality however he was treated (see Hasbun and colleagues, *Journal of the American Medical Association* 2003;289:1933). Recently, however, a small study of highly selected patients (not unlike Mr. Warner) found that early surgery may be advantageous (see Kang and colleagues, *New England Journal of Medicine* 2012;366:2466).

293 *but these rare cases tell us little:* This is a controversial area. See Ruttmann and colleagues, *Stroke* 2006;37:2094, who suggest that the risk of devastating neurological outcomes from surgery may have been exaggerated.

296 *the great majority of patients with bacterial endocarditis are cured:* This is an example of "telling the truth in the most optimistic way," as Ubel suggests, allowing patients to "prepare for the worst while allowing them to hope for the best" (see Ubel, *Annals of Internal Medicine* 2001;134:1142). The truth is that most patients with bacterial endocarditis *are* cured with "medical therapy" alone, i.e., without surgery. However, it is also true that among patients with this disease, Mr. Warner is in a very high-risk group.

Chapter 9: To the Limit

302 *His voice isn't hoarse:* Hoarseness is one of many signs that may indicate disease in the mediastinum, the central chest cavity between the two lungs. In patients with suspected lung cancer, mediastinal involvement often means that the cancer is incurable.

310 *as Stephen Jay Gould reminded us:* See Chapter 8.

310 *How, given finite resources, can we optimize:* Value in health care has been defined as (patient) outcomes relative to the costs of achieving those outcomes. As Michael Porter has explained, "Cost reduction without regard to the outcomes achieved is dangerous and self-defeating. . . . To reduce cost, the best approach is often to spend more on some services to reduce the need for others" (see Porter, *New England Journal of Medicine* 2010;363:2477 and Supplementary Appendixes 1 and 2 in 10.1056/NEJMp1011024). This "value framework" focuses on achieving and measuring outcomes that matter to patients, not merely "inputs" (the volume of services provided to patients). It also prioritizes the tracking and measurement of *long-term* costs of longitudinal patient outcomes including sustainable recovery, need for continuing interventions ("downstream effects"), and occurrence of treatment-induced illnesses. This way of thinking makes obvious sense but is utterly countercultural in medicine. For example, Porter (a professor at Harvard Business School) has noted: "No [health care] organization I know of systematically measures the entire outcome hierarchy

for the medical conditions for which it provides services, though some are making good progress." See also Lee, *New England Journal of Medicine* 2010;363:2481; Owens and colleagues, *Annals of Internal Medicine* 2011;154:174; Gusmano and Callahan, *Annals of Internal Medicine* 2011;154:207.

310 *Callahan has reminded us that several deeply ingrained values in:* See Callahan, *New England Journal of Medicine* 1990;322:1810.

311 *Many believe that the call for limits can be circumvented if:* See Emanuel, *Journal of the American Medical Association* 2012;307:39.

312 *could also decrease the quality of care:* Ibid. Notably, the converse is also problematic: Despite widespread belief to the contrary, increases in the quality of care often increase, not decrease, the costs of care. (The association between health care quality and cost is complex and poorly understood; see, for example, Hussey and colleagues, *Annals of Internal Medicine* 2013;158:27.) The key to reducing health care costs is to reduce use of (and capacity for) cost-ineffective, "low-value" health care services (see Rauh and colleagues, *New England Journal of Medicine* 2011; 10.1056/NEJMp1111662:e48; Roberts and colleagues, *Journal of the American Medical Association* 1999;281:644; Porter, *New England Journal of Medicine* 10.1056/NEJMp1011024 and Supplementary Appendixes 1 and 2; Baker and colleagues, *Annals of Internal Medicine* 2013;158:55).

312 *almost two-thirds of* all *health care expenditures:* See Agency for Healthcare Research and Quality, Research in Action, 2006:19. http://www.ahrq.gov/research/ria19/expendria.pdf.

312 *Ezekiel Emanuel and other experts have argued:* See Emanuel, *Journal of the American Medical Association* 2012;307:39.

312 *But which physicians, exactly:* It is possible that this dilemma is an example of the "bystander effect" in medical care, in which diffusion of responsibility among a large group results in failure of anyone to act. (The assumption is that "someone else" will step up and get the job done.) See, for example, Stavert and Lott, *New England Journal of Medicine* 2013;368:8.

317 *We need a twelve-lead but there's ST-elevation in lead two:* A standard electrocardiogram (ECG) captures electrical currents from twelve different locations ("leads") on the chest while a heart monitor typically receives input from only three leads. In this case, one of the monitor's three leads shows changes in the electrical waveforms that may indicate heart damage, but this requires confirmation with a standard ECG.

317 *Maybe he's embolized his right coronary:* Most heart attacks (myocardial infarctions, or MIs) are caused by a blood clot that forms inside one of the three main coronary arteries (one on the right side of the heart, two on the left) and interrupts blood flow to an area of heart muscle. In rare cases, however, the cause of an MI is occlusion of the coronary artery by an embolus—a clot (or, as suspected in this case, a bacterial vegetation) that breaks off from its origin elsewhere in the heart and then gets stuck in one of the coronary arteries. The ICU doctors, based on what they see on the heart monitor and Mr. Warner's known diagnosis of bacterial endocarditis, suspect an embolus to his right coronary artery.

321 *Ay-fib, he says to Friedman:* This is shorthand for atrial fibrillation, a common cardiac rhythm disturbance (see also Chapter 6).

322 *body cooling, they call it, post-cardiac arrest hypothermia:* Lowering body temperature to minimize brain damage during resuscitation treatments for cardiac arrest victims is one of several recent innovations used to improve outcomes for such patients (see also Chapter 8). Soon after Friedman used this technique in a widely publicized case, induction of hypothermia became common practice in New York hospitals (and ambulances).

325 *some people get what they need only because others get less:* In economic terms, this is not what rationing means. For an economist, rationing describes the process whereby "specific amounts of goods and services are allocated to consumers on the basis of criteria other than their actual preferences, willingness to pay, and income or wealth" (see Meltzer and Detsky, *Journal of the American Medical Association* 2010;304:2292). The classic example occurs during times of war when a government controls the price of certain commodities in order to supply its armies at low cost, then allocates to its citizens the remainder of these goods in an equitable manner (typically in the form of ration coupons). But, in health care, rationing refers to decisions about "which patients will receive services when not all can be served." This is different from wartime rationing of gasoline or sugar but it is rationing nonetheless. Many Americans, unaware that such rationing is a daily (indeed, inevitable) occurrence in the U.S. health care system, don't like the sound of it. Debate about this issue has been going on for a long time (see, for example, Fuchs, *New England Journal of Medicine* 1984;311:1572; Daniels, *New England Journal of Medicine* 1986;314:1380; Aaron and Schwartz, *Science* 1990;247:418; Eddy, *Journal of the American Medical Association* 1991;265:1448). Despite recent research about "waste" and "unnecessary" medical care in the United States (see also Chapters 2 and 4), this debate has focused primarily on whether (and how much) rationing will be needed for medical care that is neither wasteful nor unnecessary (see, for example, Brody, *New England Journal of Medicine* 2012;366:1949; Bloche, *New England Journal of Medicine* 2012;366:1951; Singer, *New York Times*, July 19, 2009).

325 *Lester Thurow, a noted economist, questioned:* See Thurow, *New England Journal of Medicine* 1984;311:1569. The "insurance value" of Medicare has been questioned more recently by Baicker and Levy (see *New England Journal of Medicine* 2012;367:1773).

326 *This kind of rationing—the real thing:* This has been happening for a long time; see, for example, Strauss and colleagues, *Journal of the American Medical Association* 1986;255:1143. Importantly, "real" rationing must be differentiated from "parsimonious" medicine, which "means delivering appropriate health care that fits the needs and circumstances of patients and that actively avoids wasteful care." (See Tilburt and Cassel, *Journal of the American Medical Association* 2013;309:773.) What does this mean? It means "starting with basic, proven tests and treatments; calibrating intensity of testing and treatment consistent with the seriousness of the illness and patients' goals; using good, sound judgment, like asking 'will this test change management?'; using time as an ally in the diagnostic process; tolerating uncertainty; and using interpersonal skill to allay patient fears."

327 *and make this kind of rationing even more frequent in the future:* Fortunately, evidence to date suggests that critical care specialists ration their resources wisely. (For example, the patient

Mr. Warner displaced from our ICU did well.) Typically, critical care doctors weigh patients' severity of illness, prognosis, and age most heavily when making these difficult decisions (see Sinuff and colleagues, *Critical Care* Medicine 2004;32:1588). It is important to note that such decisions can cut both ways: sometimes, when ICU beds are full, doctors refuse admission to ICU for patients they deem *too sick to benefit* from ICU care (when compared to other patients more likely to benefit). Such decisions are torturous for critical care specialists, who take great pride in thinking that no patient is too sick for them. But as demand for ICU beds continues to rise, these tough calls will only get tougher. Not surprisingly, how doctors share these decisions with critically ill patients and their families is a source of much controversy (see, for example, Young and colleagues, *Critical Care Medicine* 2012;40:261).

327 *nor is it a new phenomenon:* See Wetle, *Journal of the American Medical Association* 1987; 258:516.

327 *Why? Because they were* old: This began to change when some brave surgeons began to think outside the box. See Edmunds and colleagues, *New England Journal of Medicine* 1988;319:131.

327 *we need authoritative, rational, transparent methods to ration finite resources:* There are many ways to do this but none has been successful to date. Advance directives, appeals to "futile" treatment, and covert age-based rationing will not solve the problem (see Callahan, *New England Journal of Medicine* 1996;335:744). Insurers ration care but too often "through inconvenience" (see Grumet, *New England Journal of Medicine* 1989;321:607), i.e., by making the delivery of care onerous for physicians and patients. Partly in response to insurers' actions, private hospitals have "dumped" patients on public hospitals, sometimes with tragic results (see Schiff and colleagues, *New England Journal of Medicine* 1986;314:552). Local governments (e.g., the state of Oregon) have made attempts to ration care more rationally (see Dixon and Welch, *Lancet* 1991;337:891) but ultimately without success. Physicians have argued for decades that physicians must play an important role in such rationing (see, for example, Welch, *Annals of Internal Medicine* 1991;115:223; Ubel, HealthcarePapers 2002;2:10 @longwood essays.com), but there has been no organized, sustained effort to do so.

327 *with the notable exception of solid organ transplantation:* The most rational medical rationing in the United States involves organ transplants. Because the demand for donor kidneys, hearts, and other organs far exceeds their supply, national policies have been developed to allocate the limited number of organs among eligible patients on the waiting list. In general, these policies seem fair and reasonable: The sicker the patient and the longer she has waited for an organ, the higher her rank on the priority list. However, even in this system, the eligibility criteria and reimbursement mechanisms can seem arbitrary, even capricious. Different transplant centers use different eligibility criteria. Mr. Warner, for example, would be considered eligible for an organ transplant in some centers (despite his HIV infection and advanced age) but not in others (see, for example, Uriel and colleagues, *Journal of Heart and Lung Transplantation* 2009;28:667). Oddly, Medicare pays for kidney transplants for patients not otherwise eligible for Medicare but it does not pay for such patients to receive heart, liver, or other types of transplants. Stranger still, Medicare pays for antirejection drugs only for three years even though kidney transplant recipients generally require these (very expensive) drugs *lifelong*. This rationing of Medicare drug benefits causes some patients (who can't afford to pay for the drugs themselves) to reject their transplanted kidney three years

later. To stay alive, these patients then require chronic kidney dialysis treatments—which Medicare pays for indefinitely, but at two to three times the annual cost of the "uncovered" antirejection drugs! (See, for example, Kisken, *Ventura County Star*, July 22, 2011; Sack, *New York Times*, September 14, 2009.)

327 *Our Scylla has been described thus:* See Levinsky, *New England Journal of Medicine* 1984;311:1573.

328 *In the U.S. health care system, uncontrolled by a central budgetary authority:* See Relman, *New England Journal of Medicine* 1990;322:1809; *New England Journal of Medicine* 1991;324:195.

328 *doctors' Charybdis has been described this way:* See note, p. 325.

329 *Daniel Callahan, who recognized the inevitability:* See Callahan, *Setting Limits: Medical Goals in an Aging Society* (New York: Simon & Schuster, 1987). See also Callahan, *What Kind of Life* (New York: Simon & Schuster, 1990).

329 *Everyone shoveled dirt on its grave:* This statement exaggerates the reality. Several experts found merit in Callahan's proposals, before and after he made them (see, for example, Williams, *British Medical Journal* 1997;314:820; Daniels, *Just Healthcare* [Cambridge, 1985]; Veatch, *The Hasting Center Report* 1988;18:34). Most, however, strongly disagreed (see, for example, Levinsky, *New England Journal of Medicine* 1990;322:1813; Smith, *Ageing International*, September 1993:7; and, Dixon, *Journal of Medicine and Philosophy* 1994;19:613). Part of the complexity of this issue is that prioritization of medical treatment for the elderly varies among different socioeconomic and cultural groups (see, for example, Mak and colleagues, *Health Policy* 2011;100:219). Not surprisingly, it also varies with patients' age (see, for example, Ryykanen and colleagues, *Social Science and Medicine* 1999;49:1529).

329 *some worried that Callahan's proposal:* See Levinsky, *New England Journal of Medicine* 1990;322:1813.

329 *proposed that U.S. citizens, young and old alike:* See Callahan, *New England Journal of Medicine* 1991;324:194.

330 *Swift's proposal had appealed to intergenerational justice:* See Callahan, *Setting Limits: Medical Goals in an Aging Society* (New York: Simon & Schuster, 1987); *New England Journal of Medicine* 1990;322:1811; *New England Journal of Medicine* 2009;361:e10.

331 *Mr. Principo agreed to temporarily "suspend" his advance directive:* New York State law does not allow a physician unilaterally to "suspend" a patient's rightfully executed do-not-resuscitate (DNR) directive for purposes of performing surgery. Instead, the patient (or the patient's agent or surrogate) must consent to such a suspension. This action, in turn, makes sense only if the *patient's goals* are consistent with *both* having a DNR order and suspending it temporarily for a particular purpose (see Fins, *A Palliative Ethic of Care: Clinical Wisdom at Life's End* [Sudbury, Mass.: Jones and Bartlett, 2006]).

332 *I wrote the official order to suspend Mr. Principo's advance directive:* This could be done only after Mr. Principo's explicit consent to do so (see preceding note).

Chapter 10: Go Gentle

339 *Strictly speaking, Dr. Itrasca is correct:* Having consented to suspension of his advance directives for the duration of the perioperative period (see notes, pp. 331 and 332), Mr. Principo has given his surgeons discretion in this matter. Risks related to operative care are complex; typically, surgeons negotiate with patients their commitment to postoperative care, but this "buy-in" process is only partly understood. (See, for example, Schwarze and colleagues, *Critical Care Medicine* 2010;38:843; Mark and colleagues, *Milbank Quarterly* 2012;90:135; Raiten and Neuman, *New England Journal of Medicine* 2012;367:1779.)

340 *Mr. Principo would be like this—asleep:* Mr. Principo died peacefully two days later.

340 *they played semipro ball with the young Yastrzemski:* Carl Yastrzemski, the Boston Red Sox Hall of Famer who was born in 1939, grew up on the eastern end of Long island. There, both Yastrzemski and his father played baseball with Mr. Jackson and my father-in-law.

342 *Guilt? Yes, rarely, when a doctor has made a bad mistake:* See also Chapter 7 (and note, p. 244).

342 *Regret is the feeling that happens when:* Regret is both a cognitive phenomenon and an emotional phenomenon (see, for example, Landman, *Journal for the Theory of Social Behavior* 1987 [July 2];17:135; Power and colleagues, *Patient Education and Counseling* 2011;83:163). Differences between the feeling of regret (in the context of decision-making) and the feeling of disappointment are subtle but measurable (see, for example, Marcatto and Ferrante, *Judgment and Decision Making* 2008;3:87). Recently, "scales" have been developed to measure patients' feelings of regret about health care decisions (see Brehaut and colleagues, *Medical Decision Making* 2003;23:281).

342 *We avoid regret by purposefully defending ourselves against it:* No doubt this oversimplifies a complex phenomenon. In fact, physicians'"management" of their own feelings of regret has been studied only rarely in the clinical setting (see, for example, Sorum and colleagues, *Medical Decision Making* 2004;24:149). In contrast, cognitive aspects of medical decision-making have generated a large and growing literature over the course of more than three decades. See, for example, Weinstein and colleagues, *Clinical Decision Analysis* (W.B. Saunders, 1980); Dowie and Elstein, eds., *Professional Judgment: A Reader in Clinical Decision Making* (Cambridge, 1988); Sox and colleagues, *Medical Decision Making* (Butterworth-Heinemann, 1988); Eddy, *Clinical Decision Making* (Jones and Bartlett, 1996); Hunink, Glasziou, and colleagues, *Decision Making in Health and Medicine* (Cambridge, 2001).

343 *Regret, researchers tell us, requires two things:* Zeelenberg and Pieters (see *Journal of Consumer Psychology* 2007;17:3) have enumerated, discussed, and elaborated further (see *Journal of Consumer Psychology* 2007;17:29) on ten key "propositions" about regret. Consider, for example, their Proposition 2: "Regret is a comparison-based emotion of self-blame, experienced when people realize or imagine that their present situation would have been better had they decided differently in the past." Nevertheless, our understanding of regret remains "embryonic" (see Roese and colleagues, *Journal of Consumer Psychology* 2007;17:25).

343 *Psychologists call it "counterfactual thinking":* See, for example, Roese and Olson, eds., *What Might Have Been: The Social Psychology of Counterfactual Thinking* (Lawrence Erlbaum, 1995). See also Epstude and Roese, *Personality and Social Psychology Review* 2008;12:168, an article that reviews the results of many recent cognitive experiments investigating the influence of counterfactual thinking on behavior.

343 *Worse, in rare cases, a doctor:* The opposite situation is much more common: The patient, when conflicted or afraid—and, sometimes, in an effort to avoid regret himself—asks his doctor to take over and make the decision *for* him. In general, doctors should meet such requests with more, not less, effort to involve the patient in an authentically "shared" decision.

343 *it is patient abandonment, plain and simple:* See Quill and Cassell, *Annals of Internal Medicine* 1995;122:368 on the subject of "Nonabandonment: a central obligation for physicians."

344 *greater use of subspecialist consultants doesn't always result in higher quality:* See, for example, Fisher and colleagues, *Annals of Internal Medicine* 2003;138:273 and 2003;138:288.

344 *the scientific evidence opposing surgical treatment for patients like:* There have been no randomized clinical trials comparing "medical" therapy versus early surgical therapy for a broad spectrum of patients with infective endocarditis—and there probably never will be. See also note, p. 270.

344 *international panels of experts often publish:* See, for example, regarding infective endocarditis, Mr. Warner's problem: Baddour and colleagues, *Circulation* 2005;111:e394; Bonow and colleagues, *Journal of the American College of Cardiology* 2006;48:e1.

344 *cited this standard to deny the "appropriateness" of Mr. Principo's request:* Defining "appropriate" care is no less complex today than it was decades ago (see, for example, Wennberg, *Journal of the American Medical Association* 1987;258:2568; Fuchs, *New England Journal of Medicine* 2011;365:585). For this reason, the individual clinician's judgment and/or local institutional guidelines about what care is "appropriate" often prevail. In general, however, the legal definition of the "standard of care" is no different from the medical definition: Physicians are required to act as a "reasonably prudent physician (with the same qualifications) would act in the same or similar circumstances." (See Annas, *New England Journal of Medicine* 2010;362:2126.)

345 *these doctors adhere to "expected utility theory":* See, for example, Weinstein and colleagues, *Clinical Decision Analysis* (Philadelphia: W.B. Saunders, 1980); Sox and colleagues, *Medical Decision Making* (Boston: Butterworth-Heinemann, 1988); Hunink, Glasziou, and colleagues, *Decision Making in Health and Medicine* (Cambridge: Cambridge University Press, 2001).

345 *This approach avoids regret because:* This statement is speculative. In fact, we don't have reliable empirical data to address this issue because expected-utility decision-making is more norma-tive than descriptive, i.e., its method captures how "rational agents" *should* make decisions, not how (most) real-life doctors *actually* make decisions. For an insightful review of these differ-ences (and their significance), see Hershey and Baron, *Medical Decision Making* 1987;7:203. Notably, these authors addressed the question: *Should* expected-utility decision-makers take regret into account? Their answer: "When we make decisions for others, they experience the

major consequences (e.g., improved or worsened health) but we experience the regret, since regret is a consequence of making the choice. Thus, to take regret into account in this case is a kind of self-indulgence. . . . Thus, we suggest, regret ought to be ignored." Obviously, then, the extent to which the decision is "shared" between patient and doctor (rather than made unilaterally by the doctor "for" the patient) is a critical factor in understanding the role of regret. See also note, p. 346, below.

346 *most doctors anticipate the outcome that, if it occurred:* See Feinstein, *Archives of Internal Medicine* 1985;145:1297. Some observers have questioned the wisdom of avoiding anticipated regret. For example, Gilbert and colleagues (see *Psychological Science* 2004;15:346) concluded that "people pay a steep price to avoid future regrets, and our studies suggest that they may be purchasing emotional insurance that they do not really need." In addition, doctors must take care to remember *whose* regret matters most: their own or their patient's? When making a medical decision, doctor and patient often "see" the decision differently. For example, they weigh the "good" or "bad" of risks and benefits differently, in part because their assessments are affected by different external and internal variables (see Shaban and colleagues, *Archives of Internal Medicine* 2011;171:634; Ubel and colleagues, *Archives of Internal Medicine* 2011;171:630; Clark and colleagues, *Journal of Clinical Oncology* 2001;19:72). This becomes most evident, perhaps, when doctors become patients themselves (see Klitzman, *Patient Education and Counseling* 2006;64:61).

346 *Avoiding regret may hurt doctors in other ways, too:* Zeelenberg, for example, claims that "regret not only helps us to remember our mistakes . . . it also prepares us to behave more appropriately when we are confronted with similar choices in the future" (see *Philosophical Psychology* 1999;12:325). To make this happen, we must "decouple the aspect of regret that leads to self-reproach from that aspect that can be used to learn from the outcome" (see Inman, *Journal of Consumer Psychology* 2007;17:19). In fact, studies suggest that regret is more beneficial than other negative emotions (such as anger, jealousy, or shame) in several ways: making sense of past experiences; facilitating avoidance behavior; gaining insights into the self; and preserving social harmony (see Saffrey and colleagues, *Motivation and Emotion* 2008;32:46).

346 *the sense of privilege we feel:* See, for example, Adrian, *New England Journal of Medicine* 2012;367:2371.

346 *After the fact, for example, I can easily convince myself:* Nassim Taleb, author of *The Black Swan: The Impact of the Highly Improbable* (New York: Random House, 2007), suggests that "we humans constantly fool ourselves by constructing flimsy accounts of the past and believing they are true" (see also Kahneman, *Thinking, Fast and Slow* [New York: Farrar, Straus and Giroux, 2011]). As a result, Kahneman finds, "hindsight bias has pernicious effects on the evaluations of decision makers. It leads observers to assess the quality of a decision not by whether the process was sound but by whether its outcome was good or bad. . . . Hindsight is especially unkind to decision makers who act as agents for others—physicians, financial advisers, third base coaches. . . ." Infrequently studied in medicine, the "unkind" effects of hindsight bias may affect inexperienced physicians more than experienced ones (see Dawson and colleagues, *Medical Decision Making* 1988;8:259). See also Arkes and colleagues, *Journal of Applied Psychology* 1981;66:252.

354 *Lisa Rosenbaum, a cardiology fellow:* See, for example, "The Downside of Doctors Who Feel Your Pain" (Rosenbaum, *New York Times,* 10/31/11) and "The Art of Doing Nothing" (Rosenbaum, *New England Journal of Medicine* 2011;365:782).

354 *Lisa's grandfather wrote a book that became a hit Hollywood movie:* See Rosenbaum, *A Taste of My Own Medicine: When the Doctor Becomes the Patient* (New York: Random House, 1988).

355 *learn more about the psychology of medical decision-making:* For starters, see Schwartz and Griffin, *Medical Thinking: The Psychology of Medical Judgment and Decision Making* (New York: Springer-Verlag, 1986); Dowie and Elstein, eds., *Professional Judgment: A Reader in Clinical Decision Making* (Cambridge: Cambridge University Press:, 1988).

355 *I don't know much about medicine:* Compared to his knowledge about other things, this may be true, but Kahneman coauthored one of the most important early papers about "understanding patients' decisions" (see Redelmeier and colleagues, *Journal of the American Medical Association* 1993;270:72).

355 *an interview in the* Times *a few years ago:* See Goode, *New York Times,* 11/5/02.

356 *Kahnemanandtversky:* Ibid.

356 *that human rationality is limited:* Many others have written well about this. See, for example, Pious, *The Psychology of Judgment and Decision Making* (New York: McGraw-Hill, 1993); Hastie and Dawes, *Rational Choice in an Uncertain World* (London: Sage, 2001); Gigerenzer and Selten, eds., *Bounded Rationality: The Adaptive Toolbox* (Cambridge, Mass.: MIT Press, 2001). However, Kahneman and Tversky's work has dominated the field (see especially Kahneman and Tversky, eds., *Judgment under Uncertainty: Heuristics and Biases* (Cambridge: Cambridge University Press, 1982); Kahneman and Tversky, eds., *Choices, Values and Frames* (Cambridge: Cambridge University Press, 2000); Kahneman, *Thinking, Fast and Slow* (New York: Farrar, Strauss and Giroux, 2011).

356 *why patients are more likely to agree to risky surgery:* See, for example, McNeil and colleagues, *New England Journal of Medicine* 1982;306:1259; Kahneman and Tversky, *Econometrica* 1979;47:263; Tversky and Kahneman, *Science* 1981;211:453.

356 *why most people, when faced with a small risk:* See Kahneman and Tversky, *Econometrica* 1979;47:263; Tversky and Kahneman, *Journal of Risk and Uncertainty* 1992;5:297; Tversky and Fox, *Psychological Review* 1995;102:269.

356 *first impressions (like my own about Mr. Principo):* See Tversky and Kahneman, *Cognitive Psychology* 1973;4:207; Surowiecki, *The Wisdom of Crowds* (New York: Anchor, 2005).

356 *how hindsight distorts our view:* Ibid. See also Hawkins and Hastie, *Psychological Bulletin* 1990;107:311.

356 *Why we mistake random chance:* See, for example, Kahneman and Tversky, *Cognitive Psychology* 1972;3:430; Gilovich and colleagues, *Cognitive Psychology* 1985;17:295; Tversky and Gilovich, *Chance* 1989;2(4):31; Bennett, *Randomness* (Cambridge, Mass.: Harvard, 1998).

356 *How and why we jump to conclusions:* See, for example, Gilbert and colleagues, *Journal of Personality and Social Psychology* 1990;59-601; Kahneman, *Thinking, Fast and Slow* (New York: Farrar, Straus and Giroux, 2011).

357 *Psychologists have long believed that regret is asymmetric:* Kahneman's own thought on this subject has evolved considerably. See, for example, Kahneman and Tversky, *Scientific American* 1982;246:160; Kahneman and Miller, *Psychological Review* 1986;93:136; Kahneman, *Thinking, Fast and Slow* (New York: Farrar, Straus and Giroux, 2011). See also Landman, *Personality and Social Psychology Bulletin* 1987;13:524; Tversky and Shafir, *Psychological Science* 1992;3:358; Anderson, *Psychological Bulletin* 2003;129:139; Beike and Crone, *Journal of Experimental Social Psychology* 2008;44:1545.

358 *When Kahneman's great book was published:* See Kahneman, *Thinking, Fast and Slow* (New York: Farrar, Straus and Giroux, 2011).

359 *But decisions must be made and, when we make them:* Thaler and Sunstein have written brilliantly about the pros and cons of default decision-making in *Nudge* (New Haven: Yale University Press, 2008). As these ideas apply to medicine, see Halpern and colleagues, *New England Journal of Medicine* 2007;357:1340.

360 *we have barely begun to understand how doctors and patients:* The challenges are well known in the United States and elsewhere (see Frosch and Kaplan, *American Journal of Preventive Medicine* 1999;17:285; Barry and Edgman-Levitan, *New England Journal of Medicine* 2012;366:780; Stiggelbout and colleagues, *British Medical Journal* 2012;344:e256). In fact, there is a continuum of involvement by patient and physician, ideally guided by patients' preferences (see Kon, *Journal of the American Medical Association* 2010;304:903). In addition, the spectrum of challenges varies in different venues of care, from primary care practices (see Elwyn and colleagues, *British Journal of General Practice* 1999;477) to intensive care units (see White and colleagues, *Archives of Internal Medicine* 2007;167:461). Not surprisingly, both emotion and cognition play important roles in the process (see Power and colleagues, *Patient Education and Counseling* 2011;83:163).

ACKNOWLEDGMENTS

One doctor takes full responsibility for *One Doctor*'s flaws but I'm glad to share credit for its strengths with others. Janis Donnaud, my agent, and Leslie Meredith, my editor at Simon and Schuster, believed in this book from the beginning and made it better in the end. Mark Lachs, Cornell's Co-Chief of Geriatrics, encouraged me to write and helped me get started. Andy Schafer, the Chair of Medicine at Cornell, provided inspiration about the best that medicine can be and supported my efforts in many ways.

Most of all, I am indebted to the three extraordinary people who read this book early and often and helped me understand what it could be: my loving wife, Janice, who, among her many other talents, is a brilliant editor; my superstar daughter, Caitlin Reilly Smith, who is wise and kind beyond her years; and Art Evans, a good friend and the best doctor I know.

There is no way to thank the thousands of physicians and patients I have learned from and admired—in New England, Rochester, Chicago, and New York—during the course of my career. In a very real sense, they all wrote this book with me. Martha and Steve Richardson, together with their entire extended family, deserve singular recognition in this regard. They know the reasons why—and that, at least for now, will have to do.

INDEX

ABOUT THE AUTHOR

Dr. Brendan Reilly is the Executive Vice Chair of Medicine at the New York-Presbyterian Hospital/Weill Cornell Medical Center, where he oversees all inpatient and outpatient clinical affairs in medicine. A widely published clinical researcher and medical educator, Reilly also is the Gladys and Roland Harriman Professor of Medicine at Weill Cornell Medical College. Before his current appointments, Reilly served as the Chair of Medicine and Physician-in-Chief at Cook County Hospital in Chicago, which, during Reilly's thirteen-year tenure there, was the inspiration (and setting) for the hit NBC television series *ER*. During that time, he also held the C. Anderson Hedberg Chair of Medicine at Rush Medical College. Prior to his tenure in Chicago, Reilly served on the faculty of Dartmouth Medical School and the University of Rochester School of Medicine. He lives with his wife, Janice, in New York City and Newbury, New Hampshire.